3/10/98

To Kathy
the most caring
person I know
from
Jeane Pennock

PROFILES IN CARING

ADVOCATES FOR THE ELDERLY

PROFILES IN CARING

ADVOCATES FOR THE ELDERLY

Val J. Halamandaris

CARING PUBLISHING

519 C Street, NE, Stanton Park, Washington DC, 20002-5809

First Edition

Printed in the United States of America.

Library of Congress Catalog Card Number 90-085706
ISBN 0-9628363-0-3

Dedication

This book is dedicated to the four people who most shaped my life: To my father, John V. Halamandaris, who was the best man I ever met; to Senator Frank E. Moss, the man my father said has done more for me than he has; to Congressman Claude D. Pepper, who paid me the ultimate tribute when he introduced me as the son he would have liked to have had; and to my mother, Merry S. Halamandaris, who taught me the meaning of caring and unconditional love.

PROFILES IN CARING

ADVOCATES FOR THE ELDERLY

Contents

Acknowledgments

I have divided my acknowledgments into two parts. The first relates to those people who have helped me and encouraged me in the preparation of this book. The second is a list of people who have made significant contributions in the field of aging.

First, I would like to thank my brother, Bill Halamandaris, whose encouragement, support, research, and editorial assistance made this work possible.

I would like to thank Christopher Laxton, Rebecca Staebler, and my associate, Debra Giuliani, who spent hours poring over the manuscript to make it both accurate and readable. Carina Deans, Bernadette Hawkins, Stewart Jordan, Andrew Morrison, Dian VanDeMark, and Michelle Zook provided editorial production assistance.

J. Andrew Simmons provided art direction and designed the cover, illustrated by Kevin Chadwick.

I would also like to thank Marilu Halamandaris for her support and for her excellent photographic work, which appears in this volume and previously in *CARING* Magazine.

Kathy Gardiner Cravedi, Melanie Modlin, and Peter Reinecke of the staff of Congressman Pepper's Subcommittee on Health and Long-Term Care provided much support and assistance and deserve my recognition and thanks.

I would like to give special recognition to others whose many achievements on behalf of the elderly have been highly signficant, but whose biographies are not included within this volume. Deference should be paid to Geneva Mathiasen and Ollie A. Randall, the founders of the National Council on the Aging; Wilma Donahue and Clark Tibbitts of the University of Michigan Institute of Gerontology; Ethel Percy Andrus, the founder of the American Association of Retired Persons; Lou Glasse, president of the Older Women's League; and

Nelson Cruikshank, formerly at the National Council of Senior Citizens. James Birren, who directed the Ethel Percy Andrus Gerontology Center at the University of Southern California; Ethel Shanas at the University of Chicago; Elaine Brody of the Philadelphia Geriatric Center; Carol Estes at the University of California at San Francisco; Joshua M. Wiener at the Brookings Institution; Robert H. Binstock at Case Western Reserve University; Dorothy Rice, formerly at the National Center for Health Statistics; Paul Kerschner of the National Council on Aging; and Elma Holder, director of the National Citizens Coalition for Nursing Home Reform deserve special recognition.

Sally Hart Wilson and Paul Nathanson, formerly with the National Senior Citizens Law Center, and Bill Dombi, director of the Center for Health Care Law, have made extraordinary contributions.

Aside from those included herein, several members of Congress deserve recognition. Among those who distinguished themselves in service to the elderly were Senator Frank Church, who served as Chairman of the Senate Committee on Aging. Senator Church saved the committee when it was slated for dismantling in a 1976 Senate reorganization. He also pushed through a 20 percent increase in Social Security rates in 1972 and tied future increases automatically to the cost of living index, lifting millions of people out of poverty and providing them with the financial basis for a meaningful life. Senator John Glenn, the famed astronaut, had a brief but distinguished term as chairman of the committee, following many years of service thereon. Senator Jennings Randolph was one of the committee's more active members. Senator Charles Percy, the Ranking Minority Member of the Senate Committee, also established an enviable record fighting to improve the quality of life for the nation's older Americans.

Four other senators deserve special mention. Senators George Mitchell, John Heinz, Ted Kennedy, David Pryor, and John D. (Jay) Rockefeller IV, have all played important roles as advocates of the elderly. Senators Heinz and Pryor were both instrumental in bringing about the creation of the House Committee on Aging when they were members of that body. Both in their time have served as Chairman and Ranking Minority Member of the Senate Aging Committee and both serve on the Senate Finance Committee as well. Rockefeller distinguished himself in 1988–90 as Chairman of the Pepper Commission, the United States Bipartisan Commission on Comprehensive Health Care. Senate Majority Leader George Mitchell has demonstrated his concern for seniors as a thoughtful member of the Senate Finance Committee and as a leader of his party. Senator Ted Kennedy is undoubtedly the reigning champion in terms of advocacy for seniors; his achievements have been great and significant, commencing with his election in 1962 and continuing to the present.

In the House of Representatives, a few members deserve special mention. Congressman Henry Waxman, Chairman of the Subcommittee on Health, has done the most to help seniors, followed by Congressman Edward Roybal, Chairman of the House Aging Committee; Congressman Ron Wyden and Congresswoman Mary Rose Oakar also rank high on the list. Geraldine Ferraro deserves mention, as does Millicent Fenwick. Both made extraordinary contributions during the years they sat as senior members on the House Select Committee on Aging.

Preface

The idea for this book came to me in a taxicab in New York City. It was a scorchingly hot day. The driver scrutinized me carefully as I got into his cab with almost more packages than I could carry. Self-consciously, I tried to melt his stare and ease my guilt. With a conspiratorial grin, I told him that I was celebrating. I had a new law degree, a new love in my life, and a new job as counsel to the United States Senate Special Committee on Aging.

"Old people, you work with old people?" he asked in a skeptical, thick European accent. "What do you know about old people?"

I stammered a few lame statistics and tried hard to sound authoritative. Then, shaking his head and glaring at me in the rearview mirror he said, "Do you want to know what is the problem with old people in America, I will tell you. I am going to tell you because you are in my cab and I am the boss in here." He slammed the brakes hard for punctuation.

He pointed to a crane demolishing what looked like a relatively new building—a metaphor, he said, for contemporary American life. "In America, we celebrate youth at all costs and we undervalue experience and age. In the Old World, there are plenty of things wrong, but we celebrate the past and try to preserve our heritage; we treasure buildings that are 500 to 1,000 years old. In this country, anything that is more than 40 years old will be smashed by the wrecking ball." The same is true of people, he said.

He emphasized that in America we undervalue those people who have helped make our country great; we do not appreciate what they have done for us. "You can't know where you are going unless you know where you have been. And what is more, if you do not know who your grandfather was, you have no idea who you are," he said with simple logic.

The sad part, he said, is that we once knew this great truth. The framers of the Constitution were astute students of history. They had studied past civilizations and they built the American democracy on the collective wisdom of humanity, going back 2,000 years or more.

America, he said, was built on the time-honored and time-tested principles. Some of these have been chiseled in marble in our nation's Capitol, but even so, the lessons have been forgotten, said the man, arching his thick eyebrows and tugging at his walrus mustache.

As further evidence that we had it and lost it, he made reference to the twin statues guarding the doorway to the National Archives in Washington, D.C. He explained that one of the first things he did on reaching the American shore was take a bus to Washington for the express purpose of seeing the Declaration of Independence, the Constitution, and the Bill of Rights. "People come from all over the world to see these documents which forever liberated mankind from the yoke of oppression. And yet most Americans take them for granted," he said.

The driver reminded me that the statue on one side reads "Study the Past" and the statue on the other side of the Archives door reads, "What Is Past Is Prologue."

He said in the Old World, although it was changing there too, the elderly are still venerated because of the contribution they have made to the present generation. "In America, we take their contribution for granted. We assume our high quality of life is a birthright and we've forgotten that previous generations fought and died to make it so for us. In this country, there is little gratitude; we discard old people like empty beer cans." The unspoken premise, he said, was that the elderly have served their purpose in seeing to the current generation's comfort and enjoyment. He said this was a sad commentary, a sad waste of human potential, a disrespect for life born of arrogance and ignorance, which amounted to no less than spitting in the face of God.

As we crossed the Triborough Bridge, he asked me to consider what kind of message our contempt for the elderly projects to our young people. "What are they to think when they see their parents and grandparents squeezed dry and discarded. It cannot help but invoke in our youth tremendous anxiety about the future. Will it not signal them to live for the moment and wallow in materialism because nothing but abandonment, neglect, or abuse awaits them when they step beyond the curtain of middle age?"

Because we value life not in terms of service to others but in relationship to the acquisition of material things, older and retired people inevitably are viewed as freeloaders whose value diminishes with age. The very reverse should be true, said the philosophical taxi driver.

He then told the story about the grandfather who came to live with his eldest son and his family. The old man was unsteady of hand and eye. He broke china, spilled his soup at the table, and embarassed the son, who responded by giving the old man a wooden bowl and a wooden spoon and dictating that the old man take his meals by himself in a corner of the kitchen. Then one day, the son, who was middle-aged, came home from work to find his five-year-old child whittling in the garage. He made inquiry and the five-year-old told him that he was making a wooden bowl and spoon for his parents to use when they became old and moved in with him. The lesson was not lost. Although nothing was said, the old man was again invited to join the family at the dinner table, to enjoy his meals on china, and use silver utensils just like the rest of the family.

"What we send into the life of others comes back into our own," said the cab driver. "This is as true for a nation as it is for an individual."

What old people need is love and a reason to live. "Give them a *why* to live and they will survive any problems," he said, paraphrasing Goethe.

"Seniors need some self-respect. They want to feel needed and they want a chance to contribute. They need role models their own age who prove all the stereotypes are baloney. They need to be reminded that old age is not synonymous with disease and worthlessness. Young people need to give them a break, to give them the benefit of the doubt.

Young people must step forward to break the chain of prejudice and liberate the old people of America. None of us can escape getting older; the young people of today will be the senior citizens of tomorrow. The question then is: What kind of a life do you want not only for your parents in the future, but also for yourself?"

As he pulled up to the gate of La Guardia Airport, he quoted the Talmud in Yiddish, translating to English, telling me that the true value of a human life is the extent to which it is used to help others and emphasizing the importance of individual responsibility. "If I do not do it, who will do it," he translated. "If I do not do it now, when shall I do it."

I fumbled for the fare and thanked him. As I gathered my packages and closed the door, he hit me with a parting shot.

"Go tell that to your committee in Washington. Go ahead, take a chance. Be a hero."

I gave him a five-dollar tip, but I am indebted to him still.

On the flight back home, I decided that I would begin a search for role models, for the emerging leaders who would guide and shape the destiny of the over-65 generation—the fastest growing segment of the American population. That cab ride took place in 1969, more than twenty years ago, and I have been searching ever since.

This work was blessed by providence. For more than twenty years, I worked at the U.S. Senate or the House of Representatives, most of that time as Counsel to either the Senate or House Aging Committees. I was in a marvelous position to learn, to ask questions, to meet people, and to take note of their contributions. I have had an even greater opportunity to do so in the years that I have been out of government.

We have come far in our treatment of the elderly since those dark days thirty years ago when I first became involved with aging. In those days, ageism and age discrimination were the norm. Things are a great deal better now, thanks in large part to the people profiled in this book, which is not to suggest that all of the problems of the elderly have evaporated.

Who are the people who have done the most for older Americans?

After researching hundreds of people, I have chosen 18 who I believe have done the most to improve the quality of life for America's seniors during the last fifty years. My selections inevitably are subjective; however, I exercised my very best judgment based on painstaking and voluminous research.

In a very real sense, this book is a labor of love for me. I have known all and worked closely with most of these people. If one accepts Victor Hugo's definition that love is the ultimate recognition which we award to superbly held values, then I have no doubt that the reader will love these people as much as I have loved them. Each and every one of them is a national treasure.

While I have known each of the honorees, I did not limit the writing to the scope of my experiences. I believe that you can never truly know a person until you have read all that they have written and everything that has been written about them. Thanks to the Library of Congress, such massive research is possible. This research is augmented by personal interviews conducted with friends and associates of the honorees. Finally, in-depth personal interviews were conducted with most of those profiled, usually on videotape.

To make explicit what has been implicit, I had several purposes in mind with this book:

First, I wanted to capture for posterity the personality, the thoughts, the wisdom, and the achievements of 18 truly extraordinary Americans.

Second, this book is my way of paying tribute to the people for the sacrifices they have made and for devoting their lives in service to others.

Third, I wanted to help historians who one day will look back to see who it was that helped us make productive use of an unprecedented gift—a one-third extension of the human life span, which is one of the hallmarks of the 20th century.

Fourth, I wanted to inspire young people to emulate the examples of those whose history is told in this book. As Albert Schweitzer reminds us, when it comes to education, example is not just a factor to be considered, it is the only factor that matters.

Fifth, I wanted to give something back, to say thank you to these extraordinary people, all of whom taught me and some of whom have loved me.

Sixth, I hope this book will help focus and frame issues with respect to older Americans for the 1991 White House Conference on Aging and for the balance of the 20th century.

Many of the tributes that appear in this volume first appeared in *CARING*, a magazine for health care professionals that I helped launch eight years ago, hence the name *Profiles in Caring*. Not surprisingly, other books are planned as part of this series. All of the proceeds of this book will go to support the Caring Institute, a non-profit organization that my brother Bill and I have established along with Senator Frank E. Moss in Washington, D.C. The purpose of the Caring Institute is to help change the values of society, to return America to what it once was—the most caring nation on the face of the earth. The motto of the Institute, taken from Albert Einstein, is, "Only a life lived for others is a life worthwhile."

I invite the reader on a journey that took more than twenty years to complete. I suggest that no one can read these tributes without developing a profound respect for these modern-day social engineers who helped stamp out the prejudice and injustice perpetrated against those Americans whose only sin was to survive to a good age. The example provided by their lives proves conclusively that one life—one man or woman—can make a difference, and that, in the words of Mother Teresa, "There is joy in transcending self in order to serve others."

Val J. Halamandaris
July 4, 1990

Foreword

by Leo F. Buscaglia

It is sad that we are in a society that has such a strange attitude about aging. It seems that when we reach a certain magical number, we are expected to disappear or, at least, behave in a specific "mature" fashion.

I'm determined not to let others dictate my behavior by some predetermined code. If we want to wear a red sequined dress at 87, dye our hair purple, travel to the jungles of the Amazon, or go to the market on roller skates, then we should do it.

I cringe at titles like "Senior Citizens." The label seems only to categorize us and sets us up for lesser expectations.

We seem to have forgotten that people like Galileo, for instance, wrote his last book when he was 74. Michelangelo was 71 when he started painting the Sistine Chapel. Grandma Moses did not even turn to her art until she was 71. I love the story of Duke Ellington: He was passed over by the Pulitzer Prize Advisory Committee at 66 and he said—and I love this—"Well, God didn't want me to be too famous too young." Isn't that great? He died at 75. Pablo Cassals played at a concert at the White House when he was 85 years old. Susan B. Anthony, that wonderful lady, was president of the Suffragettes until she was 80 years old. She was arrested at the age of 52 for voting. She went into the booth and said, "I want to vote. What do you mean a woman can't vote?" She was given a new experience—jail!

There is so much we can do, no matter what our chronological age. I love the idea that George Bernard Shaw fractured his leg at 96, and you know what he was doing? He fell out of a tree that he was pruning.

I once saw Buckminster Fuller, when he was in his eighties, speak for four hours to a crowd of 4,000 with no notes, no blackboard, no audiovisual equipment, and keep everyone enthralled. He had the most wonderful vision of the future. His last words were, "I have great hope for the future. My hope lies in three things—truth, youth, and love." Like the other people I have mentioned, his life was a testimony to the fact that age is no barrier to thought, judgment, or achievement.

It offends me to hear people with self-defeating ideas such as, "You can't teach an old dog new tricks." I've taught a lot of tricks to old dogs. The challenge is ours. Living life fully is a choice and it's ours to make. We can live it happily or sadly. We can say yes to life or no, but we must take full responsibility for whatever choice we make.

We must drop the crazy self-defeating ideas and be all that God intended us to be. How dare someone die without becoming all that they were intended to be. We can change everything by making a decision. It is as easy as that.

Val J. Halamandaris has written an important book, which pays tribute to 18 wonderful people who have chosen to live life to its fullest. They have chosen to use their lives to bring comfort and help to the elderly, the ill, and the underprivileged. Through their efforts, these people have helped change America's attitudes about the elderly. As the author says, they have helped liberate the elderly and bring them freedom from fear.

The final chapter of this book, which chronicles what these 18 heroes have in common, is especially vital. More than anything else, the lives of these people bear out the wisdom of Albert Einstein's admonition that "only a life lived for others is a life worthwhile."

The lives of the 18 people presented in this book have been an adventure in loving. They remind us of the words of Thornton Wilder: "There is a land of the living and a land of the dead. The bridge is love. It is the only truth. It is the key to survival."

I urge everyone to emulate the lives of these wonderful people, to choose as they have the way of love, the way of life, forever caring, full and confident about tomorrow. We must continue to choose the way of trusting over suspicion, the way of goodness over evil, the way of enhancement over selfishness.

Life, regardless of chronological age, is God's gift to each and every one of us. What we do with our lives is our gift to God. Like the people presented in this book, let us endeavor to make our gift a truly fantastic one.

Introduction

In 1963, President John F. Kennedy rallied the nation to enact Medicare, the national health insurance plan for the elderly. He argued that there was great need, that the elderly were sick three times as often, hospitalized three times as long, at a time when they had less than half the incomes of their younger counterparts. He argued also on ethical grounds that this was the right thing to do. What was surprising, and ultimately more persuasive, however, was his argument that the legislation was needed as a matter of national defense and to preserve America's place in history.

The president justified what might seem like an extraordinary statement by quoting the historian Arnold Toynbee. Toynbee, said the president, had studied all the great civilizations of the world and had reached the conclusion that the greatness, durability, and place in history of a nation could be predicted by the application of a universal yardstick—the manner in which it cared for its aged, underprivileged, and disabled citizens. Thus, said the president, what was at stake with Medicare was nothing less than the nation's very survival and its place in history.

Senator, and later Vice-President, Hubert H. Humphrey, an historian himself, had reached a similar conclusion. He said the moral test of good government is the manner in which it treats those "on the fringes of life," referring to children who experience problems in the dawn of life, to the elderly who suffer from compound burdens in the twilight of life, and to the handicapped who he said were relegated to the shadows of life.

Toynbee, Kennedy, and Humphrey were all talking about a one-word distillation of the golden rule: caring. They knew that a nation that does not care for its children forfeits its future. They knew that a nation which does not venerate its elderly not only loses the value of its collective wisdom, but also guarantees that the lives of those in their middle years will be plagued with anxiety.

Going into the last half of the 20th century, young and middle-aged people could see that old age in America was a wasteland. In the words of Senator Frank E. Moss, it was hell to be old in America. The facts supported this conclusion.

One out of every four Americans had incomes placing them below the poverty line; most of them had not been poor before they retired. Mandatory retirement and age discrimination were common. One out of every two seniors had no health insurance or inadequate coverage. Some 30 percent lived in substandard housing without adequate plumbing, heating, or electricity. There were no meals programs, no senior citizens centers, no jobs programs, and no help with transportation. Older Americans were continually faced with a series of Hobson's choices. For example, they might have to choose between using the same limited funds to buy food or medicine or to hire a taxi to take them to a friend's funeral.

Worst of all was the verbal abuse. Bruises of the flesh heal, but bruises of the soul do not. Cruel stereotypes of the elderly were found everywhere in society, particularly in print ads and on television. Seniors were portrayed as befuddled, hard of hearing, weak, passive, and confined to rocking chairs. Epithets abounded and were equally insensitive. Seniors were disparagingly called "crocks," "gomers," "old fuddy-duddies," "no-brains," "numbskulls," "old farts," and worse. Older Americans were made to feel as if they were unwanted freaks, scavengers, and parasites who did not contribute, but lived off the work of others. Little acknowledgement was made of the fact that seniors had devoted their lives to helping build the abundance and affluence that the present generation has obviously enjoyed.

Part and parcel of the problem was the fact that the accumulation of wealth and material possessions was elevated to the preeminent value in American society. "Dallas" and half a dozen other clones at the top of the television ratings reflected and reinforced the conclusion that in America one could never be too rich, too thin, or too young. What mattered was winning and making money, not what one did for others.

Things were so bad, outsiders branded America "the no deposit, no return society"—the implication being that people in America were disposable, used up while they could be productive, and thereafter discarded like styrofoam containers.

In looking ahead at what was waiting for them in their "golden years," it should be no surprise that the last generation of young Americans decided to live for the moment and grab all they could get. Nor should it be any surprise that those in middle age were filled with stress and fear, not only because of their approaching old age, but also because they faced the struggle of caring for their own parents and trying to care for their children at the same time.

In those days, older Americans were made to feel like lepers or worse. "It is a terrible thing to have leprosy," said Mother Teresa, "but it is worse to be unloved."

Through it all, the number of older Americans kept increasing. It is staggering but true that more years have been added to life expectancy at birth in the 20th century than in all the preceding 19 centuries combined. In 1900, only four percent of the population, or one out of every 25 Americans, were age 65 or over. By 1990, life expectancy has increased from 47 to 77, a 64 percent increase. The percent of the elderly to the total population has increased from four percent in 1900 to 13 percent in 1990. The number of those over 65 has increased from three million to some 35 million in the same time period. The numbers are projected to continue their upward spiral as the "baby boom" generation begins to age. In 2030, for example, 21 percent of the population, or more than 64 million people, are expected to be age 65 or older.

The fortunate part is that America has been blessed with a group of people who could read these trends, who could isolate the problems of the elderly, and then do something about them. I call these people "Advocates for the elderly." Thanks to their efforts, life for seniors in America has improved immeasurably. Obviously, there is still far to go in meeting the needs of the elderly, particularly with respect to long-term care, but progress has been made. The question is: What happened to make the difference?

Always, it is the few people who are willing to risk everything to challenge the established order, who succeed in winning social justice for all. This is certainly true in the field of aging. History will record that there were just a handful of people, heroes and heroines, who stepped forward in the face of injustice and who won major victories on behalf of older Americans.

These people challenged the all-too-convenient stereotypes about the elderly and shattered the myth that powerlessness, dependency, and disability was a natural state among the aged.

They proved that the prevailing myths and stereotypes had their roots not in fact, but in prejudice. They had the courage to challenge ageism as an insidious evil, arguing that it was no more acceptable in American society than racism or sexism.

They proved that "ageism" was being used as a justification for limiting the rights of older Americans. This was wrong, they asserted, insisting that the guarantees in the Constitution and the Bill of Rights applied with equal force to people age 65 and older.

While their numbers were few, the eloquence of their arguments and the righteousness of their cause attracted disciples. The few multiplied into an army. Senior power was born.

The few were elevated to a position of leadership of a movement which grew and grew until it became one of the most powerful in American history. It is a movement that gathers strength every day, fed by the steady pulse of demographics and nourished by the institutional structures that the leadership put into place.

It is remarkable to contemplate that, in little more than twenty-five years, the senior citizens of America have been catapulted from near obscurity at the bottom of the American power and social structure, to the very top. What has happened, of course, is just the beginning. The power and influence that senior citizens will exercise over events in the coming years is nothing short of mind-boggling. In the year 2020, for example, the nation at large will have the same percentage of seniors to total population that the state of Florida has today—that is, almost 20 percent of the population and almost 40 percent of those who vote. The hope is, of course, that this power will be used responsibly to secure the benefit of a better life for Americans of all age groups.

In the days ahead, the emerging leaders of the senior power movement should remember that they stand on the shoulders of giants. They should remember those heroes and heroines, whose lives have been profiles in caring. As they chart out the course for the future, they would be well advised to look to the past and to the important lessons that were learned by those who came before.

Who, then, are these heroes and heroines?

Are they still living? How old are they? What are they like?

What do they believe? What is their philosophy?

Who influenced them? Who were their heroes and role models?

What did they do to bring seniors to the forefront of the American consciousness?

What were their major achievements?

What are the most important lessons they have learned?

What do they have in common?

What do they see as the major issues affecting older Americans and the nation in general over the next few years and into the 21st century?

What advice do they have for young people?

What advice do they have for older Americans?

And finally, how would they like to be remembered?

This book answers these questions. It is an effort to pay tribute to a group of remarkable people who have done the most to bring dignity and respect to older Americans. The intent is to tell their stories, as an inspiration to others. The hope is to capture their wisdom, as well as to applaud their contribution. The goal is to provide seniors with excellent examples of graceful aging and to provide young people with role models worthy of emulation.

Of the group profiled in this book, it may be fairly said that they are a treasure more valuable to the nation than all the gold in Fort Knox. They are what young boys and girls dream of being when they are young and wish they had been when they are old. Their lives prove conclusively that the American dream is not just a dream, but a reality that happens every day through positive thought, hard work, and determination. Their lives prove that it is possible to rise above poverty, ignorance, and discrimination; that one man or one woman can make a difference. But more than any of this, the lives of these extraordinary people remind us that, whether for individuals or for the nation, the solution to most problems and the way to salvation lies in the love and caring of one human being for another.

As President Kennedy reminded us, there is a great deal at stake, including the nation's future and its place in history.

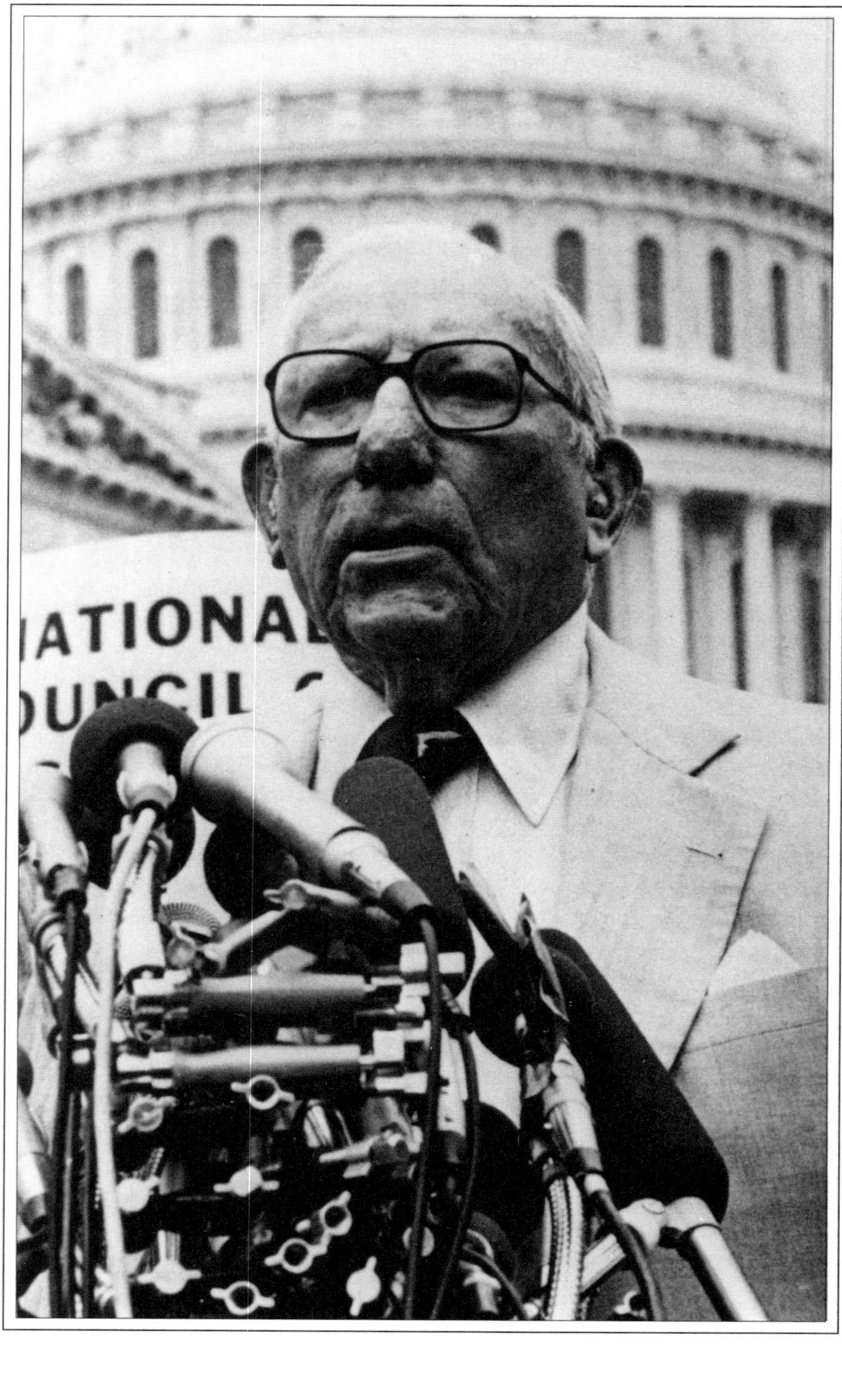

COURTESY OF SENATOR CLAUDE D. PEPPER LIBRARY

ONE

Claude D. Pepper

Claude Denson Pepper was one of the greatest public servants the nation has yet produced, ranking in his achievements with Henry Clay, Daniel Webster, Thomas Jefferson, and Franklin D. Roosevelt.

He was a farm boy from rural Alabama who overcame great hardships to become the confidant of presidents and one of the most distinguished figures ever to serve in the Congress of the United States of America.

Nothing came easy to Pepper, who worked his way through high school, the University of Alabama, and Harvard Law School, graduating always with the highest honors. He was elected to the Senate in 1935, where he fought for the rights of the underprivileged. He was hung in effigy as a warmonger when he tried to alert America to the fact that Adolf Hitler was a dangerous criminal, bent on world conquest. He single-handedly pushed "lend-lease" legislation through the Congress, giving airplanes and ships to the Allies at a crucial time, saving England and turning the tide of the war. But not for Pepper and his resolve, America might have been in the position of fighting Hitler on American soil, completely without allies. When the peace was won, he was damned by the red-baiters and the "super Americans" of the McCarthy era for introducing legislation to create the United Nations. Because of his progressive views, some people labeled him "the most dangerous man in America" and death threats hung over him like a cloud.

He lost his Senate seat in what was unquestionably the most vicious political campaign in American history. His opponents called him a communist and charged that he had "practiced celibacy" and that his sister was "a thespian in wicked New York." Even worse, he was pilloried for his stand on civil rights: photographs of him shaking hands with blacks were distributed, inscribed with racist and inflammatory statements.

He rose again, like a phoenix, to become one of the most powerful and respected members of the House of Representatives. He became chairman of the House Rules Committee, the most powerful committee in Congress, whose leader is second only to the speaker and majority leader in authority. In addition, he became the preeminent champion of senior citizens, particularly in his tenure as chairman of the House Select Committee on Aging.

His career and life spanned more than one-third of the history of the republic. He met the Wright Brothers and the Apollo astronauts, as well as Stalin, Hitler, and Churchill. His was a leading role on the stage of American politics. His influence was vast, inspiring generations of young men and women to select a career in public service. He was hero and role model to men like Hubert H. Humphrey, Hale Boggs, Paul Simon, Thomas P. "Tip" O'Neil, Lyndon Johnson, and scores of others.

He was an indomitable spirit whose whole personality was one of warmth and love and yet he was capable of fighting like a tiger for what he believed. This fact led Congressman George Danielson to christen him "the tender tiger." Every man, woman, and child in America and future generations to come—and particularly the elderly—have had and will have their lives enriched because of Claude Pepper's service in the Congress of the United States.

Early Years

Claude Pepper was born on a farm near Dudleyville, Alabama, on September 8, 1900, to J. W. and Lena (née Talbot) Pepper. When Claude was ten, the family moved to Camp Hill, Alabama, in the heart of cotton country. Times were tough, they were poor, and young

Claude went to work to help support the family. Claude's father, J. W., worked as a peace officer when he was not farming. At one time or another, he was a town marshal, chief of police, or a deputy sheriff. Claude's mother raised four children and taught them to care for others. She was very much involved in church work and she was a talented musician.

Through most of his life, Claude Pepper lived in an extended family setting. The year of his birth was only 35 years after the end of the Civil War. Both grandfathers had fought in that war and indeed, J. W. had been named for a famous Confederate general, Joseph Wheeler. Claude knew all four of his grandparents, who lived with or close to his parents all of their lives.

J. W. Pepper tried his hand at business, opening a furniture store and later a grocery store, both of which failed. The investment, however, gave Claude the opportunity to learn the mercantile business; for a time, he operated a cleaning and pressing shop out of the back of his father's store.

Claude graduated from high school in 1917. He distinguished himself academically and in extracurricular activities. The high school principal, C. C. Moseley, was one of the most influential people in his life. Moseley had traveled extensively, giving Claude books to read, and visions of far off places ripe with opportunities that became available even to young farm boys from Alabama through diligence, education, and hard work.

In the summer of 1917, Pepper became an itinerant boy entrepreneur. He bought some equipment from a man who traveled city to city cleaning and blocking hats. Business was slow and without money travel soon became impossible. Pepper returned home where a job was waiting for him. He was asked to teach at the local high school for the princely sum of $60 a month and he readily agreed.

At this time, Pepper stood five feet seven inches tall and weighed one hundred and fifteen pounds. He was teaching students most of whom were bigger and older than he was. Discipline was a problem at first until Pepper gained respect by conquering the class bully who stood six feet three and weighed two hundred and ten pounds.

For a young man, Claude Pepper was very focused. At the age of fifteen, he had written on the back of a closet door, "One day, Claude Pepper will be a United States Senator." In high school, he excelled in forensics, often regaling his classmates with spontaneous orations. His brother, Joe, remembers that during the year he taught high school, Claude would come home and practice speeches that he said he planned to deliver on the Senate floor when he was elected. His mother, Lena, when asked to comment, said wryly, "He started talking when he was nine months old and he's been talking nonstop ever since."

In 1918, Pepper enrolled in the University of Alabama. To support his college education, he worked as a steel worker, as a welder, and he shoveled coal into a furnace at a coal-fired electrical plant. It was at the university that he met and was influenced by his second great mentor, George H. Denny, president of the university. He helped Pepper to expand his mind, giving him more books to read and engaging him in debate.

Always there were obstacles. Pepper was shy and did not have many dates. His superior intellect, however, got him admitted to a college fraternity where the brothers hoped to capitalize on his work and tutorials. A fraternity brother called an affiliated sorority one night to negotiate a blind date. Pepper was eavesdropping on the line when the girl said she'd go out with anyone in the fraternity but Claude Pepper and then went into a diatribe about how homely, short, and misshapen he was. Pepper burst onto the line, telling the girl to mark the day because he intended to be a United States senator and he wanted her to remember all the White House balls and other grand social events that she was going to miss because of her intemperate conduct.

Pepper graduated Phi Beta Kappa in 1921 and set out for Harvard Law School. He waited on tables, ran the cafeteria, and emptied coal ashes in the power plant for three years to earn his tuition. He found time to compete on the track team and graduated in the top five of his class. He met his great friend, Thomas J. Corcoran, on the steps of the Harvard Law School; it was a friendship that would produce dividends for the nation. It was at Harvard that Pepper met his third great mentor, Roscoe Pound, Dean of the Harvard Law School. "Harvard had a great effect on me, it opened my eyes," said Pepper in his autobiography.

After law school, Pepper turned down a high-paying job at a utility company, preferring what he called "public interest employment." He became a professor of law at the University of Arkansas. Among the students he inspired was William J. Fulbright who went on to be elected to the United States Senate and served for many years as chairman of the Senate Foreign Relations Committee.

Pepper moved to Florida in 1925, because he thought the state had a great future. He took a position with Judge W. H. Davis, who was practicing law in Perry, Florida. He became a partner in that firm and at the same time plunged headlong into politics. Pepper explained:

> I entered public life because my early years in the destitute South convinced me that life for human beings should and could be much better than it was. What could make it so? Neighbors, churches, and private enterprise all had roles, but they all had limits, too, and those limits fell far short of providing security, health care, and some comforts of life for the many. It seemed to me that government policies and action were required to help in this nation's "pursuit of happiness" for its citizenry.

In 1929, Pepper was elected to the Florida state legislature. One of the first bills he introduced exempted older people from paying for fishing licenses. The bill was passed and this quick success, fueled by Pepper's oratorical skills, made him something of a celebrity. But Pepper lost his bid for reelection, in part because he had a tougher opponent, but also because he refused to vote in favor of a resolution proclaiming the superiority of the white race and condemning Mrs. Herbert Hoover because she had hosted a black congressman's wife at the White House.

Pepper said the loss was a blessing in disguise. It opened up a more direct route for him than he could have foreseen. At the age of 33, Pepper ran for the U.S. Senate seat held by Park Trammell. Pepper appeared to have won the race until, as one historian put it, "the Tampa vote came in 'hot' for Trammell." In those days, Floridians had to pay a poll tax if they wanted to vote. Those who could not pay sometimes found that people were willing to give them money, and pay the poll tax for them, as long as the recipient agreed to vote the way the benefactor wanted. It was generally agreed that Trammell's 4,000 vote victory margin had either been bought or stolen, but Pepper did not protest.

Two years later in 1936, Senator Trammell died. Within weeks, Florida's other senator, Duncan Fletcher, also died in office. Pepper filed to fill the seat held by Senator Fletcher. "With a memory of the stolen 1934 election still fresh in their minds, Floridians apparently felt that I had earned the seat; no one filed against me," said Pepper.

But there were more good things in store for Pepper in 1936. On December 27, Mildred Webster, the great love of his life, agreed to be his wife. A full-scale wedding took place at the First Methodist Church of St. Petersburg on December 29th, barely 36 hours after they had become engaged. The couple took a honeymoon in Cuba and moved into an apartment in Washington, D.C., early in January of 1937, ready to begin their life together.

For Pepper, winning Mildred's hand may have been more important than winning the Senate post. He had suffered all of his life with an inferiority complex as far as his physical appearance was concerned. Cruel words from fellow classmates had been burned deep into his soul. In his own eyes, he was surely the most homely man alive. Mildred was a beauty. Pepper never forgot the first time he saw her on the steps of the State Capitol in Tallahassee and how she looked in the yellow gown that she wore. It was love at first sight, but this was not unusual. "Everyone who met Mildred fell in love with her," remembers Tip O'Neil. Mildred accepted a date with Pepper to go to the Speaker's Ball in 1929 and dated Claude off and on for six years. If only he could get Mildred to love him, he thought, then he could do just about anything. And things pretty much worked out that way. With Mildred at his side, Claude felt complete and at peace with himself for the first time. "I have never known such happiness," he wrote in his journal.

Mildred was a wonderful asset. In addition to her stunning good looks, she was a perfect hostess. She had an excellent knowledge of politics and could more than hold her own on the campaign trail. She was outgoing, vivacious, and bright—one of the few people who might have been as bright as he was. They were a team. She was the catalyst he needed to fulfill his potential and he gave meaning, position, and security to her life. "We were both deeply devoted to each other," he said. "I could not have been more fortunate in my choice of a mate."

Senate Career

Claude Pepper hit the U.S. Senate like a buzz saw. His maiden speech chastised his colleagues who were becoming disenchanted with Roosevelt's New Deal policies. He drew a Biblical analogy concerning the lost tribes of Israel who left Egypt in search of the promised land. When they got where they were going they hesitated, said Pepper, and "the resultant judgment of retribution" is all too well known. "All of them who were then more than twenty years of age, left their bones to bleach in the wanderings of the wilderness." Pepper went on to say that Roosevelt had brought the American people to the brink of the promised land. He closed by saying he had no intention of wandering in the wilderness and urged his colleagues to move full speed ahead.

The usually reserved Senate broke its rules and applauded the speaker. As a matter of fact, they gave him a standing ovation. Newspaper stories lauded both the speech and the speaker. Typical of those was the following from the columnist, Drew Pearson:

> The speech was one of the greatest of its kind ever heard in the chamber. First speeches by newcomers are usually very dull and cautious affairs. Pepper's address shattered this precedent. It was extraordinary in brilliance of delivery and stunning effect. . . . Few paid much attention to him when he started. Five minutes later all eyes were riveted on him and the Senate was as still as a tomb. History was being made and the Senators and the press gallery knew it. A new leader was taking his place.

Pepper became FDR's point man in the Senate. His friendship with Thomas Corcoran made him an insider at the White House. Time and time again his booming voice would ring out against the injustices and oppression of the times. The unfriendly *New York Herald* at one point blasted Pepper: "When the White House has an important balloon to send up, it invites Senator Pepper to supply the necessary oratorical helium."

In defense of Roosevelt, Pepper noted that they were ideological soul mates; both had a passion to improve the lot of the common man. In 1928, Pepper had sent Roosevelt a letter suggesting that the modern Democratic party should be founded on this populist rock and that FDR should be the head of it. Roosevelt listened and this is exactly what transpired.

Pepper's defense of Roosevelt's policies became the main issue in Pepper's 1938 campaign. Pepper received national attention and appeared on the cover of *Time* magazine. The caption reads: "The Florida fighting cock who will be a White House weather vane." Pepper won and by extension so did FDR. When the clouds of war appeared ominous in Europe, Pepper personally went to see what Hitler was doing. He attended the Nuremberg Nazi Congress and was greatly alarmed at what he saw and heard. He quickly came to the conclusion that Hitler was a madman with serious intentions of taking over the world by force of arms.

When Pepper arrived in London, he met Joseph P. Kennedy who was then Ambassador to Great Britain. It became evident to Pepper that Kennedy was not seeing to business. Kennedy did not see Hitler as much of a threat. The ambassador also felt free to criticize President Roosevelt, not only in private but before British nationals, as well.

Pepper returned home and told FDR what he had seen of Hitler and of Kennedy's less than distinguished performance. Kennedy was recalled to Washington, causing enmity with Pepper that would surface later. More to the point, Roosevelt began making plans for all-out war. But this was easier said than done. The isolationists still held a firm control over Congress and public opinion. No American mother was comfortable with the thought of her son dying on European soil, absent extreme threat or provocation. Indifference, denial, and appeasement were the tenor of the times.

Pepper set out to help FDR. He developed an idea called "lend-lease." It was an exchange of military bases for ships and plans. The idea was to give American planes and ships to the British while the ones that they had ordered were reinserted into the American arsenal as soon as they were built. FDR told Pepper this was a marvelous idea, but could offer no public endorsement. Undeterred, Pepper introduced the bill which provoked a fire storm of reaction. He was blasted by politicians, both inside and outside of his own party. True to his beliefs, Pepper asked for an immediate vote in the Senate Foreign Relations Committee. He lost by a margin of 22 to 1. But he persevered and two years later, the bill was passed and the military hardware was released to Britain, earning Pepper the everlasting gratitude of Winston Churchill.

A group calling themselves Mothers of United States of America were less grateful. They hung Pepper in effigy from a tree on the Capitol lawn. The dummy which hung from the rope sported a sign which read "Claude 'Benedict Arnold' Pepper." Congressman Danielson, then an FBI agent, was assigned to protect Claude Pepper and several other congressmen from threats of assassination. "He did not know it at the time, but I followed Claude Pepper around day in and day out, seldom letting him out of my sight."

Pepper's response was totally in character. He said:

> Knowing these women, like all other Americans, are sincere in their patriotism, placing America first and Hitler last, I feel that their hanging me in effigy is a splendid demonstration of what we are all trying to preserve—freedom of speech and freedom of action in the American way of doing things. I only hope that the spectators and those who hear about this business will feel that I also love America and that I am sincere in my daily efforts to defend the United States in liberty, the right of free speech and free action.

In time, the number of Pepper's supporters grew. A little known congressman named Lyndon Johnson contacted Pepper. He said he wanted to help Pepper and FDR. The two men worked closely thereafter toward this objective. Pepper urged full preparation for war, including compulsory military service. He took the Floor of the Senate on May 6, 1941, asking a series of rhetorical questions:

> How many sheep does a sheep-killing dog have to kill before he is branded as a sheep-killing dog? How many more nations besides the 14 he has already destroyed does Herr Hitler have to take to become the sheep-killing dog of the earth, to be destroyed like that dog which has castigated himself as unfit to live?

Pearl Harbor proved to the nation that Pepper and Roosevelt had been right. The isolationists grudgingly gave in and the nation prepared for war. Pepper was one of the few people in America who was consistently briefed on the war effort. Roosevelt had learned to value Pepper's counsel. Pepper encouraged Roosevelt to run for an unprecedented third term. He made an impassioned seconding speech for the President after his name was placed in nomination by the convention and he campaigned with the President on several occasions. Clearly, a warm friendship had developed between the two men.

Pepper wrote in his notebook:

> Roosevelt's first hundred days, I am convinced, saved the country from collapse and preserved our form of government. . . . The bank holiday, the National Recovery Act, the Works in Progress Administration (WPA), Public Works Administration (PWA), the Agricultural Adjustment Administration—each met a specific national need, but together they engendered a new American spirit. People who thought their country was going down the drain quickly realized that it need not. They took their cue from the man in the White House, who cheerfully called on them to gather around their radios for some reassuring "fire-side chats." His calm, confident voice insisted that "the only thing we have to fear is fear itself." Roosevelt was like a mechanic giving a jump-start to an automobile with a near-dead battery. His pictures showed a jaunty, smiling president (most Americans were not even aware he was disabled), a welcome contrast to the glum, starchy Hoover. FDR clearly believed in the future, and Americans who had doubted there would be one came to believe in him.

"A president was running the country the way I thought it should be run," wrote Pepper. "Now we had a caring Federal government that worried not about the Rockefellers and the Du Ponts but about the elderly indigents, poverty, peoples' health and housing and even about former plowboys."

Pepper describes FDR as the caring president. He says that experience with polio made him a better human being. It gave him compassion and sensitivity to other people's problems. "He had a soul sweetened by suffering," said Pepper.

Throughout the war years, Pepper was on hand to help clear the way for FDR. At the same time, he introduced a long list of legislative initiatives. Many of these were in the area of health care. He won approval of legislation to create the National Cancer Institute in 1937 and in time won approval of measures creating 12 of the existing 13 National Institutes of Health. These institutes have helped find cures for many life-threatening and chronic diseases with which mankind is afflicted. He also introduced legislation that created the World Health Organization.

He was shocked to find that one out of every four young men called to the army in the draft were unfit. He reacted by introducing legislation to create the Senate Subcommittee on Wartime Health and Education. He chaired this committee for six years. The committee is credited with a number of milestones. For example:

- It was the first to recommend a national health insurance system that would enable all Americans to obtain the health care they need.
- It was the first to recommend home care as an essential component of any future health care system.
- It was the first to recommend "capitation," the use of a set fee in financing a future health care system.
- It was instrumental in establishing that the federal government hadto play a major role in financing research aimed at preventing and curing disease.

Serving on the Senate Committee on Military Affairs, he became an expert in military preparedness. Florida can thank Claude Pepper for the forts, airfields, rocket facilities, and bases which were placed in the state. Pepper's efforts on the Senate Commerce Committee undoubtedly helped spur the Florida economy further as a center of industry, trade, and tourism.

He introduced legislation to create an international organization dedicated to preserving peace and a ban on nuclear weapons even before World War II was over. He told one interviewer his logic: "I believed the seeds of the third world war were present at the end of the second, and the advent of nuclear weaponry made that possibility all the more horrible. I wanted to do everything in my power to keep the two giants, us and the Soviet Union, from becoming enemies."

He introduced and won passage of the first minimum wage law guaranteeing workers at least twenty-five cents an hour.

Senator Pepper advocated equal rights for women, sponsoring legislation to correct the inequities which existed even then. In a January 1943 speech, he said:

> When the Declaration of Independence was written and those moving words that "all men are created equal" were incorporated therein, to lift the hopes and the hearts of the oppressed everywhere in the world, I do not believe that Thomas Jefferson was thinking only of mankind which happened to be masculine in sex. I think he spoke about human beings and therefore that it is in accordance with the principles of the Declaration of Independence to say that women are born equal with men in the rights of citizenship and civil prerogatives. I hope therefore, that this may be the last hurdle which it will be necessary to surmount: that the race to bring equality, complete freedom, independence and liberty for women shall at last be won.

The bill was blocked by a Senate filibuster. At the same time, he fought for and won enactment of legislation to abolish the poll tax. In his statement of introduction, the Senator said:

> To those who say the abolition of the poll tax is an unwarranted interference with state prerogatives to establish voter qualifications, I can only say that when the states are acting properly in the prescription, fitness to vote, aptitude to vote, they are unlimited in their power. However, when they go beyond the scope of proper qualifications and impose onerous burdens, then it becomes the duty of Congress to correct the situation and to preserve the right of every elector to vote.

Roosevelt's death had a profound effect on Pepper. Others lost a president; Pepper lost a president, a dear friend, a fellow poker player, and a soul mate. As an aside, Pepper was fond of telling how FDR would pay off his penny-ante poker losses with checks that no one would cash for obvious reasons. Shortly before the president's death, Pepper had extolled the president's virtues, calling him one of the greatest Americans who ever lived. He said in a Senate speech:

> I have tried to hold up the hand of the commander in chief. I have tried to help him help the people of this nation through a depression which nearly destroyed us, and through the dark days when the threat of Hitler and the dastardly Japanese was looming on the

> horizon and many people did not see the danger. I have tried to help him win this war and to lay the foundation for a permanent peace. When the selfish interests, when the blind or bitter isolationists, when members of his own party even have pressed daggers to his side, I have done what I could to help.

Harry S. Truman, the man who succeeded Roosevelt, had served in the Senate with Pepper, but Pepper was of the opinion that he lacked presidential stature. He liked Truman, but went so far as to say that out of all the men who served with him in the Senate chamber, Truman would have been considered the least likely to become president. The one thing that Truman had done to distinguish himself was that he chaired a committee on the Senate to investigate defense contractors suspected of fraud, overcharging, or shoddy workmanship. He had "dared to take on the military-industrial complex and caught many people in the act" says Pepper, "thus, Truman lost some of his anonymity."

During a 19-nation tour of Europe and the Middle East following the war, Pepper flew to Moscow and met with Joseph Stalin. Pepper came away with the impression that the U.S. had badly treated the Russians at war's end. He believed that the Russian Army was exhausted and that Stalin wanted peaceful coexistence with the U.S. On his return, Pepper took the side of the Henry Wallace Progressives in opposing the military phases of the Marshall plan, which supplied arms to Greece and Turkey where communist revolts were being suppressed. In 1948, Pepper wrote to Dwight D. Eisenhower, urging the general to run for the presidency on the Democratic ticket, opposing Harry Truman. Some say Truman never forgave Pepper for either his opposition to the Marshall plan or for urging Ike to run. Still worse, Pepper had allowed his own name briefly to be put forth for president, believing Truman could not beat Governor Tom Dewey. But Truman did win, surprising everyone including himself.

Pepper maintained that President Truman was a realist and understood that this was all part of the political game; that he did not hold a grudge. Others hold that Truman was angry and bent on revenge, to the point that he recruited and supported a candidate to run against Pepper in the 1950 election.

The 1950 Campaign

Men who do great things make great enemies. Pepper was no exception. In his constant efforts to advance the lot of the common man, the poor, and disenfranchised, Pepper made more than his share of enemies. There was the National Association of Manufacturers which was still smarting from his victory on minimum wage legislation. The American Medical Association was worried that Pepper's plea for national health insurance would be heeded and upset their existing fee-for-service structure. Edward M. Ball, trustee of the billion-dollar Florida Du Pont interests, was angry because Pepper fought a tax increase which had been earmarked for defense contractors. Conservatives were angry because he helped remove the poll tax and because he advocated federal action to stop discrimination and assure civil rights for blacks. Joseph P. Kennedy, still smarting from Roosevelt's rebuke based on information provided by Pepper, contributed about $150,000 to get Pepper defeated. Kennedy told Tip O'Neil that he thought Pepper had a real chance of being nominated for president and defeating him in the Senate race was a way to derail the prospect. Then there were people who thought that anyone who had met with Stalin must be a communist.

All of these people and groups conspired to oust Pepper from the Senate, to break his wings so that the fighting cock would never fly again. Their timing was excellent. The national mood was one of uneasiness characterized by a political march to the right and paranoia personified by Senator Joseph McCarthy and further fanned by the House on Un-American Activities Committee.

But there was more to the story. The pendulum had swung back in favor of the isolationists. Pepper's views for a United Nations were out of sync with those who would have cut off all ties with the world and take refuge in Fortress America. Big business and big money were sick and tired of the New Deal idea that they should be taxed to pay for elevating the blacks, the poor whites, and the downtrodden. Others were sick and tired of FDR and anyone identified with him. Pepper saw the warning signals. His choice was to stand by his convictions or to recant, become a political opportunist, an intellectual chameleon and thereby win reelection. It is to his credit that he decided to stay with his principles at any cost.

In the campaign, Pepper was labelled "Red" Pepper, a "pinko" and a "sympathizer with Communism." He was smeared not only as an apologist for Joseph Stalin, but as a southerner who fraternized with blacks and who advanced their interests at the expense of whites. He was labelled anti-business, but the charge was more vicious—that he was the puppet of union gangsters.

Pepper's enemies scoured the countryside to find the right opponent who could make use of the weapons and the war chest they had assembled. They found their man in "Gorgeous George" Smathers, a congressman and friend of Pepper's. Pepper gave Smathers his start, campaigned for him, and was largely responsible for his election to Congress. Friendship notwithstanding, Smathers viciously and effectively used the arsenal which had been assembled with no notion whatsoever of fair play.

The following lines allegedly attributed to Smathers provide some impression of the kind of battle that followed:

> The leader of the radicals and extremists is now on trial in Florida. Arrayed against him will be loyal Americans. . . . Standing against us will be certain northern labor bosses, all the socialists, all the radicals and all of the fellow travelers. . . . Florida will not allow herself to become entangled in the spiraling spider web of the Red network. The people of our state will no longer tolerate advocates of treason. The outcome can truly determine whether our homes will be destroyed, whether our children will be torn from their mothers, trained as conspirators and turned against their parents, their home and their church. I stand for election on the principle of the free state against the jail state.

According to *Time* magazine, the most famous and purposefully confusing lines in the campaign were delivered by Smathers at a gathering of northern Floridians:

> Are you aware that Claude Pepper is known all over Washington as a shameless extrovert? Not only that, but this man is reliably reported to practice nepotism with his sister-in-law, and he has a sister who was once a thespian in wicked New York. Worst of all, it is an established fact that Mr. Pepper, before his marriage, practiced celibacy.

Smathers denies making either statement attributed to him. What is certain is that Pepper's opponents arranged for an article to appear in the *Saturday Evening Post*, authored by Ralph McGill, self-proclaimed oracle of Southern liberalism. McGill later expressed regret for writing the article, saying he was tricked into doing so, but the damage had been done. The article called Pepper "a spellbinding pinko supported by leftist friends." As if this were not enough, a little book, red in color, called "The Red Record of Senator Claude Pepper," was distributed during the last weeks of the campaign. Reportedly, during the last week of the campaign, nine tons of the material blanketed Miami, Pepper's strongest base.

Through it all, Pepper fought back, always taking the high road. He never mentioned Smathers by name. Although he had information in his possession which would have impeached Smathers's integrity, Pepper refused to use it, insisting he would continue to campaign on his record and on the issues. He refused to sink to the other men's level. Pepper reached out to President Truman at the last minute, but received no help.

The smear campaign worked. Smathers won by 67,000 votes. A conservative publication distributed nationally is reported to have commented: "Republicans joyfully saw the result as a harbinger of a national conservative trend . . . a blow to the Fair Deal nationally and a warning of the communist issue which Republicans are surely to raise this fall."

"McCarthyism claimed several senatorial victims in 1950," said Pepper. "Besides Frank Graham, former president of the University of North Carolina and myself, McCarthyism engulfed the majority leader and majority whip of the Senate, Scott Lucas of Illinois and Francis Myers of Pennsylvania; Millard Tydings of Maryland, a decorated war hero and chairman of the Senate Armed Services Committee; Elbert Thomas of Utah, chairman of the Education and Labor Committee; and Elmer Thomas of Oklahoma, chairman of the agriculture subcommittee of the Senate Appropriations Committee."

Pepper wrote in his diary at the time, "We lost—or did we win?" In his autobiography, he concludes that he gained more in defeat than he would have had he won. He reasons that had he stayed in the Senate, he would have continued his preoccupation with foreign affairs and perhaps lost the opportunity to help people as much as he was able to do so in his House career.

Transition

The loss was a bitter pill for Claude Pepper. The vicious nature of the campaign, the betrayal by a friend, and the seeming repudiation of his values were a heavy burden to carry. He had a sense of being cut down in his prime. Had he won reelection, he would have become chairman of the Senate Foreign Relations Committee. Pepper wanted this post in order to continue his work toward achieving a permanent world peace.

The transition from confidant of presidents back to law practice in Tallahassee was difficult for Pepper. He was not only starting all over again, but starting in the hole because he had massive campaign debts to pay. "I had to fight my way up slowly. I never let it get me down. Mildred would not have let me if I had been inclined to do so," he said.

He borrowed money for furniture and opened a small office, but things were slow. Pepper was discouraged. "I have never admitted the word or thought failure in the lexicon of my thinking but it strikes me occasionally that it might be possible," he wrote. Slowly, the clients came and they got results. He began to get major clients and he won tough cases. Buoyed by these results, he opened a law office in Miami and one in Washington, D.C. He chose good people to work with him. One partner became a U.S. senator, another governor of Florida, and a third became a U.S. circuit court judge. Unlike many who had come to Washington, Pepper had been too busy pursuing the national interest to feather his financial nest. Now for the first time, Pepper was making big money.

But Pepper did not abandon his interest in public service which he said offered greater rewards than making money. "I know loving the law as I do that my best service can be rendered in politics, that is where I belong," he wrote in his diary. He campaigned for Stevenson in 1952 and 1956, considered challenging Smathers, but decided against it and finally in 1958, he made a come back attempt, narrowly losing to Senator Spessard Holland in the Democratic primary.

Two years later, Pepper became involved in the presidential campaign. The election of John F. Kennedy and the political themes he sounded from election day forward were vintage Claude Pepper. Kennedy's election over Richard Nixon must have sounded like the "all clear" signal following an air raid warning. The migration of thousands of ethnics and older Americans to Florida, swelling the numbers of the 1960 census and creating a new congressional district in Miami, must have looked like the arm of fate beckoning Pepper back to Washington. He ran in 1962 and won overwhelmingly.

"Once I had dismissed the thought, believing that a former Senator would not be happy in the House. But I had to ask myself: Do you want to be in government for prestige or so that you can accomplish good things? The answer was the latter," he wrote in his journal, adding that the goodwill from his losing effort in 1958 helped him win the election of 1962. He headed back to Washington "to do something that meant something."

House Career

Claude Pepper was elected to Congress in 1962. His service in the Senate, his well-known abilities, and the friendships he had made were among the reasons he was appointed to the House Committee on Rules. The Rules Committee is the traditional route to power in the House of Representatives. It decides which bills get to the House Floor, the length of debate, and whether or not amendments are in order. Members who serve on this committee can earn IOUs from the leadership and the White House.

Pepper used his position on the Rules Committee to advance the body of legislation known as the Great Society as proposed by his old friend, President Lyndon B. Johnson.

It is no exaggeration to say that he broke a crucial impasse and cleared the way for passage of the Civil Rights Act. Nor would Medicare have been passed without his advocacy.

Claude Pepper had very little difficulty getting reelected to the House with each successive term. He was the consummate politician whose constituent services were legendary. He was listed in both the Washington, D.C., and Miami telephone books and he took calls from literally anyone who called him day or night. He maintained an open door policy in his office and anyone that wanted to see him was given the chance to do so.

Beginning in the late 1960s, members of Congress were provided with electronic signing machines to ease the oppressive burden of constituent mail. Pepper refused to use one. He said it was too impersonal. He sat down at his desk late in the afternoon on every day and signed all of his mail personally, often inscribing detailed additions in his own hand.

Pepper also kept in touch. He was always on the go. He was never content to sit in his office in Washington or to sift through whatever information his congressional staff gathered on his behalf. He was always probing, always challenging, always collecting data for himself, and forever talking about the problems of the individual people that he had met in his journeys. Perhaps more than anyone else, Pepper had his fingers on the pulse of the American public. What was remarkable was that he was equally comfortable as an insider, as part of the Democratic leadership of the House, and as an outsider who represented the interests of a broad group of constituents.

Pepper was a celebrity from the first day he took the oath as a member of the House of Representatives. He was amazed to find in the House of Representatives so many people who had been inspired by his career in the U.S. Senate.

Pepper soon found that he enjoyed service in the House of Representatives even more than he enjoyed service in the Senate. "I loved the Senate," he said. "I dearly loved the House of Representatives."

Pepper gave several reasons for preferring service in "the People's house." Among them are the following:

- It is much easier to campaign in a geographically limited congressional district than crisscrossing an entire state.

- A representative gets to know more of his constituents personally because they are fewer and all live nearby.

- The House is a friendlier place than the Senate, its 435 members being allegedly less important, and thus less self-important, than the 100 senators.

• It is even easier to achieve one's legislative goals from a House seat than from a supposedly loftier perch in the Senate. Senators can talk a bill to death by filibustering; House rules forbid the filibuster and sharply limit debate.

• A representative belongs to fewer committees than a senator. Thus he can know more about legislation and wield more influence on conference committees trying to reconcile differences in bills passed by both houses.

• Addressing the House on important occasions is like making a speech before an audience. Addressing the Senate is like talking to a grade-school class when most of the students are out for recess and those who aren't are unruly.

Pepper said that he was pressed on several occasions to again run for the Senate, but that he was not the least bit tempted. "The opportunities to achieve my legislative goals were so numerous that I no longer yearned to return to the Senate." He noted that he was rising in seniority in the House and had what was considered to be "a safe seat." This meant that he could do what was thought right, without fear of political repercussions.

Pepper often reiterated that his loss of a Senate seat had been a blessing. It gave him an opportunity to step back, to think, and to be in touch with "the common people." Had he won, he would have been chairman of the Senate Foreign Relations Committee and likely continued his service on the Senate Armed Services Committee. "Those committees do not save many souls," he said.

Pepper's service in the House is often associated with his chairmanship of two select committees. Select committees are organized by the Congress to investigate a particular problem. They have investigative authority, but generally no authority to report legislation to the Floor of the House. Typically, such committees have a limited life and go out of business when their purpose is accomplished.

In 1970, Claude Pepper was appointed the chairman of the House

Select Committee on Crime. The committee was in business for six years. The committee's work was unusual in its quality. Serious efforts were made to trace the infiltration of organized crime into the world of entertainment, sports, and law enforcement. Legislation was created giving law enforcement officials new tools to use to fight the Mafia; this legislation has had a major impact over the past 20 years. Pepper's committee examined the problem of airline hijacking and introduced legislation to require the use of metal detectors at all American airports. As a result, the incidence of air piracy within the United States has virtually ground to a halt. Obviously, crime was not eradicated in America, but major inroads were made. The operations of major crime figures in America and abroad were exposed for public view and a number of racketeers went to jail. At times, Pepper was under enormous political pressure to refrain from investigating one area or another, but he never flinched. He followed his conscience wherever it took him and let the chips fall where they may.

The House Select Committee on Aging

In large part, Pepper's career in the House is associated with his service on the House Select Committee on Aging. Pepper advocated the creation of the committee as far back as 1969 when a young Congressman, now Senator, David Pryor, first suggested that one be established. But House Speaker Carl Albert hated select committees and would not hear of the idea. Undaunted, Congressman Pryor rented a trailer which he parked in the House parking lot and unilaterally created what he called the House Trailer Select Committee on Aging. Congressman Pepper joined Congressman Pryor as did Congressman, now Senator, John Heinz. Working together, the three men were successful in winning approval for the measure. The House Select Committee on Aging was created in 1975. Pepper was the second ranking Democrat who ascended to the chairmanship of the committee in January of 1977. Pepper chaired the committee for a dozen years, giving up the helm only to become chairman of the House Committee on Rules. Even so, he retained the chairmanship of the Aging Committee's Subcommittee on Health and Long-Term Care.

Under Pepper's leadership, the House Aging Committee became one of the most celebrated of congressional committees. The committee reflected its chairman in that it was constantly in action and constantly exploring new frontiers. Membership on the Select Committee became a plum that was sought by virtually every member of Congress. Its membership increased from 20 to more than 60. It was and is the largest committee in Congress; one out of every seven members serves on it. Because of its size, Pepper's leadership, the quality of the staff, and the fact that it made news, the committee was inordinately successful.

In 1977, Pepper undertook to shatter the myth that powerlessness and incompetence is a natural state of aging. He conducted hearings to examine stereotyping of the elderly in the media. He brought a host of vital and vibrant role models to testify before his committee, including R. Buckminster Fuller, Averell Harriman, Ruth Gordon, and Jack Albertson. "Older Americans have fought this country's wars, built its cities, reared its children, and tilled its soil," he said. "They have a right to our deepest respect. They deserve much—and need much. The stereotypic notion that aging is inevitably associated with feeble-mindedness, frailty and the inability to produce or continue to contribute should not persist."

A few years later, he brought before the committee half a dozen witnesses, all of whom were over 100 years of age, most of whom were continuing gainful employment or otherwise making meaningful contributions to society. Among them was Harry Lieberman, 104 years old, otherwise known as America's Chagall, who started painting when he was in his nineties. Also included was Dr. Charles Parnell, who was 102 and continued to maintain a family practice in New Jersey.

What Pepper proved through his hearings and through his example is that age is no barrier to achievement. These hearings were predicate to the enactment of legislation in 1978 that eliminated mandatory retirement with respect to service in the federal government and raised the mandatory retirement age in private business to 70. In 1988, Pepper succeeded in winning enactment of legislation that banned all forms of mandatory retirement. Said Pepper in the public debate,

"Ageism is as odious as racism and sexism. Mandatory retirement arbitrarily severs productive persons from their livelihoods, squanders their talent, scars their health, strains an already overburdened Social Security system, and drives many elderly people into poverty and despair."

He added, "To say that the aged must retire in order to make room for younger workers is sheer tomfoolery. A man has got no more right to another man's job than to another man's wife."

In one of his tours, visiting senior citizens in the greater Miami area, he found hundreds of seniors who simply did not have enough to eat or who did not have the ability to make their own meals. Pepper introduced and won passage of amendments to the Older Americans Act which created the current nutrition and congregate meals programs for senior citizens.

In his frequent visits to nursing homes, he found the quality of some such facilities left a great deal to be desired. He conducted hearings which documented voluminous examples of horrific abuses. The House Aging Committee proposed major reforms, which Pepper was successful in getting enacted, working in concert with Senator Frank E. Moss.

Next, Chairman Pepper tackled the problem of home health care. Pepper had been an advocate of in-home health services as far back as 1942. Pepper believed that such services were necessary to support seniors and the disabled in their own homes as a means of postponing or preventing institutionalization. He found that the current Medicare and Medicaid programs were not covering home care services to the extent that Congress intended. Every state, for example, was required by Congress to provide home care under the Medicaid program and yet most did not do so. In fact, more than half of all the Medicaid payments to home care were paid out by one state, New York. Pepper was able to win legislation that removed an impediment in the law requiring a minimum three-day hospitalization as a prior condition to receiving home health services. When Pepper and the entire House Aging Committee met with President Carter in 1977, Pepper listed this as a top priority to be accomplished. Pepper was an incrementalist. He took the legislative gains that were possible in the area of home health care in 1977 and returned to the issue in 1987. Because of Pepper's continuing interest, no single issue dominates the history of the House Aging Committee more than the topic of home health care.

On a related point, Pepper in 1983 won passage of an amendment to Medicare that created coverage for hospice services. He understood hospice to be a form of home care services directed at providing medical intervention, palliative care, and support for those who are terminally ill. He believed in helping people live to the end of their days and that they should be allowed to die at home in the company of friends and family.

A single letter that he received from a constituent led to the committee's most publicized hearings on abuses in the sale of health insurance to the elderly. Pepper documented example after example of senior citizens who were induced to purchase four, five, and in one case as many as 74 duplicative health insurance policies in supplementation of Medicare. He brought forth witnesses who had spent more than $50,000 in the purchase of such worthless insurance and who literally sold their homes in order to make the payments. As a result of a thorough and devastating committee report, the Congress enacted what amounts to federal minimum standards for the sale of such so-called "Medi-gap" insurance.

A telephone call in the middle of the night led to hearings on private pension abuses. Pepper documented that billions of dollars, which properly belonged to retirees, was being stolen by the unscrupulous. Similarly, he conducted hearings on home repair frauds, funeral abuses, and hearing aid frauds, and exposed so-called work-at-home schemes, which victimized the elderly. In other highly publicized hearings, Pepper exposed diploma mills that sold phony medical degrees, as well as graduates of these phony schools, who were practicing medicine and in some cases even performing surgery on their unsuspecting patients. As always with Pepper, it was not enough merely to expose these abuses. He insisted on appropriate legislative reforms.

The loneliest time of his life came in 1978 when his beloved Mildred died of cancer. For a time, he plunged into the depths of depression, but ultimately bounced back with new resolve to do something about what he called "that great monster, cancer."

In thinking about what he could do, Pepper remembered Roosevelt and the Manhattan Project. He reasoned that if only the world's greatest scientists could be brought together and locked in a room for a period of time, they might collectively come up with the cure for the dread disease. Pepper called for and helped chair the International Symposium on Aging and Cancer, which was conducted under the wings of the National Institutes of Health. The conference is credited with pioneering new methods and identifying promising new areas of cancer research.

With First Lady Rosalynn Carter, Pepper tackled the problem of mental health care among the elderly. He proved that Medicare is shortsighted in that it fails to cover much in the way of cognitive impairments. He helped cut through the garbage-can term, "senility," which was so often and so easily applied to the elderly of the nation. He brought to the attention of the nation the fact that much of what passes for senility is really a condition called Alzheimer's disease. He was successful in getting money appropriated for a dozen research centers to investigate the cause of this devastating disease.

Pepper was instrumental in creating the first World Assembly on Aging, which was conducted in Vienna in 1978. His reputation had preceded him and he was greeted there like a head of state or a rock star. The conference laid the groundwork for international cooperation and research in gerontology.

In 1981, Claude Pepper took on Ronald Reagan, the most popular president since Franklin D. Roosevelt. He pointed out that, in his campaign speeches, President Reagan had promised not to cut Social Security and yet in 1981 the president called on the Congress to reduce Social Security by $62 billion. "I was alarmed at the difference between Reagan and his rhetoric," said Pepper. Pepper marshaled a powerful coalition of senior citizens which appeared at the White House Conference on Aging and demanded that the president withdraw the proposed reductions. In the end, Pepper forced the creation of a bipartisan commission, which, under his guidance, developed a plan to keep Social Security solvent well into the next century. "No single function of government affects as many Americans as profoundly as Social Security," said Pepper. "It provides a solid bulwark for the old, the poor, and the disabled, protecting them from what Roosevelt referred to as the 'hazards and vicissitudes of life'.... If Social Security is to continue to withstand periodic attacks and remain a strong and enduring expression of our national resolve, then all Americans must understand that Social Security is not a problem to be solved but rather a solution to be preserved."

It was the first and the most important defeat for President Reagan, who promised thereafter not to make further intrusions on Social Security and this time he kept the promise. Thanks to Pepper, it became political suicide for anyone to advocate reduction in Social Security payments. Pepper campaigned for more than 70 candidates for the House and Senate in 1984, holding up the hand of each candidate and having them recite a pledge that they would never vote to reduce Social Security. Pepper was at the height of his political power. This was recognized by *Time* magazine. He was one of the few Americans to be featured twice on the cover of *Time*.

In 1984 through 1987, Pepper toured the country, conducting hearings under the umbrella of an organization that was created around him and loosely called "Pepper's People." The purpose of these hearings, press releases, and rallies was to build interest in the creation of a national health insurance program, including home care coverage for catastrophic illness. "My one great wish is to live long enough to see the day when this great and prosperous nation can give every man, woman, and child, regardless of age or ability to pay, every bit of the health care he or she needs. I think this is part of the American dream," he said in a highly publicized speech.

In another speech, he said:

> The sleeping giant of American politics, the senior citizens of America, some 28 million strong, have awakened, they are hurt and they are angry, they have been double-crossed, deceived, and betrayed. I am here to tell you that they will no longer tolerate such abuse and continue to turn the other cheek. They have left their rocking chairs and taken up placards. The elderly of America do not come on bended knee as supplicants to the highest Houses of power. We do not plead for benevolence from those who occupy the seats of the mighty. We seek justice and we come to demand our rights.

By 1987, Pepper had heard enough. He had reached the conclusion that long-term care was the most desperate problem affecting America and that home care was the best solution. On a train, headed for a Democratic party leadership retreat, Pepper sat with a legal pad and drew up the outline of his long-term home care legislation.

Views on the Issues

Claude Pepper knew he had cancer in 1987. With time being so scarce, he chose to husband his energies to work on what was most important to him. The first goal was to insure the creation of a national memorial to Franklin D. Roosevelt and in this he succeeded. The second was to bring about the enactment of a national long-term care legislation based on home care and in this regard he came up a few votes short.

The enactment of long-term home care legislation was Pepper's last great obsession. In the debate on his bill, H.R. 3436, which took place on June 8, 1988, Pepper pleaded his case:

> Mr. Speaker, members of the House, this is a day for which I have waited and worked, and I might say prayed for 50 years, a chance to do something to lighten the burden upon the masses of the people of this country, trying to help those saddled with a long-term illness. . . . I ask you, as we sit here in the comfort of this Chamber today, do not forget those people back home . . . think about the people who are affected, think about what it will mean to the people of this country less fortunate than we . . . . And so I ask you, my colleagues, when you go home tonight and you close your eyes and you sleep and you ask, "What have I done today to lighten the burden upon those who suffer," at least you could say, "I helped a little bit today; I voted to help those who needed help." It may not answer all the problems, and it does not, but it will give comfort. It will cool the brow of many who suffer. It will give hope to many who almost are despaired.

The Pepper bill would have amended Medicare to provide coverage for a broad range of in-home health care services. The services would have been available to those who suffered from either physical or mental disability. Individuals who needed help in performing two or more of the essential activities of daily living, such as getting out of bed, getting dressed, and feeding themselves, would be eligible to receive assistance. The help would have been available to the 4.1 million Americans who suffer from Alzheimer's disease, the 6.5 million seniors who suffer from heart disease, stroke, crippling arthritis, as well as a similar number of middle-aged people who are victims of accidents. The bill would also have helped some 3 million chronically ill and disabled children who are born with cerebral palsy, epilepsy, and other chronic diseases. As far as Pepper was concerned, the real issue in long-term care is not age but disability.

Pepper had worked out an inventive but reasonable financing scheme. He proposed removal of the $45,000 cap, which was then the limit on earnings susceptible to the Social Security tax. Only three percent of all Americans make more than this amount. Pepper reasoned that 97 percent of all Americans paid the tax (seven percent) on all their income to fund Social Security and Medicare and he could see no reason why the wealthiest Americans could not do likewise. In short, Pepper's proposal would have made the Social Security tax more progressive. It would have raised the necessary revenue not only for the present, but into the distant future.

A coalition of some 140 major organizations supported Pepper in his view that long-term care was the greatest problem facing America going into the last decade of the 20th century. Some 167 members of Congress agreed, but it was not enough to get past technical objections imposed by a jealous committee chairman. Pepper vowed to bring up his bill again. He also structured a high-powered bipartisan commission made up of six congressmen and six senators, all key players with respect to health care. In addition, President Reagan appointed three representatives to the panel. Pepper was named the first chairman of this commission which was created for the purposes of fashioning recommendations to the Congress as to how it should address the problem of long-term care, and the fact that some 37 million Americans do not have any health insurance coverage at all. The latter problem was less significant to Pepper because most of these people eventually find coverage in the Medicaid program.

Following Pepper's death, the commission was named in his honor and Senator John D. "Jay" Rockefeller IV was named its chairman.

The commission passed its recommendations with respect to health insurance for the uninsured by the slim margin of 8 to 7. However, the long-term care recommendations passed by the margin of 11-4, a strong mandate which essentially echoed the principles of Congressman Pepper's bill.

At Congressman Pepper's funeral and at the Capitol Rotunda ceremony, Majority Leader George Mitchell told the public and most of the assembled House and Senate: "The best way that we can honor Claude Pepper is to fulfill his one unmet dream, to enact his long-term home care legislation."

Dozens of senators and congressmen pledged themselves toward this end. They remember the fact that he kept to himself the fact that he was dying when the disclosure of this fact would have swept his bill into enactment. They also remember that in the debate, in which proponents and opponents each had half an hour, Pepper yielded 15 minutes of his side to members of Congress that he knew would use the time to oppose him. They remember that Pepper was right when he told them President Ronald Reagan's Catastrophic Health Protection Act was bad legislation and that it would be repudiated by the elderly. In short, they remember the class of the man, his great vision of the future, and an unerring ability to discern what was important and right for the nation's senior citizens.

Several bills have been introduced in the Congress to provide comprehensive home care coverage in order to meet the long-term health care needs of the nation. To Pepper, this was the single most important issue not only for the elderly, but for all Americans. Both the Democratic and Republican parties in their 1988 presidential platforms committed themselves to the enactment of such a plan, but only the future will tell whether Pepper's great dream will be realized.

Insights and Perspectives

What was he like, this man of legends? He was five feet, eight inches tall, always well dressed, usually wearing a three-piece suit with a Phi Beta Kappa key stretched across his vest.

He was blessed with good health. He had an operation in 1976 to replace a calcified heart valve. The story goes that upon awakening from the anesthesia, Pepper jokingly reprimanded the surgeon for not making him 30 years younger and better looking.

He was always a firebrand. He shook things up. He had the energy and stamina of a teenager. However, he was temperate in his habits, allowing himself only one glass of wine with dinner. He had two eccentricities—he liked hot soup and crackers with every meal and he had a passion to read Prince Valiant in the Sunday comic section.

It was not unusual for him to work 15-hour days even in his 89th year. By metabolism, he was nocturnal. He worked late into the night reading or writing in his journal. Predictably, he did not like getting up in the morning, although he did so on a regular basis. If adjectives could describe Pepper, genteel, gracious, lovable, and aggressive would be high on the list. He had a certain star quality. He was like a blossoming flower—the longer one knew him, the more he revealed himself. He was equally at home talking to construction workers and Harvard lawyers.

He had a wonderful sense of humor, which he often turned on himself. Some of his jokes were older than he was, but he told them with such gusto and enjoyed them so much himself, they never failed to get a laugh.

Pepper retained an essential curiosity about life and an enthusiasm for getting at the root of problems and finding solutions. He managed to stand up for what was right with the rigidity of the Rocky Mountains and somehow find the flexibility and resilience to make room for new ideas. He had the ability to adapt to his changing environment. He was very balanced in his sense of time. He was able to draw on the past without dwelling on it, to make the most of the present and savor every moment, and at the same time to look many years into the future. He often said that every day on earth is a blessing and it must be savored as such.

He had a keen mind and a vast store of knowledge. He could hold his own with scientists on subjects as diverse as nuclear physics or genetic research. He had a wonderful memory and he had lived long enough to see the same set of circumstances present themselves several times and he knew what solutions did and did not work.

He was one of the most moral men in Congress. He set a standard for himself that was a little higher than most people seemed to be able to meet, but he did not seek to impose his standards on others.

He never lost sight of where he came from. He approached life with the gratitude for the blessings that he had received and he tried his best to share these gifts with those who were less fortunate. He was an exception to the old adage that power corrupts. Claude Pepper, like fine wine, got better with age. He was great fun to be with and had a gift for transforming even the most mundane occasion into a celebration.

He had a wonderful gift for the language. His oratorical powers were second to none. He had the uncanny ability to move people with the English language.

Pepper had known hunger and tried to help people obtain food. He had been jobless and tried to help people find employment. He knew what it meant to be without a shelter and he tried to help people find a home. He knew how tragic it was for children to go without an education and he did his best to help make it available to them. He had known great pain and tried to bring comfort and caring into people's lives. He had seen hopelessness and fear in the eyes of the elderly and tried to bring them comfort and security. He had seen farmers and small businessmen go broke and he did the best he could to give them every opportunity for survival.

> "I seek a better life not just for the elite but for all. I reject the notion that those who are underprivileged have earned their fate and hard work inexorably leads to success. I believe that health and economic security and—to the degree possible—happiness of its people is the proper concern of the government. . . . No one and nothing except government is big enough and powerful enough and universal enough to make life bearable for the masses of our citizens. Voices cry out from high places "let the private sector do it." Fine if it can and will, but the truth is, it will not and can not.

In his book, *Pepper, Eyewitness to a Century*, he puts forth what he called a fundamental dichotomy which has been at the heart of domestic political structures since the beginning of the Republic. One view which he ascribed to Ronald Reagan is that government is the enemy and that anyone can become rich and successful if they are willing to work. Those who do not are lazy or unwilling to work. The second point of view, which Pepper represented, is that government should make opportunities available to all members of society and lend a helping hand to the handicapped, poorly educated, sick, forgotten, or those who were down on their luck, in order that they may become productive and contributing members of society.

"America should be in center stage among the nations of the earth," said Pepper, "standing up for what is right and opposing what is wrong and trying to build the institutions that will preserve the peace and the happiness of mankind." Related comments follow.

On the Role of Government

> I've always tried to make government the friend of the people. The government of the United States belongs to the people of this land and whenever their troubles, their disasters and their needs impel its use, it is available. It is the mightiest institution on the face of the earth and it can be a hand that will lift up the people if they call upon it.

On Public Life

> Compassion, genuine concern for one's fellow man should be at the heart of every man or woman who assumes the awesome responsibilities of public office.
>
> Fundamentally, there are two types of men in public life. Those who in their hearts want to serve the people and those who in their hearts want to serve the special interests and the privileged few. I have fearlessly aligned myself in Washington for those fighting from day-to-day to better the lot of the common people in America; trying to raise their wages and see that they get fair working conditions, to give needed capital to little as well as big business, to provide better health care facilities, more adequate educational opportunities for the children of today, better homes for the poorly housed, jobs for the unemployed, a larger mental and spiritual horizon for the forgotten and neglected, a deeper, richer, fuller life for all the men and women in America.

On the Democratic Party

> The welfare of the majority lies in the triumph in the principles espoused by the Democratic party. I want it to be the liberal party of this nation. I want it not to compromise upon that matter. We must stand for principle and not election always. We must be so firm in

> our allegiance to a unitarian political philosophy that the people of this nation shall know upon whom to call when they are convinced that this philosophy is right.

Learned and Believed

When asked about his philosophy of life, Congressman Pepper said simply, "Make it better." He believed that every human being should devote his or her life in service to humanity in order to make life just a little bit better for others.

He believed that one person can make a difference. He often referred to his lonely battle to secure passage of lend-lease legislation or measures to abolish mandatory retirement as examples of how one person can succeed against the greatest odds.

He believed in taking action. He put it this way in a 1941 speech:

> Give me the young man at Arcola, and at Lodi, who went forward in the face of the enemy's hail of bullets, and not the shrinking man at Waterloo. So long as life lasts, men hope to go forward and upward in their course, to dream dreams, and eventually to soar beyond the summit of the highest clouds.

He believed the only limit on human accomplishment was the ability to dream. He knew that the idea was father to the deed and in Sandburg's words, "that nothing happens but first a dream."

He believed that nothing was impossible and that, in fact, the impossible was often more easily accomplished than the remotely possible.

He believed in the importance of standing up for principle. "Be true to yourself," he used to say, "and you can be false to no man."

He believed that a person should live as if every day were his last and yet at the same time live as though they would live forever.

He believed that one should not sit idly in the face of injustice. Indignation, outrage, and action are appropriate responses, he said.

He believed with Einstein "that only a life lived for others is worthwhile" and with Mother Teresa that "there is joy in transcending self in order to serve others." He once said, "I have no desire to affluent living. I could have made more money by practicing law but money does not mean that much to me. I would rather try to get a bill through

Congress that would help people to do something to make our country a little bit better."

He believed with Helen Hayes that "to rest is to rust."

He was an advocate of aggressive aging, of involvement instead of retirement.

He believed in the importance of keeping alive the child within each person. He agreed with Huxley that "to carry the spirit of childhood into old age is the secret of genius."

When asked what was the great secret of the universe, he said, "Love one another and do unto others as you would have others do unto you."

He believed with Father Brook "that when one reaches out to help another human being, he touches the face of God."

When asked who were the most important mentors in his life, he mentioned educators C. C. Moseley, George H. Denny, and Roscoe Pound, as well as Franklin Delano Roosevelt. He said that Roosevelt left the country three great legacies. First, he showed by his example and leadership that the government of the United States belongs to the people and that this great institution will lift up the people if they call upon it. Second, he left a legacy of compassion and genuine concern for one's fellow man. Third, he left America on center stage in world affairs.

When asked what advice he would have for young people, he said: "I have advised young people to fashion their lives and to live in such a way that when they come to the upper ages of life, they will be able to look back and say that they did something to make it possible for other people to walk on higher ground, to live a little healthier, happier, and better lives."

When asked for his advice to seniors, Pepper told an *Associated Press* reporter:

> Keep on doing what you've been doing all along, but maybe at a slower pace.
>
> I was playing golf one day when I noticed my partner's clubs were lighter than mine. I tried his and I found I could handle them easier. So I changed to less weighty clubs.
>
> So that's what you do in life. When you come to a time when there's a need for any sort of change, simply lighten your clubs and change your behavior a little bit, and go right ahead.

Honors and Awards

During the course of his career, Claude Pepper was showered with awards. He received literally rooms full of plaques and other memorabilia. Foremost among these awards was the Presidential Medal of Freedom, the nation's highest civilian honor, which was bestowed on him on May 25, 1989, by President George Bush. Other honors include the following:

Honorary Degrees: LL.D., McMaster University (Canada), 1941; University of Toronto (Canada), 1942; University of Alabama, 1942; Rollins College (Florida), 1944; D.Sc., University of Miami, 1974; Doctor of Fine Arts, International Fine Arts College, 1982; Doctor of Humane Letters, Mt. Sinai Medical Center (New York), 1982; Doctor of Humane Letters, University of South Florida, 1982.

Awards: National Parkinson Foundation Award for Public Service, 1965; Alianza Inter-Americana Award, 1966; Mary and Albert Lasker Public Service Award, 1967; Eleanor Roosevelt Humanities Award, 1968; Veterans of Foreign Wars Award, 1968; Professional Air Traffic Controllers Award, 1970; Volunteers of America Ballington and Maud Booth Award, 1978; Florida Democratic Party Hubert H. Humphrey Statesmanship Award, 1979; National Retired Teachers Association Andrus Award, 1980; Ze'ev Jabotinsky Centennial Award, 1980; Democratic Club of Miami Beach "Man of the Year" Award, 1980; Ollie A. Randall Award of the National Council on Aging, 1980; Retired Senior Volunteer Program Award, 1981; the Presidential Award of the Western Gerontological Association, 1981-82; Florida Gold Coast Chamber of Commerce "Man of the Year" Award, 1981; B'nai B'rith "CHAI" Award for outstanding contributions to community service, 1981; Burden Center Alice Brophy Award for Services to the Aging, 1981; Home Health Care Humanitarian Award, 1982; National Education Association Award, 1982; American Institute for Public Service "Jefferson Award" for Greatest Public Service Benefiting the Disadvantaged, 1982; Fraternal Order of Eagles Franklin Roosevelt Award, 1983; American Academy of Achievement Golden Plate Award, 1983; B'nai B'rith John F. Kennedy Profiles in Courage Award, 1983; The University of Alabama Hugo Black Award, 1984;

the Alabama Gold Medal of Honor, 1985; the Fraternal Order of Eagles Social Security Award 1985; the Franklin D. Roosevelt Four Freedoms Award, 1985; the Lifetime Achievement Award from the Foundation for Hospice and Homecare, 1986; the Claude D. Pepper Award of the National Association for Home Care, 1987, and the Allied Signal Award for Achievement in Aging, 1988.

In accordance with an Act of Congress passed November 21, 1988, Building 31 of the National Institutes of Health was christened the Claude Denson Pepper Building on May 10, 1989. The Pepper Building, on the NIH campus in Bethesda, Maryland, is the main administration building and the seat of the 13 individual Institutes of Health. Pepper, who sponsored or cosponsored legislation creating 12 of the 13 Institutes, was hailed as the "legislative father" of NIH by its director, James B. Wyngaarden, M.D.

In 1985, Florida State University honored him and his wife through the creation of the Mildred and Claude Pepper Memorial Library. The library is a depository of all the Congressman's papers as well as thousands of photographs, books, and newspaper clippings and film. It contains an accurate replica of both Claude Pepper's senatorial and congressional office. Congressman Pepper also raised money in his lifetime to endow an eminent scholars program and a chair in social gerontology. The Mildred and Claude Pepper Foundation was also established to continue this work.

Finally, pursuant to an act of Congress, Claude Pepper's body lay in state in the rotunda of the nation's capitol on June 1-2, 1989. It was an honor granted previously to 23 Americans in the history of the republic, including only six members of Congress.

As Seen by His Colleagues

"Claude Pepper gave meaning and definition to the concept of public service," said President George Bush. "He fought for the poor and the elderly in his own determined way. Those who agreed with him were proud to follow his banner. Those who disagreed with him always respected him. He was a gentleman and noble human being."

"For longer than the rest of us," said Jim Wright, former Speaker of the House, "he was a moving force in American life. He was always a voice of the voiceless and a helping hand for the helpless."

Former President Jimmy Carter, said: "Pepper was a master at using his influence in government for the benefit of those most in need."

"I have learned that the thing that really counts in political life is wholeheartedness, integrity, and true desire to do what you say you are doing. Of all the people I have known in Congress, Congressman Pepper most clearly brought that lesson home to us," said Congresswoman Millicent Fenwick.

"I always say he was the greatest Roman of them all. The finest American who ever lived," said Congressman Jake Pickle.

"If I were to write *Profiles in Courage* I would place him at the top," said Congressman Gus Hawkins.

"No single person has had a greater impact on the public life of America," noted Congressman Tony Coelho.

"He set the standard by which members of Congress can judge their lives and their performance and there is no finer tribute than that," said Majority Leader Richard Gephardt.

"He was what public service was all about. He was trying to make life better for the people. He was what we wished more people in politics would be like," said former Congresswoman Geraldine Ferraro.

"I think of Claude Pepper whenever I see a combination of passion and compassion, true dedication and devotion and true patriotism. Our lives are better and our country is richer because of this wonderful human being," said Senate Majority Leader George Mitchell.

Remembered

When asked how he would like to be remembered, he said: "I hope when I have come to the end of my journey, I can look back and see that I have made a difference, that I have made the road a little lighter for those who follow after me."

In his autobiography, he said: "Providence has given me a life of personal satisfaction and fulfillment that comes from knowing one has been able to make life a little bit better for others—for many others. This is something that those who spend their lives trying to maintain and expand entrenched privileged will never, ever know."

When asked the same question by Morley Safer as part of a CBS "Sixty Minutes" tribute, Pepper volunteered that he had written his own epitaph. When pressed by Safer, he said: "He loved God and the people and tried to serve both."

Claude Pepper devoted his life to making life better for others. It is hard to say which of his achievements most benefits individuals and the nation. He played a key role in blunting Nazi aggression and in doing so preserved freedom not only in America, but throughout the world. He was a major factor in the enactment of the Civil Rights Act of 1965, which many historians say was the most important piece of legislation to be enacted in the 20th century.

Equally important, he gave Franklin D. Roosevelt the blueprints he needed to position the Democratic party as the advocate of the common man. Pepper was a populist, a New Dealer before there was a New Deal. He fought for old age pensions in the Florida legislature a dozen years before Social Security was created. He was not only architect but chief defender of these policies. In 1981 when Social Security was in its greatest jeopardy, he stepped forward to save it.

His achievements in health care were vast. He looked at health care as a basic civil right and as a matter of national defense. America could not defend itself, he reasoned, unless its citizens were healthy and fit. He lived to double the average life expectancy at the time of his birth and he wished the same blessing on every person in America. If the 20th century will be remembered for two world wars, television, the computer, and man's landing on the moon, it will also be remembered for the progress that was made in medical research. The average life span was increased in the 20th century more than in the previous 500 years. It is true, but hard to imagine that one man, Claude Pepper, is primarily responsible for this achievement. Pepper conceived and pushed through congressional legislation the World Health Organization and which created 12 of the 13 National Institutes of Health, the finest medical research facilities the world has ever known. As in the case of his intervention with Lend-Lease legislation, it was not only America that benefited, but the entire world.

Another of his most important achievements is the inspiration of generations of American leaders. He served as role model and mentor to many young Americans. He was what every young boy dreamed of being when young and wishes he had been when old.

Another huge contribution was his work to insure freedom at every level for the citizens of the United States and to keep them free from fear. He used his full energies to keep people "free from oppression, free from the fear of illness and poverty, free from the fear of discrimination, from the fear of ignorance, and from the fear of opportunity foreclosed." To put things in a positive context, he did his best to empower human beings, to remove obstacles, to give people a maximum number of choices and opportunities. He worked tirelessly for social justice, social mobility, and equality of opportunity. He was a great champion of the underprivileged.

The *Almanac of American Politics* says of him that he was "a pivotal figure in politics and in American history for a longer time than anyone else." He was an original, a true genius who never forgot his roots, who worked hard to make it possible for other children of humble backgrounds who apply themselves to become senators, representatives, or presidents.

His most lasting legacy, however, will be his work on behalf of older Americans. "Claude Pepper treated the elderly with the respect they deserved and the gratitude they merited," said Bob Hope. "He never let America forget that we are strong today because of the contributions of those who came before. He convinced the nation and seniors themselves that they were a valuable asset and that they were as much a part of the American present and future as they were a part of the past."

Claude Pepper helped shatter the myth that senility, decrepitude and powerlessness are a natural state of aging. Through his example, he proved that people could continue to grow, to learn, to live vigorous and productive lives, to handle challenges of great complexity and continue to exercise excellent judgment well into their eighth and ninth decades and beyond. By his life and his example, he totally redefined the concept of aging in America, shattering stereotypes and opening a new world of opportunity for the millions of America's senior citizens, past, present, and future.

It may be oversimplification, but a philosopher once wrote that the careers of truly great men and women can be capsuled in one phrase. For example, with respect to Abraham Lincoln, most people will say, "He freed the slaves." With respect to Claude Pepper, historians might say, "He liberated the elderly of America and brought them freedom from fear."

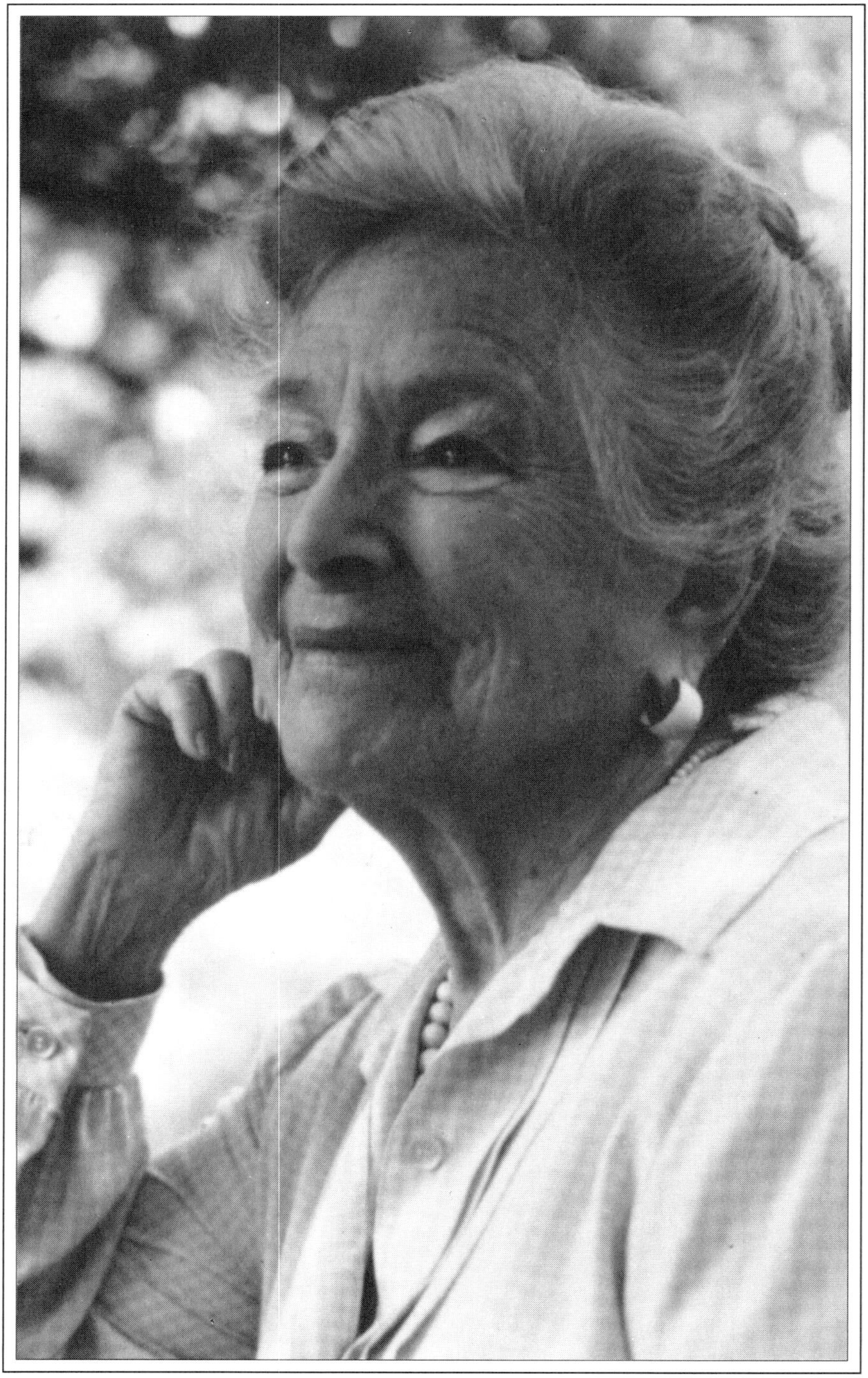

COURTESY OF HELEN HAYES

TWO

Helen Hayes

Helen Hayes is known and loved internationally as the "First Lady of the American Theater." It is a reputation she richly deserves. She is universally acclaimed by her peers and laymen alike as the best ever to set foot on a stage.

Over the years, she has brought joy to countless millions who have viewed her performances, not only in the theater, but through the magic of movies and television.

What is less known about Hayes is the fact that she ranks second to none as an advocate for the nation's senior citizens. Throughout her life she has fought against ageism and against the notion that seniors should be out of sight and out of mind. She has fought hard to protect the solidarity of the family and to keep the elderly in independence in their own homes instead of placing them in institutions. Through her portrayal of heroic figures, such as Queen Victoria, she has been able to demonstrate that aging is not necessarily a time of weakness, powerlessness, and senility. In her own life she has survived crises which would have broken a less resilient person. Having come through it all in grand style, Hayes, going strong into her ninth decade, not only serves as a role model, but is working aggressively to impart her knowledge to others.

Through her syndicated radio program, "Our Best Years," Hayes reached millions of senior Americans and their families every week. She dispensed comfort, caring, and wisdom in equal measure.

Hayes has used her celebrity to open the doors of Congress. She used her high degree of credibility to argue for social justice. She fought side by side with Congressman Claude Pepper to bring about the enactment of legislation that prohibited the dismissal of aging workers simply on the basis of chronological age. She has fought for nursing home reform and to bring about the enactment of a national program of long-term care based on home care.

Hayes describes herself as a curious person. "I was born inquisitive and I shall die inquisitive," she says. She admits to being a perfectionist. "Mother yearned for quality and set her sights on perfection. It was a contagious fever and I caught it." Hayes admits that the fact that, at five feet, she is short stuck in her craw until she decided to overcome it. "I became the tallest five-foot person in the world." Throughout, she has maintained a positive outlook on life: "I have always been concerned with the whole of life and not the fragments; the positive and not the negative; the words and not the spaces between the lines. I am a triumph of the familiar over the exotic," she comments wryly.

She is an advocate of continuing education, quoting Benjamin Disraeli, who said, "The more extensive a man's knowledge of what has been done, the greater will be his power of knowing what to do."

Out of all of the roles that she has played over the years, nothing more suits her than her present role as a premier spokesperson and advocate for the elderly. No doubt a good portion of her success and acceptance comes from the fact that she is playing herself: not acting out lines written for her, but putting into action what she actually thinks and believes.

Few people have made a greater contribution to enriching the nation than has Helen Hayes. She deserves the respect and commendation of good men and women everywhere.

Early Years

Helen Hayes was born in Washington, D.C., on October 10, 1900. Her father, Francis Van Arnum Brown, was a manager and salesman for a wholesale butcher. Her mother, Catherine (Hayes) Brown, can be credited with developing young Helen's interest in acting and dancing. It is reported that Hayes made her first amateur performance as a pupil in Miss Minnie Hawkin's dancing school, where she impersonated a Gibson Girl at the school's May Ball. Hayes joined the Columbia Players, an acting company based in Washington, and made her professional debut at the age of five as Prince Charles in *The Royal Family*. Hayes came to the attention of producer Lew Fields, in whose production *Old Dutch* she first appeared on Broadway at the age of nine. She was a smash hit from the beginning. She appeared in several other productions on Broadway before returning to the Columbia Players and to school. She completed her education at Washington Sacred Heart Academy in 1917.

Since that time, Hayes has collected honorary degrees from Smith College, Columbia University, the University of Denver, and Hamilton and Elmira Colleges, both in New York. In 1952, she received a Doctor of Fine Arts Degree from St. Mary's College in Princeton, New Jersey.

Hayes loved her father, who she describes as the "gentlest, kindest, dearest man who ever lived." He had a passion for baseball, often taking young Helen with him to Griffith's field to root for his hapless Washington Senators and for their ace pitcher, Walter Johnson. Helen loved this time with her father, but increasingly she was pulled away from him by her mother's ambitions and the theater.

She describes her mother as a driven, hard-charging, enthusiastic person who was full of determination. She was a wonderful companion who "charted our course, keeping things shipshape, leaving Father more and more in our wake," she says. "I hated her for making Father unhappy. This is when I learned that it is possible to love and hate in concert."

Hayes married playwright and producer, Charles MacArthur, on August 17, 1928. The marriage brought her great happiness, a daughter, Mary, and a son, James. Mary died of polio in 1949, marking what was the most difficult period in Helen's life. Characteristically, she pulled through by throwing herself into her work and by forming a foundation to raise money to find a cure for the dreaded disease. The discovery of the Salk vaccine in 1952 understandably was one of the most gratifying events in her life. Asked how she survived this ordeal, Hayes told *USA Today* in a 1987 interview:

> One night, when I was desperate, I put on the light. I was so

afraid I'd do something awful, like take too many sleeping pills. This was not long after Mary died. I picked up my book of Psalms, and I just opened it at random, and there was this one that said: "I waited patiently for the Lord, he inclined unto me, and heard my plea." And I thought, all right, patience, patience does it. Well, this woman quoted this, and she said, "You say patience, patience. But how can I find that patience?" So I wrote her and said, "I think maybe that wasn't the right word for everybody, but maybe determination that I will not let this destroy me. And, maybe that fit. You'll have to fight. You have to fight just as hard as you know how, more than you know how."

Her husband, Charles, who collaborated with Ben Hecht in writing the prizewinning play *The Front Page*, also wrote and produced a long string of other literary and movie hits before his death in 1958. Again, Hayes was devastated.

"There is a secret to surviving tragedy," she notes. "It is not to keep to oneself." She credits Charles with teaching her how to be confident in that most "audacious act" of loving mortal things. "They leave you. They perish. But one must love again; one must adventure endlessly in loving, never fearing loss or pain."

James G. MacArthur, her adopted son, is now an established actor perhaps best known for his part in the long-running CBS television series "Hawaii Five-0." He has two children—a son, Charles, and a daughter, Mary.

Hayes has been a star of stage, screen, radio, and television, but the theater will always be her first love. "Quiet laughter in the theater is the sound of heaven," she says.

Theater Career

Talk to people on Broadway, and they will tell you that they will never forget Helen Hayes. Everyone has his or her favorite play, favorite role or one performance that was especially important to them. Hayes's career in the theater shows incredible versatility and energy. She has played everything from slapstick comedy to Shakespeare. In the end, she may be best remembered for her historical portraits of famous people. Properly so, since she began her professional career playing a prince and in her time has played both queen and empress.

Critics have especially acclaimed Hayes's performance in the play *Dear Brutus* by Sir James Barrie, which was later recreated for television. Others remember *She Stoops to Conquer* or her dazzling performance as Cleopatra in George Bernard Shaw's *Ceasar and Cleopatra*. Returning to Broadway after the birth of her daughter, Hayes received national acclaim for her portrayal of the tragic Mary Stuart in Maxwell Anderson's *Mary of Scotland*, which he wrote especially for her.

In 1935, Hayes played the lead in Laurence Houseman's *Victoria Regina*, which played on Broadway and across the nation for four years. Ms. Hayes played the role of Queen Victoria 969 times and with such grace that one critic said, "Many count the play as one of the happiest experiences in all of modern theater." In the play, Hayes, as the British queen, aged 80 years within two and a half hours. Her appearance in this play brought Hayes the Drama League of New York City's Medal for Most Distinguished Performance in 1936.

Another highlight, in 1944, was her portrayal of Harriet Beecher Stowe in the play *Harriet*, which ran for 377 performances. Her first London performance was in 1948, where she starred in Tennessee Williams's *The Glass Menagerie*. In 1950, she played in Joshua Logan's *The Wisteria Trees*, based on a book by Anton Chekov, and two years later in Mary Chase's *Mrs. McThing*. Other credits include *The Skin of Our Teeth* by Thornton Wilder, *Harvey* by Mary Chase, and O'Neill's *Long Day's Journey Into Night*.

Hayes shares with Ethel Barrymore the distinction of being the only actress for whom theaters have been named in New York. This was done on November 21, 1955, the 50th anniversary of her first appearance on stage. In that year, she won the Antoniette Perry Award as Best Actress for *Time Remembered*.

When asked if she missed the stage, noting that she has not appeared since 1971, Hayes answered in the negative. She reported that she had suffered a very serious asthma attack during a performance in Washington, D.C. Physicians finally came to the conclusion that she was allergic to the theater and ordered her to quit. "Seriously," she added, "theaters are full of dust, pollen and mold, and all those things to which I was allergic."

Movies and Television

Helen Hayes always preferred Broadway to Hollywood, but that didn't stop her from making memorable movies. It is fortunate that she appeared in a dozen or more films so that future generations will have the opportunity to see her.

Hayes started acting in silent movies and she was in some of the first talkies while still a teenager. In 1932, she won an Oscar for her performance as Best Actress in *The Sin of Madelon Claudet*. Other highlights include *Farewell to Arms* (1956), adapted from the Hemingway classic, *Anastasia*, in which she portrayed the Dowager Empress and which co-starred Ingrid Bergman and Yul Bryner, and *Airport* (1971), for which she won the Oscar as Best Supporting Actress. Hayes is the only actress to be batting 1,000 on Oscars—she has won every time she has been nominated. She shares with Ingrid Bergman the honor of being the only actress to win both the Best Actress and the Best Supporting Actress Award.

Her television appearances have been many. She was the recipient of an Emmy award in 1954. Americans will remember her from her visits in conjunction with CBS-TV's much-heralded "Omnibus" program. From 1972-74, Hayes played in a TV series called "The Snoop Sisters," in which she helped solve one mystery after another.

In 1982, Hayes narrated and helped produce a film for public television entitled "No Place Like Home," which contrasts the quality of life of those Americans placed in nursing homes with those who are receiving health care and supportive services at home. The film is a powerful indictment of the bankrupt nature of American social policy which invests billions of dollars to place infirm seniors in institutions, but only a tiny fraction of this amount to maintain them in independence in their own homes.

"No Place Like Home" clearly touched a nerve. It set off a tidal wave of discussions in every community in the nation. Special screenings were arranged for House and Senate committees and Hayes was summoned to testify before the Senate Committee on Labor and Public Welfare. Understandably, the film won its share of awards, including the Robert F. Kennedy Award, the Gabriel Award, and the American Film Festival Award. Hayes was honored as well, receiving the highest awards from both the National Association for Home Care and the National HomeCaring Council.

Radio

Hayes began in radio with a series of 15-minute talks in 1930. She had a major part in various network programs thereafter. One highlight was in 1939 when she starred with Orson Wells on CBS. From 1940-41, she produced and acted in "The Helen Hayes Theater." In 1940, she won an award as the Best Radio Actress. During the Second World War, her program "This Is Helen Hayes" promoted the nursing profession and helped recruit nurses for the army and navy.

From 1982 through 1986, Hayes hosted a weekly radio program directed at the nation's elderly, whom she prefers to call "maturians" because it sounds more militant. Hayes noted in a 1982 interview that she was proud to be taking over this show from broadcast great, Lowell Thomas. "I am devoting my life to helping maturians cope with the events in their lives," she added.

Transcripts from this highly regarded radio program provide an excellent summary of her views on the issues as noted below.

Views on the Issues

Helen Hayes has strong views on just about every topic of importance to the nation's elderly. Her attitude throughout is highly positive:

> This is a great time of my life, the best in many ways. I can do what I want, when I want, go where I please—as often and as long as I like. I'm accountable to no one and no one need check in with me. The world is my playground, my workroom, my stage, and my responsibility in a small measure, too. I've been given much. I owe a great deal. What I like about the eighties—mine and the century's—is that this decade is so full of change. The best part of it is that the miracle of modern medicine prolongs health and life so that "old" does not have to sound like punishment. What we need now is to have the social sciences catch up with the medicine men.

Attitudes toward the Elderly

Hayes has fought ageism just as she has fought against other kinds of discrimination in society. She says that part of the problem is our "adoration with youth." She adds that it may well be that the camera is at the root of the youth cult. "How utterly lovely are the young images jumping out at us from every magazine cover, television screen and billboard. Look in the mirror and you think you are from another planet. But the image there has the benefit of life instead of the mastery of makeup." Fortunately, she concludes, attitudes are changing. "The more older people stay in the mainstream of life the more accepting generations will be with each other."

Should Seniors Rest or Continue Activities?

Hayes says she is at odds with behavioral psychologist B.F. Skinner, who believes in making concessions to growing old, giving the old brain a chance to rest. "I, of course, refuse to slow down, lie down or back down. To rest is to rust. Skinner says, 'It's characteristic of old people not to think clearly, coherently, logically or particularly creatively.' To that, I say simply 'bosh'!" Hayes is opposed to abdication. "New horizons, new ideas, new activities, new points of view; there is life after sixty-five," she exclaims.

Advice on Successful Aging

Hayes advises seniors to enjoy life, to adopt a positive attitude, to set goals for themselves, to keep busy, and to do as much as they can to help others. Maintain as much independence as you can, she advises. "You will come to the inevitable conclusion that you are, if not in command, certainly in charge of supervising how you age. What goes on with your body is to some degree related to what goes in. Enthusiasm, productiveness, stimulating activities, intellectual progress—these are the ingredients for avoiding the retirement blues."

On Retirement

Hayes advises seniors to retool, not retire:

> Choose a path that will lead to an occupation—part- or full-time—mentally, physically and financially suited to your needs.

Teaching, I think, should be one of the avenues open to maturians—using what we have spent a lifetime acquiring to broaden the experience of the young. If you're looking to invest in your future, do it by investing in your mind. Life begins at retirement not because your job is finally behind you but because the world is suddenly open to you and you've prepared yourself for your debut.

On the Fear of Involvement

We seem to live in a society so complex that we don't know how to relate, and we've stopped trying. We are afraid to *touch*: We fear involvement and responsibility. There was a time when families cared for each other's children, when adults could admonish someone else's child and not fear the wrath of the parent. Now we have turned away from each other, and the results are devastating.

The touch of another being isn't just a human necessity. It activates the biological mechanisms which help the body heal itself. It makes the mind like itself. Not just young lovers' heart rates change when they hold hands. It happens even to patients in a coma when they are stroked . . . perhaps our collective minds would ease and our bodies would benefit if we, as a nation, could get past the antiquated idea that touch must be either a sexual signal or an act of aggression.

Sex and the Elderly

This subject, sex, and especially senior sex, which engenders hundreds of callous jokes, is a subject that too many of these people never giggle, laugh, or smile about when they are with each other, alone. We grow old and we think we're no longer lovable. Why? Because our skin doesn't fit as well, or the bounce is gone? Nonsense.

Hayes says that she can see no reason why at the very time of life when loving should be most enjoyable, least encumbering, seniors should give it up. "What is respectable for the young is not decadence in the old. The only obstacle to love are those you invent yourself."

On Nursing Homes

Hayes says that nursing home reform is "one of the most pressing social problems that we face." She has visited her share of such facilities, some of which have not had much to recommend them. "Just opening the front door or stepping off the elevator on certain floors can waft a message never to be forgotten. Sound, sights, and smells to scare off the bravest." "Many women," she says, "wind up in nursing homes because they thought there was no alternative. Responsibilities overwhelm them. Financial insecurity limits their lives. Loneliness depresses them. Fear of illness or crime drives them to despair." She adds that reform will only come "if the public realizes that we must apply pressure, remain informed, vigilant, and actively involved."

On Home Care

Hayes is a strong supporter of home care. It is less expensive and it keeps families together, she notes, adding that recovery is faster in our own surroundings than shut away in a hospital or other institution. She adds, "Science has taught us to lengthen life. Now we must learn to make a longer life worth living. Older people deserve choices that let us live out our days as we wish. We've seen people making such choices all over America, and we realize what we might have known from the start: For most of us, there really is no place like home."

On Age-Segregated Housing

Hayes opposes age-segregated housing. She favors, instead, measures which insure the solidarity of the American family. "I have always been of the opinion that separating the generations is a gross injustice to all concerned."

On Hearing Losses and Other Disabilities

> When the president dons a hearing aid, he's not betraying a weakness; he's showing a strength. By his action he says it's perfectly all right to have a disability. President Franklin Roosevelt, on the other hand, didn't let the public know for a long time that he had paralysis.
>
> Fighting as hard as we can against a disability is essential; we don't want to give in and give up. But denying it, for reasons of pride or prejudice, is a whole other matter. Many people, especially the elderly, don't like to admit to hearing loss and would rather suffer than succumb. Not hearing well enough is debilitating and dangerous.

On Mental Health

Hayes says recognizing the link between "mind and disease is as old as tribal medicine." She urges her counterparts accordingly to think positive thoughts:

> We all remember from our school days those experiments in conditioning by the Russian physiologist Pavlov, which have long been accepted as the first in the field. He demonstrated that the body will respond to mental stimulation. If I say to you "lemon juice," you probably can feel a change in your mouth, a tingling, can't you? Scientists are making great strides in understanding how this works. Eventually it will help us to fight disease, to stay well. We have learned, for instance, that great and continued stress or shock lowers the immunological activity of the body, making us susceptible to illness.

On Exercise and Therapy

Hayes notes that seniors are under great stress. "Living alone—at any age—can be hazardous to your health," she says. "The best prescription against anxiety and tension is physical exercise. A long walk, scrubbing the floor, throwing a bowling ball, or cutting the lawn is as effective as any tranquilizing drug—and has only beneficial after-effects, at a price you can't beat."

Those who need counseling, of course, should seek it, she advises. However, she believes the chief benefit of therapy comes from the rapport between two human beings. "It all comes down to caring and comforting—those things we can give each other."

On Work and Play

Hayes hopes that the Judeo-Christian work ethic is not so ingrained in our upbringing that it makes us feel guilty when we don't work or aren't otherwise engaged in some serious pursuit. If we overwork and underplay, we tend to feel depressed. She argues for a balance between work and leisure. "If we overplay and underwork, we feel we're ignoring our responsibilities. Play should be a routine part of our days. It's mandatory, not elective."

At the same time, Hayes feels that many young people today are raised with the idea that work is something to be avoided:

> We neglect to teach our children the pleasure of work and we rear them in an environment that doesn't encourage or admire hard work for its own sake. To get away with a minimum amount of work is the ideal. Leave it to machines, robots, services, gadgets, electronics, automatons. If we continue to fail our children, this negative approach to work will also stifle creativity and progress.
>
> The satisfaction of working to the limit of one's capacity has to be reinstilled in our society. Those of us who are older and remember the time when everyone worked, children included, have a lot to contribute.

On Fear of Failure

"The most marvelous life training course I can think of is the theater. In this business you learn early in life the advantages of failure. Failing has its benefits: you become more elastic and less rigid and self-effacing if you learn to accept it as an essential aspect of living." She adds that self-doubt and fear of failure are the "leg irons that keep us chained to the wailing wall of unaccomplishments."

On Education

Hayes is a strong advocate of continued education. She recalls the Jewish children who brought forth for their first lesson the ancient Talmud and found a bit of honey placed on the book in order to taste the sweetness of knowledge. "The activity itself," she adds, "pursued not just in school, but rather, throughout a lifetime, is the payoff. We must create a learning society—one devoted to the joys and rewards of continuous learning, as distinct from the one shot passing of some exam."

On Voting and Senior Power

Hayes believes that Gray Power is destined to play an ever-increasing role in American politics.

> Declining birth rate and advancing longevity—the seesaw is tipping to our side. An older electorate is better informed, more

experienced. Today's candidates are sensitive to the voting strength of maturians. One out of nine voters is now in the 18-to-20 age group. The concerns of the older voters go beyond their own welfare, beyond the current tendency to reduce governmental services and benefits, beyond temporary stopgap legislations. They care about the rest of the world, about their progeny, about the health of the planet. Gray Power in the voting booth is formidable, if it is predicated on continuing involvement by an informed constituency.

On the Appropriate Role for Seniors

"The job older people have—a job they need not compete for—is to be Aging Activists," says Hayes. "Now we must acquire a cheerful attitude, stop griping, and take charge of things. Claude Pepper [couldn't] do it alone. We are a formidable statistic. Just before 'they' start whispering about how we are the cause of a staggering national indebtedness, let's pay our dues with actions—in politics, in volunteerism, in charitable works. It's not enough to grumble and grouse and write a few letters of complaint. More important is the support we can and must give each other."

Books and Other Honors

Helen Hayes is also a scholar and a writer, having written nine books. She believes that she should leave behind for others a little of the thoughts, values, and philosophies which helped her in her impressive career. Her first effort was a book called *Star on Her Forehead,* which she coauthored with Mary Kennedy in 1949. This was followed by *A Gift of Joy* in 1965, *On Reflection* with Anita Loos in 1968, *Twice Over Lightly* in 1972, *A Gathering of Hope* in 1983, *Our Best Years* in 1984, *Loving Life* in 1987, *Where the Truth Lies* in 1988, and *My Life in Three Acts* in 1990.

Hayes's leadership abilities were recognized when she was selected vice-president of the Actors Fund in 1975. She also served as president of the American Theater Wing and of the American National Theater and Academy. In 1956, she was chosen as chairman of

National Citizens for Eisenhower. In 1978, she received the Medal of the City of New York, the Medal of Arts of Finland, and the American Exemplar Medal from the Freedoms Foundation. She also received the Laetare Medal from the University of Notre Dame in 1979. In 1985, she received the Lifetime Achievement Award from the Foundation for Hospice and Homecare, and in 1986 she was awarded the nation's highest civilian award, the Medal of Freedom, by President Ronald Reagan.

Summary

In 1900, when Helen Hayes was born, life expectancy was 47. The fact that she has lived into her ninth decade is in and of itself a wondrous achievement. The fact that millions of others have made this journey in longevity along with her is equally remarkable.

During her lifetime, Hayes has seen the nation change from the horse and buggy to the computer revolution. Almost every major invention that Americans now take for granted, from the airplane to the computer, was developed since 1900 when she was born.

Throughout her career, Hayes has demonstrated a marvelous ability to embrace this change while remaining true to her values. Through good times and bad, she has somehow kept her wonderful sense of equanimity.

Ralph Waldo Emerson writes that there is a fraternity of the best made people in all walks of life who have achieved and made extraordinary contributions to others. Hayes has her own list of heroes, including Congressman Claude Pepper, Buckminster Fuller, Bob Hope, Katherine Hepburn, Charles Schulz, famous Broadway producer George Abbott, and Victor Kugler, the man who provided Anne Frank and her family with a place to hide in Amsterdam. "To put your life willingly on the line isn't possible for everyone," she says, but "I think one must be emulating someone." Hayes adds that she studied biographies early in her life in the hope of finding the key to greatness.

Whether Hayes found the key to greatness in the writings or the example of others, or whether she found it within herself, there is no disputing the fact that she found it. Claude Pepper expressed the sentiments of many who know her in telling about an audience that he had with Pope John Paul II in 1982. He said:

> Last September, I was in Rome waiting for an audience with His Holiness, the Pope. I was ushered into a small private room, where I beheld this vision, this beautiful lady coming towards me with open arms. I thought His Holiness had sent down an angel to escort me. It was Helen Hayes.

Hayes once wrote that there were times when she felt that the absorbing work of the theater deprived her of other things in life. "I have learned that I was wrong," she told *Parade* magazine, "for what God has given me through my profession has made me sometimes able to help others—and myself. Certainly, it has made my life rich and meaningful."

The millions of Americans who will readily agree that she has helped enrich their lives can only cheer when Hayes adds, "As an active maturian, I myself intend to keep working until . . . well, perhaps the turn of the century, which I plan to celebrate on my feet."

❧

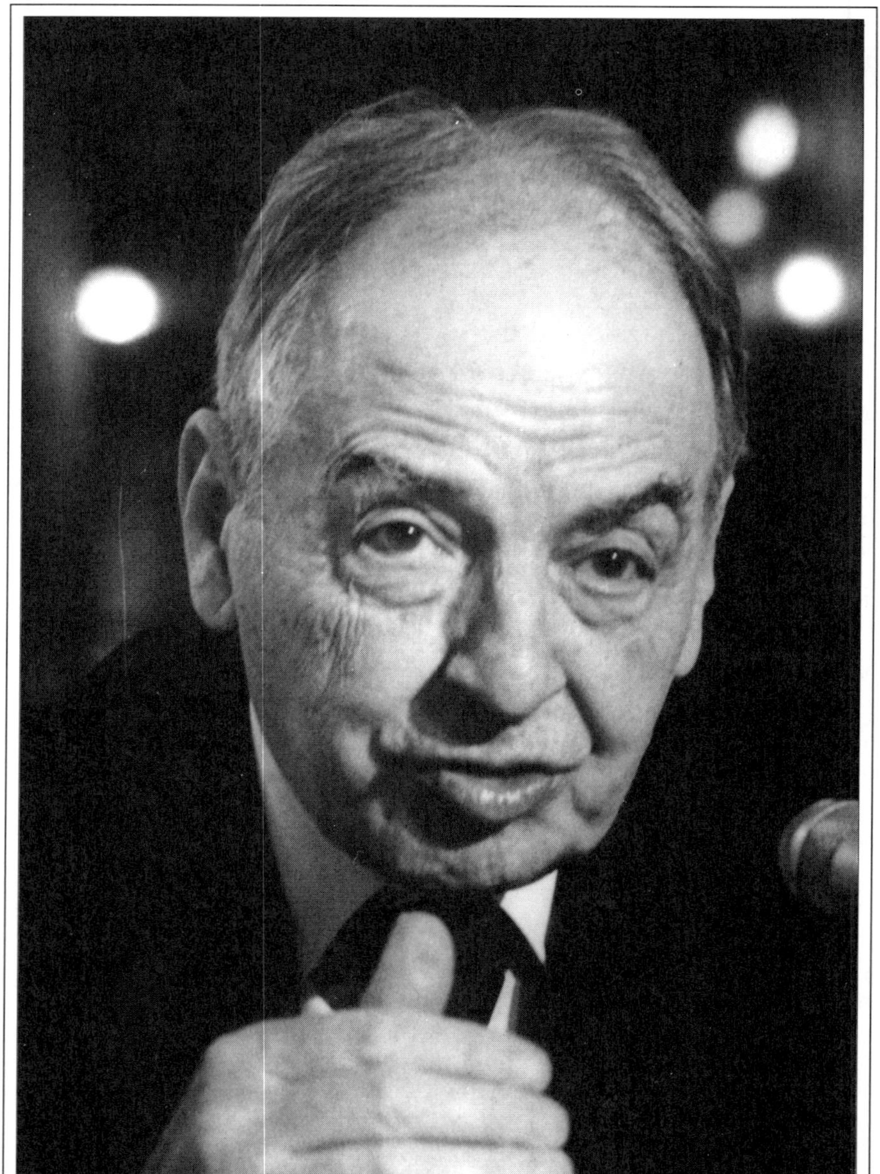

MARILU HALAMANDARIS

THREE

Arthur Flemming

Dr. Arthur Flemming is a tall man both in stature and in service to the American people. For more than 85 years, this modern Lancelot has crusaded for peace and social justice. He has battled each of the five horsemen of the modern day Apocalypse; ignorance, prejudice, hunger, pestilence, and disease have all felt the sting of his sword.

Unlike the Lancelot of old, Flemming has conducted his campaign without losing sight of his values or compromising his integrity. He is the very essence of morality.

Flemming is one of the most complete human beings God put on the earth. He is a man of ideas and a man of action. He is both teacher and doer. He is a man of intellect and a man of emotion. He is at once the personification of a highly efficient Washington lawyer and at the same time the best and most charismatic evangelist. He is a man of great gentleness and a man of great power. He can whisper in quiet tones to comfort a sick child and bring a crowd of 5,000 to their feet with a fiery speech that matches the best of William Jennings Bryan.

He is the kind of speaker that the greatest of speakers, such as his student Mike Vance, rank with the best that they have ever heard. What makes him so effective is that he is such a wonderful human being. He is the personification of the Emersonian admonition that what you are speaks more loudly than anything you say.

He is a complex man with interests as diverse as arms control, the environment and civil rights. For more than 60 years, he has worked to improve America's educational system. When it comes to human rights and civil rights, no one has done more than he. The same could be said for his efforts to improve the quality of life for the nation's senior citizens.

Flemming believes firmly in the importance of attracting the best young people in America to government service. His contribution toward the establishment and protection of the civil service system in America is unequalled.

Any examination of his career reveals a pattern of excellence and achievement beyond the highest expectations of others. Excellence was the fuel that propelled him to higher and higher posts. His basic integrity, combined with his intellect and his burning desire to make a difference, brought about his elevation to some of the most important and sensitive positions in government.

He has been the friend and confidant of seven presidents, representing both political parties, which have come to rely on him and value his good counsel and judgment.

Arthur Flemming is truly a man of the people. He has devoted his life to serve humanity and he vows to continue the fight until the very end of his days, moving at a pace that would put men one-fourth his age to shame. While his achievements have been many, he continues to look to the future toward his most impressive goal: bringing health care and especially long-term care to the American public. If the past is prologue, Flemming will achieve this great goal and go on to set and reach still others of similar import to the nation.

Years from now, when historians rank the impressive individuals who have served the nation as secretary of the Department of Health, Education and Welfare, there is little doubt but that Flemming's name will appear at the top.

Background

Arthur Flemming was born in 1905 in Kingston, New York, located about 90 miles north of New York City on the Hudson River. His father was a lawyer with a thriving practice who also was very much involved in the life of the community. The elder Flemming, for example, served as Judge of the Surrogate Court, as a corporation counsel and president of the school board. His mother was the daughter of a Baptist minister. Like her husband, she was very much involved in civic affairs, especially matters pertaining to the local Methodist Church.

Arthur attended public schools and graduated from high school in Kingston, a wonderful city in which to be raised, he remembers. Much of Arthur's early life centered around the local Methodist church and when it came time for him to go away to college, he considered two schools—Wesleyan in Middletown, Connecticut, and Ohio Wesleyan located in Delaware, Ohio.

He postponed the decision for a year, while he worked as a reporter with the *Kingston Daily Freeman*. "I had been working there during the summers and I decided to postpone my college education in order to get the experience of working there for a year. It was an education that I always valued greatly. I was fortunate to be working directly with the Managing Editor and I learned a great deal from him and I certainly learned much about the city and the county and life in general."

The year was 1923. Young Flemming decided to attend Ohio Wesleyan because of the school's excellent reputation in forensics. Flemming had enjoyed excellent success in debate as a high school student and the opportunity to participate in what was reputed to be one of the best debate programs in the nation fascinated him.

At the university, Flemming did exceptionally well, not only in forensics but in virtually everything else that he tackled. He was voted president of the class and was also successful scholastically. It was at Ohio Wesleyan that he developed his affection for government and political science.

In 1927, Arthur graduated with his B.A. degree and headed for Washington, D.C. It was a year to remember. Lindbergh crossed the Atlantic, Babe Ruth hit 60 home runs, and Warner Brothers made the first talking movie.

His first impression of Washington was that it was "a small, sleepy, segregated, southern city." Calvin Coolidge was in the White House and his work style was very much in tune with the city; the President was known to take two-to four-hour naps each day. Flemming says Washington was a kind of bucolic environment, mostly farmland, and that government was small if not non-existent. "President Coolidge was not about to expand the federal government; that was not part of his political philosophy."

Flemming took a job as a part-time professor in government at Washington's American University where he was also the coach of the debating team. A year later, he received his master's degree in the field of international law.

He left A.U. in order to take a job with a news magazine that is now *U.S. News and World Report*. At the time he worked there it was called *U.S. Daily* and then *U.S. News*. He worked as a reporter for almost five years covering major events in Washington, including President Franklin D. Roosevelt's press conferences. On the side, he went to law school at the George Washington University and obtained his law degree in 1933.

Flemming has fond memories of President Roosevelt. He remembers covering White House press conferences, which were held every Tuesday and Thursday. "It was a fascinating experience to see the President in action, to listen to him as he shared his dreams and aspirations for the nation in what was a very difficult period in our history."

Flemming notes that he studied Roosevelt's style and noticed among other things that he never answered hypothetical questions, saying: "That is an iffy question and I don't answer iffy questions. I have trouble enough explaining what I have done and what I am going to do. If I answer a hypothetical and the real situation comes along, I might have to explain why I acted differently than the way I responded to a hypothetical question."

Flemming rates FDR high on both substance and style.

> I would give him very high marks from many points of view. I saw him come in and go through those first 100 days and launch the New Deal programs. One of the great things that he did was to start the country going down the road of social insurance by recommending Social Security to the Congress. Social Security was the product of a Task Force which he set up upon taking office. It was chaired by his Secretary of Labor, Mrs. Francis Perkins, the first woman to serve in the Cabinet of the President of the United States. I think he gave the nation tremendous leadership at the time and that the nation was fortunate to have him as a leader during the difficult period of the Depression and the War.

When asked as a former debate coach to rank the presidents from the point of view of communication skills, he ranks Roosevelt first by a wide margin. He notes that President Ronald Reagan also "has some ability along that line," but adds that Reagan does not have the depth of Roosevelt, who was "more inclined to do his homework."

On December 14, 1934, Flemming married Bernice Virginia Moler and began a family that soon included two daughters and three sons.

Law degree in hand, Flemming returned to the American University where he was named the first director of the School of Public Affairs. "I had two or three other faculty members, but not much in the way of financial support," remembers Flemming, who nonetheless built an effective department. He served as director from 1934 to 1939.

At American University, Flemming developed an in-service training program for federal employees in the areas of personnel administration, organization, and supervision. The program was started with money supplied by the Spelman Foundation and proved to be very popular because of a U.S. General Accounting Office ruling that said agencies could not spend money training their own people. American University filled the void. In this way, Flemming became acquainted with the chief personnel officers at all of the federal agencies. In 1939, Harold Smith, the Director of Budget under FDR, recommended Flemming for a post on the U.S. Civil Service Commission, a post that by law had to be filled by a Republican. Flemming was only too happy to accept. "It has always been a source of pride to me that I received my first Presidential appointment from Franklin Roosevelt," says Flemming.

From Civil Service to Cabinet

Flemming served on the U.S. Civil Service Commission from 1939 to 1948. The commission had responsibility, among other duties, for overseeing the recruitment of government employees. The commission and the civil service system were put into effect as a reaction to what had been a much-abused patronage system. The idea behind civil service was that individuals working for the government ought to be selected on the basis of merit. The Congress said there was a need for a career civil service of the highest possible standards where jobs were secure, not subject to the political winds that batter Washington with each election.

Important as it was, the position soon took on greater significance. World War II was on the horizon and President Roosevelt asked Flemming to assume responsibility for the Commission's defense and, later, war-time activities including the job of coordinating with the Defense Department. The president appointed a War Manpower Commission and named Flemming as a member representing the government as an employer. Flemming was also appointed as Chairman of the Labor, Management and Agriculture Committee of that commission with the responsibility of helping move people from non-defense to defense work. The work of the Manpower Commission, of course, ended with World War II in 1945, but Flemming's appointment to the Civil Service Commission continued three years into President Truman's term.

Flemming tells an interesting story about his dealings with President Truman. He said he picked up rumors that the president might want him to resign from the commission. He asked advice from a powerful member of the House of Representatives who told him to see the president directly. Flemming made an appointment with the president and no sooner walked in the door but that Truman called him up short. "They tell me that somebody around here is trying to tell you that I want your resignation. There is not one damn bit of truth to that. I don't know anything about Civil Service and I hear that you do. I want you to stay." Some years later, when Flemming was considering leaving the commission, the two men had a chat about politics and politicians, including General Eisenhower. "I knew Ike wouldn't run against me," he remembers Truman saying. "We are too good of friends." The year was 1948 and both parties had tried to court Eisenhower to run for president. Eisenhower ultimately decided not to run on either ticket.

In 1948, Flemming left Washington, D.C., to take the post as president of his alma mater, Ohio Wesleyan, but soon thereafter war broke out in Korea and President Truman set up a Cabinet-level Office of Defense Mobilization. Flemming was asked to help out on manpower issues. "For two years during the Korean hostilities I commuted back and forth. I spent four days in Washington and three days back in Delaware, Ohio," remembers Flemming. "When President Eisenhower was elected, I was the only Republican in the office so they made me acting director."

Simultaneously, Sherman Adams, who headed up the president's transition team, sent for Flemming and informed him that he was being appointed to a three-member Committee on Government Organization. He said that former President Herbert Hoover had recommended him highly. He made it clear that the advisory group was part-time in nature, but expected to continue throughout the administration. The other two members of the group were Governor, later Vice-President, Nelson Rockefeller and President Eisenhower's brother, Milton.

President Hoover had gotten to know Flemming when they worked together as members of the first Hoover Commission. Created by Congress in 1947, the 12-member Commission on Reorganization of the Executive Branch had the mission of trying to find ways to make the executive branch run more smoothly. President Truman, who was always an advocate of involving retired political figures, appointed former President Hoover to chair the commission. Parenthetically, another member of the commission was Joseph Kennedy, patriarch of the Kennedy clan.

The commission was presented with the fact that, in the 20 years from Hoover to Truman, the executive branch had increased from 250,000 employees to two million and annual appropriations went from $3.6 billion to $42 billion.

Flemming asserts that President Hoover was vastly underestimated by the public: "He was a brilliant man and of course he very much appreciated the opportunity that President Truman gave him to come back into public life. A rather close relationship developed between the two presidents. President Hoover did an excellent job of running the commission and the results were highly beneficial to government."

The commission concluded that because of the depression and the war, the federal government had swollen to become "the biggest business on earth" and a poorly run one at that. The problem was that there were over 1,800 agencies, bureaus, or departments in the executive branch, often with overlapping functions. The purposes of the entities were not always clear and the individuals who headed them were not always accountable to anyone, much less to the president. The commission developed a list of 51 recommendations, 39 of which were enacted into law by the Congress. The result was the consolidation and the simplification of the organizational chart of the department. The president's hand was strengthened, in the sense that he was given greater flexibility and at the same time more staff under his direct control to help guide the burgeoning executive department.

President Eisenhower also honored Flemming by nominating him to be the director of the Office of Defense Mobilization, a Cabinet-level post. This meant that he was also, by law, a member of the National Security Council. In short, the two most important advisory groups in the executive branch are the Cabinet and the National Security Council and Flemming served on both.

Flemming accepted the post and set out to break the news to the trustees of Ohio Wesleyan. They surprised him by saying they would wait for him. They would install an acting president and hold a place for him on his retirement from government. Flemming served in the posts from 1953 through 1958. Along the way, he found time to serve on the second Hoover Commission, this time appointed by President Eisenhower. Finally, he returned to Ohio early in 1957, but destiny again intervened.

Health, Education and Welfare

The year was 1958. Marion Folsom, the highly regarded former Kodak official who was one of the architects of the Social Security system, had been appointed to serve as Secretary of the Department of Health, Education and Welfare. Folsom suffered a minor stroke and decided he must step down. The responsibility of running the second largest department in the government was just too much.

Flemming had scarcely dusted off his desk at Ohio Wesleyan when President Eisenhower sent for him and offered him the post.

> I was a little torn because my own college had given me a leave for four years. There was no way I could ask them to extend the leave of absence, but I finally decided to accept. I returned to Washington and ran into an old friend, a fabulous servant of the people named Mary Switzer, who welcomed me to what she called the most exciting department in the executive branch. I quickly found out she was right.
>
> Every morning when you woke up you knew you had the opportunity to do something during the day that would help X number of people, sometimes it would be several hundred and sometimes it was several million. I could hardly wait to get to work. I didn't want to miss out on one opportunity to help.

Flemming has high words of praise for President Eisenhower who, he said, was the "best practitioner of consultative management" that he had ever seen. He said that, contrary to popular rumors, Eisenhower was not a laid-back president; he was directly involved. He set the agenda, encouraged full debate at Cabinet meetings, participated in them vigorously himself, and then after he had heard from everyone, the president made a decision that he most often announced on the spot. In other cases, he would say that he wanted "to sleep on the issue" and a decision would follow the next day. He said that Eisenhower always insisted that action minutes be prepared and circulated after he signed them so that all present in the Cabinet meetings would understand what decision had been made. Flemming noted that President Eisenhower had developed this management style in running World War II and later when he set up NATO. "Remember, he was dealing with some highly developed egos, people like Churchill, Montgomery, and de Gaulle and the only way to manage was on a cooperative, consultative basis."

Flemming said that Eisenhower knew how to delegate. Once a decision had been made, he left it to his subordinates to follow through while at the same time he remained accessible and interested in the results. He was also willing to take the heat and stand by his people. Flemming remembers with fondness that President Eisenhower was initially skeptical about a program that Flemming had proposed to provide federal aid to higher education. After a long and contentious debate by the Cabinet, Eisenhower agreed with Flemming's proposal and once he made up his mind, he threw the full weight of the presidency behind the proposal, refusing to yield in the face of a storm of criticism.

Kennedy to Carter

In 1961, John F. Kennedy was sworn in as president of the United States. In this same year, Arthur Flemming became president of the University of Oregon, a post he held until May of 1968. "We fell in love with the Northwest and the university was at a very exciting stage. The enrollment was about 8,000 when we arrived and grew to about 15,000 before I left."

But Flemming was never really out of government. He recalls that in 1961, Senator Jacob Javits, Republican of New York, called him and asked if he would chair a special committee to help bring about the enactment of Medicare. He explained that President Kennedy had promised during his campaign to pass such a law, but had failed twice in the Senate. The senator wanted to help and said that he, Senator Anderson, and President Kennedy had agreed that what was needed was a commission of citizens that would take a fresh look at the problem. The senator wanted to know if Flemming would agree to chair such a group. He agreed to do so.

> We worked on the report for about a year and a half and presented it to President Kennedy in his office in 1963, one week before his assassination. The President reacted very positively to the report. I happened to be the last person out of the Oval Office. The President asked if I was going to testify and present the findings of our report to the Congress. I said: "Certainly." He expressed appreciation and underlined again his conviction that action was needed.

The Flemming report was well received by the Congress and it did help break the impasse. Of course, Medicare was not enacted until 1965, during the Johnson Administration. The fact that Flemming enjoyed an excellent reputation with President Johnson also helped to spur the Medicare legislation along. Flemming had known LBJ for dozens of years, when the lean Texan was first elected to Congress. Some years later, he witnessed LBJ's election to the Senate and his promotion as Majority Leader. During most of his term, President

Eisenhower had to deal with a Democratic Congress that included Lyndon Johnson as the Majority Leader in the Senate and Sam Rayburn as the Speaker of the House. Flemming, like the president himself, enjoyed an excellent relationship with both men. President Johnson later appointed Flemming to an Advisory Committee on Labor Management Relations.

In 1968, the year that LBJ left the White House and Richard Nixon defeated Hubert H. Humphrey, Flemming moved from Oregon to St. Paul, Minnesota. In that city, he accepted the job as president of Macalester College. The liberal arts college had received a significant sum of money from Minnesotan Dewitt Wallace, publisher of *Reader's Digest*, in large part because his father had previously been president there. "It is a very good school and I had a good experience there," remembers Flemming.

> But near the end of my third year, the invitation came from President Nixon whom I had known when he was vice-president in the Eisenhower Cabinet. I was asked to be a consultant to the president on aging and to serve as a full-time chairman of the Second White House Conference on Aging. I was delighted to accept.

By any objective measurement, the 1971 White House Conference was by far the most efficient, constructive, and successful of the three conferences that have been held to date. The reason, of course, was Flemming's dynamic leadership. The great majority of the recommendations made to the Congress were enacted into law. Among the major reforms were: a suggested 20 percent increase in Social Security benefits, tying future increases to increases in the cost of living, establishing the Supplemental Security Income (SSI) program, pension reform, increased support to building housing specifically designed for the elderly, federal support for transportation for the elderly, and nursing home reform.

Shortly after the completion of the conference in November 1971, President Nixon appointed Flemming as U.S. Commissioner on Aging. The commissioner, within the Department of Health, Education and Welfare (now Health and Human Services), has overall responsibility for programs involving the elderly.

Two years later, there was a vacancy on the U.S. Civil Rights

Commission. It was not a full-time job and under the law, the president could appoint someone to the post who already had another federal job. "I was asked whether or not I would be interested and I said I was. I served as chairman of that commission from 1974 all the way through the Ford and Carter Administrations until I was involuntarily retired by President Reagan in 1982. I suppose they didn't like the kind of findings and recommendations that they were getting from the commission."

Flemming has a very positive impression of President Jimmy Carter, particularly for his record on civil and human rights. When asked the question, which president has done the most for civil rights, he answers President Johnson, if the test is the enactment of landmark legislation. But if the test is implementation, then Flemming credits President Carter. "President Carter was in a class by himself in the sense that he practiced what he preached. He had his own affirmative action program that was clearly reflected in his appointments to the judiciary where he appointed a great number of women and minorities to federal judgeships. In addition, he kept the pressure on his cabinet officers."

Flemming tells the story of one cabinet officer who insisted on appointing a WASP, even though his agency had a very poor equal opportunity record. President Carter, when made aware of the fact, rejected the appointment, sending a scorching handwritten memo to the cabinet officer, that said: "This is personally embarrassing to me." As Flemming said, "The point is that President Carter set a standard which he held up to others and, of course, it was very consistent with his emphasis on human rights generally. I think he made a real contribution to the cause of civil rights in America."

SOS and Long-Term Care

In 1981, Flemming was invited to join with former Secretary Wilbur Cohen as co-chairman of an organization Cohen had earlier founded entitled Save Our Security. SOS was a coalition of some 120 national organizations that was organized to stave off cuts in Medicare and Social Security.

The two former secretaries, one a Democrat and one a Republican, cut a wide swath on Capitol Hill. Between the two of them, they boasted more than 75 years of experience in government service. No one could question their objectivity or their motives. No one could speak with more authority on problems of the elderly. The two men worked with Congressman Claude Pepper and Robert Ball and effectively blocked the serious threat to cut the heart from the Social Security program. In 1982, they turned their attention to deflecting proposed cuts in Medicare benefits. Flemming remembers:

> Wilbur felt, and I agreed, that the suggested cuts in Social Security and Medicare amounted to breaking the compact that the Congress had made with the elderly. We thought the result would be that the elderly would lose faith in the programs and in government generally and that is why we decided to combat these efforts.

But Flemming has never been one to limit his effort to stop something from happening; he is a positive man who likes to devote his energies to making things happen. From 1986 to 1990, he served as chairman of the National Health Care Campaign, and worked towards bringing comprehensive health care, including long-term home care, to all Americans.

When asked what advice he would give the next secretary of the Department of Health and Human Services, he responded:

> I would urge him to use his position to lead a crusade designed to get the Congress to enact a national health plan that would guarantee the universal right of access to adequate health care at a reasonable cost to all Americans.
>
> To me this is the overriding domestic issue of our time. It is tragic, but there are about 37 million Americans who do not have any health insurance coverage. We need a national plan that is comprehensive, by that I mean which includes preventive measures and coverage for both acute and long-term care.
>
> I feel it is fiscally irresponsible for us not to take this step. Our neighbors to the north in Canada put into effect a plan that provides access to all of their people. They are providing comprehensive care for something like 8.6 percent of their gross national product. We are spending 11.1 percent of our GNP, we have all kinds of gaps in coverage, and we have 37 million people on the outside looking in. Why the difference? Canada has an adequate cost-containment

program. We do not have anything resembling an adequate cost-containment program and we will not have one until we have a national health plan.

While Flemming favors the enactment of a comprehensive national health insurance plan covering all Americans and all ranges of services from preventive to acute care and long-term care, he will take whatever incremental improvements he can get. He supported the Catastrophic Health Protection Act of 1988 because he believed it would bring important new protections to the elderly. Like others, he did express reservations about several aspects of the bill, including its failure to cover long-term care.

In order to help cure the defects of the so-called Catastrophic Health Protection Act, which has since been repealed, Flemming worked long hours and traveled throughout the country, heading a campaign which resulted in thousands of letters, thousands of phone calls, and hundreds of personal visits in support of the Pepper/Roybal Long-Term Home Care bill.

In fact, Flemming recalls that he and Wilbur Cohen were having dinner with Congressman Claude Pepper when the Congressman first outlined this proposal. "I turned to Wilbur as we were leaving Congressman Pepper's office and said, 'Wilbur, the Congressman is on fire on this issue, let's give him all the support we can marshal.'"

In arguing for the bill, Flemming pointed out that there is a genuine need for long-term care, which is approaching the crisis stage. He added that something must be done because the polls universally show that the American public wants action. He notes that 83 percent of the American public favors home care as the best solution to the nation's long-term care problem and favors financing the new federal entitlement program by lifting the $45,000 cap on Medicare payroll tax.

"I am delighted to have been a follower of Claude Pepper in connection with so many great issues. But I particularly appreciate the opportunity that I have had to be a follower of his in connection with his home care bill. This is true because the passage of this bill, this breakthrough in the area of long-term care will give the whole nation a shot in the arm. It is going to replace despair with hope," said Flemming at a March 1988 rally.

Honors

Flemming has received dozens of honors over the years. Among them include the Navy's Distinguished Civilian Service Award for his work on the Navy's manpower survey board in 1944; the Daughters of the American Revolution's Award of Merit for outstanding service and worthy accomplishments for the protection of our constitutional republic, 1956; Reserve Officers' Association of the United States in recognition of outstanding service for National Defense Objectives, 1956; the Presidential Medal of Freedom, the highest civilian award, presented by President Eisenhower, 1958; the President's Committee on Employment of Physically Handicapped Commendation, 1961; the National Geriatrics Society Man-of-the-Year Award, 1972; the National Association of Retired Federal Employees Award for tireless work to secure a better life for America's older citizens, 1972; the Department of Health, Education and Welfare—Region III Humanitarian Award in recognition of his outstanding service to humanity, 1973; the National Black Caucus on the Black Aged, Inc., award for outstanding service to the aged, 1974; Department of Health, Education and Welfare Arthur J. Altmeyer Award for outstanding contributions to economic security, 1974; the National Council on the Aging Ollie Randall Award, 1975; the American Association of Retired Persons Andrus Award, 1980; National Coalition on Aging, Inc., award in recognition of personal commitment and outstanding service toward the spiritual well-being of older Americans, 1981; and the Leadership Conference on Civil Rights Hubert Humphrey Civil Rights Award, 1982. In 1988, he was selected one of the ten most caring Americans by the Caring Institute for his "lifetime of public service and his constant crusade for social justice through service to seven presidents, concern for government employees and example of being a public servant." In 1989, he received an award that meant a great deal to him—the first Annual Claude Pepper Award, given each year to the person who makes the greatest contributions to the elderly and disabled. Two major awards came in 1990. He received the Creative Achievement Award from the Creative Thinking Association of America, given to Flemming and two other people who were selected as having the most profound and positive effect on America for the balance of the 20th century. Later in the year, he also received the prestigious Allied Signal 1990 Achievement in Aging Award for his leadership in health related to aging.

What He Has Learned

When asked what he has learned, he stresses the importance of having good values. He points to Congressman Claude Pepper as someone who was always in touch with his values. "I always have the feeling that he kept focused on the individual or some family that he was picturing in his mind. We all can get caught up in abstractions and forget what is really important, which is helping people."

When asked how he maintains his vitality, he answered: "By keeping involved. I have long felt that non-involvement leads to very rapid mental, physical, and spiritual deterioration and I think the scientific literature will bear me out on this."

Flemming says he believes that the Social Security program proved a point:

> We as a national community have demonstrated that we have the capability and capacity to pool our resources through payroll contributions in such a way as to protect our people, wherever they may live, from, to quote FDR, the "hazards and vicissitudes of life." They know these resources, which they have helped to accumulate, will remain inviolate and that they will have a vested, earned right to draw on this when needed.
>
> Now that is one legacy that my generation has handed down to our children and grandchildren and great grandchildren. But I can see no reason why we shouldn't be able to hand down the same kind of legacy in the health care area. As older persons, we are members of families and we know that our present health care system is not doing well by our children and great grandchildren. We would like to see that corrected for future generations.

Flemming said he has learned how important it is to have a cause and for every cause to have a leader. "But over the years, I have also learned that it is equally important, if you are going to take full advantage of the opportunities that come to you in life, to be a good follower."

"I don't believe in demonstration projects," he said. "They are the worst kind of discrimination. They are great for the people involved in the demonstration but they are terrible for all the people that are on the outside."

Flemming recited a story told to him by President Eisenhower, who was making the point that one should not presume to make decisions for other people. "He was talking to me one day about Ohio Wesleyan. He said, 'You know I have always had a desire to be the head of a small liberal arts college. Near the end of my term as Chief of Staff of the Army, persons talked to me about a number of positions. But no-one talked to me about being the head of a liberal arts college. Shortly after I went to Columbia as president I was having dinner one night with a good friend who was chairman of the board of a liberal arts college. He said, 'You know, about a year ago, we were trying to persuade ourselves that we should go down to Washington and talk with you about becoming president of our college.' I said, 'Brother, I was sitting right there waiting for you. If you had come in with an offer, you would have gone out with an acceptance.'"

Flemming says he has learned how important it is to surround oneself with good people. He said that is why he has worked so hard on behalf of the career civil service, to make it into something that would serve the nation into the foreseeable future. He added that he was very disturbed by the fact that President Reagan has been highly critical of public servants. "The effect has been to drive good people out of government and to make it very difficult to challenge bright, younger people to come into the civil service."

Finally, he said that one particular interpretation of the commandment, "Thou shalt love thy neighbor as thyself" has always meant a great deal to him. He acquired this definition from a pastor in London. The pastor said in a sermon that the commandment imposes no obligation on people to like their neighbor. "I breathed a sigh of relief when I heard that, because I knew a few people whom I had found it hard to like. But after all, you can't be commanded to like somebody. That is a feeling that has to come from within. Also, it is obvious that the commandment does not require us to approve of everything that our neighbor says and does. The commandment does, however, place a common responsibility upon us to help our neighbor achieve her or his highest possibilities." He added:

> I think that all of these issues with which I have been involved in my life, whether we are talking about civil rights, education, aging, or health care, are issues that involve our trying to help our neighbors to have the opportunity of achieving their highest possibilities.

Remembered

When asked how he would like to be remembered, he modestly demurrs, "I will leave that to others." But there is no doubt about it: Flemming will be remembered by the nation and by the millions of families whose lives he has touched. He has left a legacy not only in the form of his achievements, but also in the example that he offers to others. Congressman Claude Pepper once described him as "a great and noble general, a modern-day Moses who will lead the nation's elderly out of pain and bondage into the promised land of full health-care security." Senator Frank E. Moss called him the "consummate man of the people."

But it is too early and perhaps inappropriate to try to fully capture Flemming's career in one sentence or in one article. This is true because this book is necessarily limited to an exploration of the past and the present. Flemming seems to get better with age. Although his achievements have been monumental, he rarely looks back. He is a man of the future. He looks forward to the days and the years ahead with such excitement and conveys such a high sense of expectation it motivates all who know him to ask: What great works will he produce in the coming years? What dragons will he slay? And what grave injustice will he correct? There is a certain unspoken understanding among those who know him that his best work and the things for which he will be most remembered are yet to come.

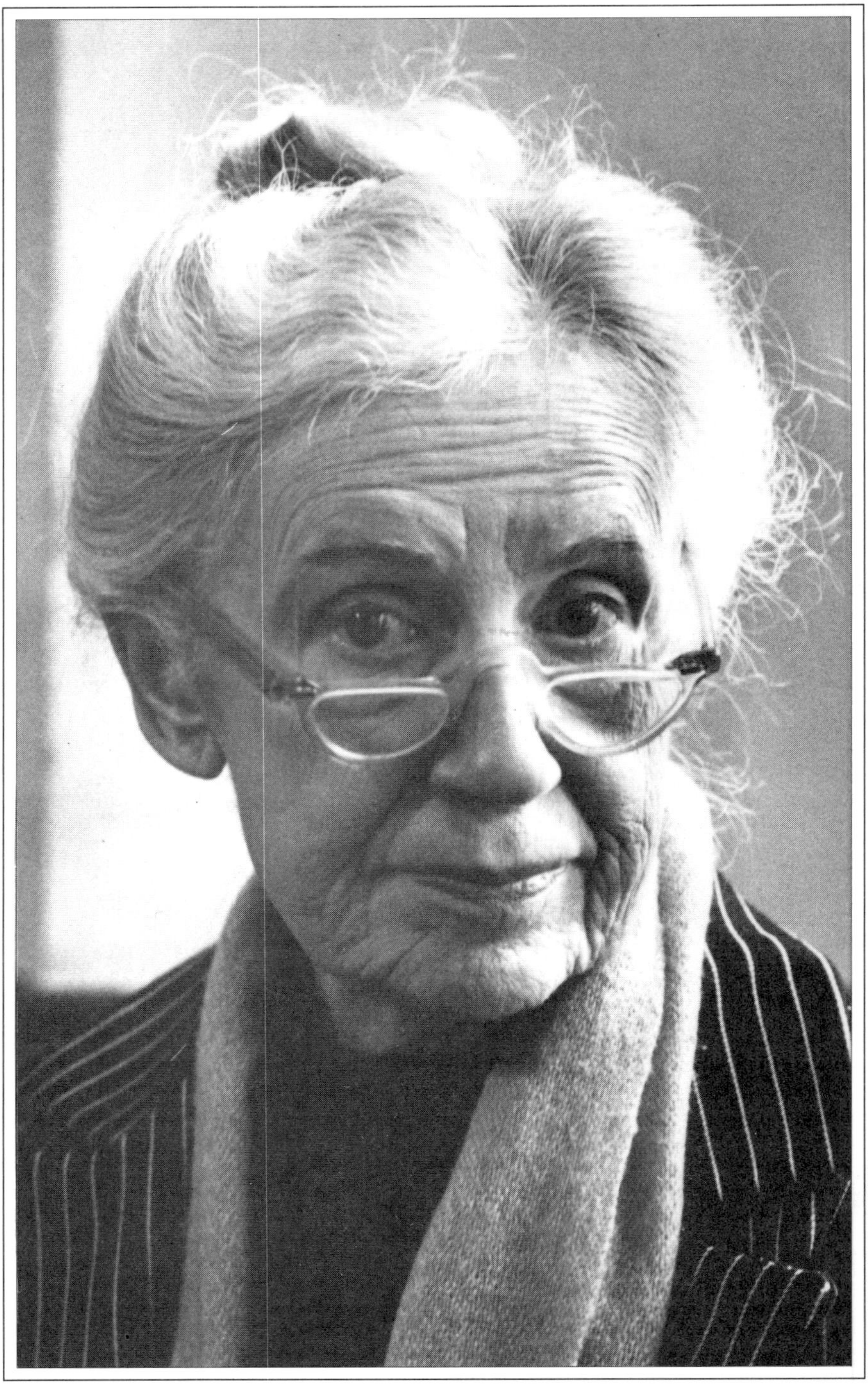

COURTESY OF MAGGIE KUHN

FOUR

Maggie Kuhn

When historians of the future look back, they will find that a handful of people were responsible for sensitizing the American public to the needs of the coming tidal wave of older Americans. They will find that a small number of people began fighting against "ageism" long before most people realized there was such an evil.

Among these people will be Margaret E. Kuhn, known as Maggie to most of the nation. No one person has done more to demonstrate the importance, the power, and the human dignity of the elderly than she. By her positive example, she has given hope to millions of older Americans that they can continue to serve as active and productive members of society. She has proven age is no barrier to contribution. She serves as a role model also for younger Americans who are wondering what to do with their lives.

It is noteworthy that Kuhn did not come to the attention of the American public until she retired. By that time, she had already devoted a lifetime to improving relations among the races. She fought against racial discrimination, nuclear war, and sexual discrimination against women. But what attracted public attention was the fact that she challenged the disengagement theory popular through the 1960s, which held that people after the age of 65 should do as little as possible. She issued a call to arms entreating her fellow seniors to put aside their golf clubs and knitting needles and become political activists.

"Do not go gentle into that good night, / old age should burn and rave at close of day; / Rage, rage against the dying of the light," could well have been Kuhn's theme song. In 1970, she shattered the myth that protest movements are only for the young, when she formed the Gray Panthers. It was an organization which began with a small cadre of militant senior citizens who had courage enough to march on Congress and state capitols, demanding their rights. In short order, the few became an army, a formidable alliance of the young and old joining hands to fight the evil of ageism. Kuhn defined ageism as the notion that people become inferior because they have lived a specified number of years.

By her example, Kuhn, together with her Gray Panther colleagues, helped shatter the myth that old age is synonymous with powerlessness, decrepitude, and weakness. She shattered other myths—that old age is bad, that it is a disease, that it is synonymous with senility, and that it is sexless. "We need to counter the old dehumanizing images of old age with new ones that enable us to be comfortable with our bodies. We need to continue to grow, learn and keep our minds and spirits vibrant as long as we live. We are not wrinkled babies succumbing to trivial, purposeless waste of our years and our time. We are a new breed of people. We are redefining our goals, taking stock of our skills and experience and looking to the future."

As the ultimate expression of the phrase "Senior Power," Kuhn was a paradox. She was quiet and shy and yet she could be as aggressive as a bulldog in the pursuit of her goals. A small woman with a fragile appearance, she had the strength many times that of steel. Her calm demeanor hides an internal volcano stoked by outrage at the injustices perpetrated in society.

Through her exemplary life and living example she proves conclusively that old age is not a defeat, but a victory; that it is not a punish-ment but a privilege.

Years from now when historians call the roll to determine which people have done the most to advance the interests of the nation's seniors, Kuhn will rank near the top. No one is more deserving of the respect and admiration of her fellow citizens than Margaret E. Kuhn: she is an extraordinary human being.

Background

Maggie Kuhn was born on August 3, 1905, in her grandmother's house in Buffalo, New York. Her parents were living in Memphis, Tennessee, when her mother became pregnant, but her mother refused to have her child there in protest against the rigid system of racial segregation that was practiced in the deep South at the time. It was the first of many protests in which Kuhn participated.

Her mother took the long and tedious journey back home where Margaret Eliza (Maggie) was born. Her earliest memories include images of her maternal grandmother, for whom she was named.

Maggie's grandmother was her early role model. "She lived in a big, old, comfortable shabby house where people came for friendship and love. There were people who were married at Grandma's, people were born there and funerals were held at her home. She was a very deeply concerned and caring person. I am glad that I had the privilege of knowing her," says Kuhn.

But there were others who helped form her character. Her father gave her strength and grit. She remembers her father as a very strong and extremely hardworking individual. He did not have much in the way of formal education, yet he taught himself higher mathematics, Latin, and Greek. He started as a mail clerk in an office and soon worked his way up to managing several offices for what was to become the respected international business credit and reference firm, Dun and Bradstreet. She recalls that her father had a very deep sense of community and a social conscience.

She notes that her mother, too, had this same community spirit. She was an activist far ahead of her time; a tough but compassionate individual. It took a good deal of courage for her mother to be strong, because her father was very much the man of the house, a strict taskmaster with very firm values and ideas of his own.

Her mother's sister, whom Kuhn lovingly remembers as Aunt Pauline, was also a strong influence on her life.

> I adored her. She taught me to read. She was a suffrage leader in western New York. Like many young girls of that time, she married young and had a child early, only to have her husband killed. He was

an engineer on a train and died in a wreck. So Aunt Pauline and her child moved in with grandmother.

The accident had occurred because someone had failed to throw a switch and the train derailed. Unfortunately, the courts failed to award any compensation in this very famous 1872 case, which established what was known as the "fellow servant rule." The ruling was later struck down by the U.S. Supreme Court. Under this ruling, the court said that it was a fellow employee who was at fault in causing the accident by failing to throw the switch. It said, therefore, that the employee was responsible and not the railroad. The railroad was excused of all responsibility and Aunt Pauline and her child did not even receive funeral expenses owing to the wrongful death of their husband and father. The event provided the impetus for Maggie's aunt to become a political activist, advocating women's rights and fighting for other social causes. Her conviction rubbed off on her young niece.

When Maggie was still at an early age, her family moved to Cleveland where she graduated from West High School. She obtained her B.A. from Flora Stone Mather College, Case Western Reserve University in Cleveland, graduating in 1927. She had intended to become a teacher of French or English, but events pushed her in another direction. The problem was that a person had to get straight "A's" in school in those days to be accepted as a member of the teaching profession. Her perfect record was spoiled by what she refers to as "an altercation" with a teacher.

Kuhn was in the middle of her apprenticeship, doing her student teaching. She was given the assignment of planning a grammar lesson. This exercise was dull, so Kuhn tried to inject some interest by devising a relay race. The first students to the blackboard were permitted to write sentences, others who finished next were to select the subject and the verb, slower people the modifiers. "It got very exciting at the end," remembers Kuhn. Inevitably, a fight broke out among the students. Kuhn could not get them to stop, so she hurled an eraser at the largest troublemaker in the class just as the teacher entered the back door to check up on how well she was doing. "That ended my teaching career on the spot," she says.

Employment and Forced Retirement

Her first job was with the Cleveland YWCA where she started as an assistant clerk in 1928. She worked her way up into more and more responsible positions. Her good work came to the attention of the national staff of the YWCA who offered her a job. She accepted and moved to New York.

In 1946 she accepted a new post with the National Alliance of Unitarian Women in Boston. Following this employment, she moved to the United Presbyterian Office of Church and Society. She later served this same organization as director of the Division of Church and Race.

In short, Maggie Kuhn worked for more than 43 years fighting for social justice and peace. After so many years of service, she unfortunately became a victim of injustice in the form of mandatory retirement.

The year was 1970 and Kuhn had just turned 65. She was commuting from Philadelphia to New York, working in the central office of the Presbyterian Church to help improve relations among the races. She was told abruptly one day that her services were no longer needed.

The group threw her a farewell party and gave her a sewing machine, suggesting that a hobby like this would be good in her retirement years. Obviously, they did not know her very well. Kuhn said that she and five other friends were struck with the injustice of it all. They were contemplating the $64 million question: What do you do with the rest of your life after retirement?

"We decided we needed each other to find the answer and we started what became known as the Gray Panthers." The group started out in protest of the Vietnam War, but quickly turned to a spate of other social issues. They sought to bring together the young and the old to influence public policy.

She never unpacked the sewing machine. She was pleasantly surprised that rather than retirement being the end of something, it served as an important beginning. Rather than being constrained or limited by increasing age, Kuhn was liberated. It was a new age in which anything was possible. Kuhn remembers: "This is the age of liberation and we struggled—for liberation in terms of racial justice, for the long struggle against sexism, and now we turned our attention to the struggle against age discrimination." The Gray Panthers were born.

Gray Panthers

Kuhn's blazing rhetoric soon caught the attention of the media, which resulted in an appearance on the "Today Show" with Barbara Walters. She was an instant celebrity. She developed an immediate following of hundreds of people all across America who were moved by her words and wanted to help with her cause.

Twenty years after its founding, the Gray Panthers has increased from 6 to 60,000 members and supporters. There were over 80 Gray Panther networks in the United States in 1990.

The Gray Panthers have an impressive agenda. They have been working to help improve the quality of nursing home care and to increase the availability of home care and hospice as alternatives to institutionalization. They have worked to increase—or at least stop cuts in—Social Security and Medicare benefits. They have worked to abolish mandatory retirement.

Kuhn believes home care and hospice are particularly important. "We have been working for home health care for a long time. It is a service which allows seniors to stay independent in their own homes, where they want to be," she says.

The organization is now very much concerned with problems facing Third World nations. It has placed a great deal of importance on helping bring about the enactment of a comprehensive health insurance program for all Americans. Of special interest to the group are problems facing older women.

In preparation for her leadership role, Kuhn returned to school, attending graduate school at Temple University, the University of Southern California, the University of Hawaii, the San Francisco Theological Seminary, and the University of California at San Francisco, where she was chosen as Distinguished Senior Scholar at the Aging and Health Policy Center.

She is a prolific writer, having served for many years as the editor of *Social Progress*, now called *Journal of Church and Society*. She has written a book entitled *Maggie Kuhn on Aging* and has begun work on her autobiography. She has been the subject of two documentary films. One was called *Aging in America* and the other *Maggie Kuhn: Wrinkled Radical.*

Kuhn has played a leadership role in a number of important organizations. She began at an early age. When she was eight, she joined the local chapter of the Audubon Society and began a life of caring for God's creatures great and small. She served on Ralph Nader's Retired Professional Action Group in 1973. She was a member of President Carter's Commission on Mental Health between 1978 and 1980. In 1982, she was selected as a delegate to the United Nations Forum on Aging and a year later she was a delegate to the World Assembly for Peace and Life Against Nuclear War. She served on the board of the National Senior Citizen Law Center, the Institute of Medicine and Community Health, and the National Advisory Board for Health Policy. She is also a member of the board of trustees of the Foundation for Hospice and Homecare.

Honors

Her good work has been rewarded in many ways. She was chosen to deliver the alumni address at her 50th College reunion in 1976. In 1981 this school, Case Western Reserve, honored her with their Distinguished Alumni Award.

She has received honorary doctorates from Swarthmore College, Moravian College, Simmons College, Antioch College, Albright College, Marycrest College, Grinnell College, and the State University of New York.

Among the awards given Kuhn are the Humanist of the Year by the American Humanist Association, the National Freedom Award of Roosevelt University in Chicago, the Distinguished Service Award in consumer advocacy by the Speech and Hearing Society, the Unitarian Woman's Annual Award for Ministries to Women, the 1977 Annual Peaceseeker Award of the United Presbyterian Peace Fellowship, the Global Award, the Presidential Citation of the American Public Health

Association, the first annual award for justice and human development by the Witherspoon Society, the annual award by the Philadelphia Society of Clinical Psychologists, and the Lifetime Achievement Award from the Foundation for Hospice and Homecare.

Kuhn has been honored in still other ways. She was selected as one of the first people to visit the People's Republic of China in 1976. Two years later, she was chosen by the U.S.– China Peoples Friendship Association to serve as tour leader for another visit.

The Woman's Way Organization of Philadelphia recently presented her with their Lucretia Mott Award, named after the famous women's suffrage leader. In 1978, *World Almanac* chose her as one of the 25 most influential women in the United States. In 1983, the *Ladies Home Journal* chose her as one of the 100 most important women in America.

Kuhn is frank to say that she is fueled by outrage and injustice. She can't understand how other people can stand by and do nothing in the face of inequity or obvious wrongdoing. She employs burning rhetoric to gain attention to the problem and then offers solutions in quiet, cool, soothing tones. Asked where she got her fire inside, she said that part of it may have come from "adolescent revolt." She adds, "I guess that some of it comes from my ethical and moral commitment and my commitment to people. I am a people person. People are the only thing in the world that matters."

Views on the Issues

Maggie Kuhn has strong opinions on the important issues of our time. She has a lifelong passion for ending the arms race; she describes herself as a pacifist. She has worked most of her life to protect the environment against air and water pollution. She has been an outspoken advocate of civil rights, fighting all manner of discrimination, whether it is on the grounds of race, creed, color, religion, or sex. It goes with-out saying that she is a strong supporter of the women's movement since both her mother and sister were pillars of the women's suffrage movement. However, what is of most concern here is Kuhn's views on the issues relating particularly to older Americans. A summary of some of these views follows below as taken, in part, from personal interviews and from *Maggie Kuhn on Aging*, a dialogue edited by Deiter Hessel.

On Mandatory Retirement

Kuhn and the Gray Panthers established as one of their top objectives the enactment of legislation barring the dismissal of employees for no reason other than the fact they had reached the arbitrary age of 65. She argued that forced retirement damages self-esteem and leads to feelings of uselessness, damaging people both physically and psychologically. "The maintenance of an institution that forces older people out of their work roles requires perpetuation of an agist belief system. This system requires that all groups buy into the concept that old people are less able than young and ought to enjoy leisure time, even if they do not want it," said Kuhn. Claude Pepper pushed legislation through the Congress in 1982, that barred forced retirement before age 72, and in 1988 won passage of an amendment barring mandatory retirement at any age.

On Health Care

Maggie Kuhn is an advocate for national health insurance. She wants people to have the care that they need, but has grave concerns about the medical-industrial complex. "We don't need to elaborate on the health crisis: the shortage and the expense of quality health care, the abominable distribution of it, its fragmentation and ultraspecialization—all converge at this particular period to make health a national issue, affecting not only the elderly, but people of all ages. What we have is 'sickness' care. We spend more for the treatment of disease than any other nation—close to 12 percent of the gross national product." She advocates a greater emphasis on "wellness" and preventive medicine.

She adds that medical schools do not emphasize geriatrics; students are taught to read machines but not to touch the body. Care is highly specialized and fragmented so that it is difficult for anyone to have a full view of the patient and his/her needs. Medical students may come in with idealism, but the system drains it out of them. "They get caught in pressures to acquire quickly a large, lucrative practice where they think the dollars are going to flow. They have succumbed to another value system which makes it difficult for them, as human beings, to be human."

She strongly encourages members of the clergy, senior citizens, and all Americans to become health care advocates. It is her perception that once admitted to a hospital or a nursing home, patients lose many of their constitutional rights. She believes that volunteers should help monitor the care of the patient, assist the patient, assist the family, act as liaison with the medical personnel, spend time with the patient on a person-to-person basis to determine his or her well being and to receive and follow through on complaints lodged by patients or family.

On Sex

Kuhn notes that society is uncomfortable with the notion of seniors having or wanting sex. "It's assumed that sex is a no-no—that sexual competence, interest and the ability to attract members of the opposite sex are lost when one gets old. Such mythology must be eliminated from the thinking of people and from the practice of society." She notes that couples are often broken up when they are admitted at the same time to a nursing home or that attendants sometimes are not sensitive as to their need for privacy. She adds that society finds it acceptable for an older man to have a relationship with a younger woman, but not vice versa. Older woman should be encouraged to take younger sex partners, she says. "The overall mind-set has to be changed in order to open to people of both sexes the opportunity to establish deep friendships and loving relationships until the very onset of rigor mortis."

On Education

Kuhn believes that seniors should be encouraged to return to school. Church should play a central role in this respect, she believes. Seniors should be put to work as teachers, she says, teaching their life experiences to younger people. She notes that there is a natural alliance between the old and the young, pointing to such programs as Foster Grandparents. The mind, like our muscles, needs exercise, she contends; what is used continues to develop even in old age.

On Senior Centers

Maggie Kuhn has harsh words for "Golden Age Clubs" and senior centers, which have as their purpose socialization and leisure activities for the elderly.

> I call them glorified playpens. That's extravagant language and I mean it to be. They trivialize old age, assuming that all that people want to do in their old age is to play—just one round of merriment after another. Many of my peers have been conditioned to believe that they deserve to play after so many years of hard work.
>
> How does this prepare anyone to deal with the angst that is within us all about growing old? The sheer terror of not having enough money, of acquiring some crippling disease, cannot be dispensed with fun and games. One man said to me with some disgust, "I have made ashtrays for everyone that I know. Can I give you this ashtray?" This is not to downgrade play, but play in these terms is such a waste. Play does not help to develop new positive images of strength.

On Retirement Communities

> They are playpens. They are very safe. Playpens are meant to be safe and comfortable. The people are out of the way of the rest of society. They are self-contained. Some come complete with guards, a moat, barbed wire, hospitals, a club room and a community church. It is just gruesome. There is this facade of congeniality, but there is very little evidence of true community.

On Bingo Games

"It is a very easy way to get a big warm-body count. Nothing interferes with the game. We are perpetuating mindlessness."

On the Subject of Retirement

> I believe that you don't retire from life, which is what retirement now means, but that you recycle and redirect your goals. This is a

component of continuing education. A special effort ought to be made to extend continuing education to provide opportunities for retired people to become involved again in the life of their community.

I believe we stand precariously on the brink—we have the capacity to destroy our society or to heal and humanize it. Many new ideas are to be tested. Each of us has some influence, a platform. America suffers from rampant ennui. Old people often have an exaggerated case of inertia linked with cynicism, loneliness, and despair. Much of the despair will lift when we realize that the power ultimately is in the people.

We are the stewards of our lives. We are the futurists! How do we keep ourselves alive and contributing to our society?

On the Primary Needs of the Elderly

"Most of the things the older people need, all people need: food, clothing, shelter, medical care, adequate income and a purpose for living. We should not lose sight of the fact that many people who have never been poor become poor when they are old." She believes that the method society has chosen to deal with these needs is often wasteful. She rejects paternalism in favor of self-reliance. "It is true that some people are hungry for attention and are quite ready to be cared for on their way to wrinkled babyhood. Service programs can help people feel less pain and anxiety but they do not deal with the root causes. Services are really novocaine shots unless they sensitize people to the need for social change," she says. It is for this reason that she has chosen to work directly on the attitudes and values of society.

On Long-Term Care

Kuhn has been an outspoken critic of nursing homes. She realizes the need for good homes and has worked to insure that care delivered there is of high quality. As noted, she is an advocate of home and community-based care:

Though day-to-day skilled nursing care is necessary for some people, and some nursing homes offer excellent services, we must not continue to institutionalize people who should be enabled to stay in their own homes or in homes where they could share communal living with people who care for each other. All of us have to build our own parachutes, and intergenerational living may be one of them.

On Employment

Maggie Kuhn believes in the importance of work, whether paid or volunteered. She suggests that several seniors might try taking and sharing one job. "In our old age we are free to try new things, to innovate, we're free to burst out of our old, wrinkled skins and to be creative. We are the elders and should be society's futurists. We ought to be testing new instruments, technologies, concepts, ideas and styles of living. We have the freedom to do so and we have nothing to lose."

"I think we should become healing agents in society. I'm enormously struck with what antibodies do in the human body to combat disease and put down infection. I would like to think of us as releasing healers—to help heal a sick society in whatever way we can." For example, she suggests seniors set up speaking bureaus and travel from city to city to speak to the seniors. She says seniors should be builders of coalitions, act as watchdogs and guardians of the public interest. They should act as consumer advocates, and whistle-blowers—as energizers, enablers and liberators."

On the Importance of Oral History and Life Review

Old people ought to be encouraged to develop a sense of history, says Kuhn. They should be encouraged to review their own history, valuing their own origins and past experiences. "With rapid technological change, we are made to feel that our experience is useless. If we could stimulate a life review, we would see what we have lived through, the ways in which we have coped and survived, the changes we have seen—all of this is the history of the race. Older Americans have lived through more changes than any other human group. If we do not see the value of this experience because of our society's foolishness and our lack of insight as to what makes human beings really human, we will have done great damage to ourselves and to those who come after us."

Advice and Reflections

Asked what advice she would offer to future generations, she says that we must find a way to work together. She believes that the secret is an alliance of interest between the youth and the senior citizens of America. She tells young people, "Find an old friend, an old person who can be your friend. And you and that old person can give each other a great deal of good advice and you can be teaching and learning from each other every step of the way, and both lives will be enriched and made more exciting and viable because you've been together."

When asked for her reflections on turning 80, she responded as follows:

> I feel a certain sense of achievement. I am a survivor. I've had cancer. I have deteriorating retinas. I have arthritis which makes my gait uncertain, my hands are crippled and my knees stiff. But I am thankful because I still have all of my mental faculties. I do hope that nothing happens, because to lose one's faculties is the ultimate human tragedy. You can deal with all kinds of physical infirmities and triumph over them but the loss of a mind, brain damage, is something of another matter.

She says that her commitment to peace and justice and people is stronger now than ever before. She says that now is the best part of her life. Of all her achievements, the one that ranks on top with her is founding the Gray Panthers. She offers this sage advice to seniors:

> It seems to me that all of us at any time in life, but certainly in late life, can only survive and thrive when we have a goal, a passionate purpose that we're going to devote some time and energy and thought to. It is important that this objective be beyond ourselves. I am not talking about something like perfecting our golf game. That's not the goal. I am talking about having a goal that bears on the public interest, the common good. We are the elders of the tribe, and the tribal elders are concerned about the tribe's survival, not their own.

Asked how she would like to be remembered, she recited her favorite epitaph: "Here lies so-and-so, under the only stone she left unturned." She added, "I am proudest of what I have done in late life—the fact that we have forged a successful national coalition of old people and young people working together and that we have moved to bring about a new kind of political awareness, building coalitions that transcend special-interest politics."

Her choice of the best and the brightest members of Congress reflects her strong feeling of the bond between the old and the young. Her favorite congressman, whom she admired for his integrity and his example, is Claude Pepper, the former chairman of the House Rules Committee and the Subcommittee on Long-Term Care of the House Select Committee on Aging, who was the oldest member of Congress before his death in 1989. Her second choice is among the youngest members of the U.S. Senate, Senator John Heinz, Ranking Minority Member of the Senate Aging Committee. She says she admires Senator Heinz for his forthright and exemplary leadership on issues of aging. She also admires Congressman Ron Wyden of Oregon, one of the youngest members of the House, and himself a longtime member of the Gray Panthers. Her standard is not only that they work to serve the elderly, but that, like her, these men share a great social consciousness.

Summary

Maggie Kuhn has much in common with the Founding Fathers who wrote the Constitution and the Bill of Rights. At the age of 65, she wrote and issued her own declaration of independence. It was a protest against ageism and what she called the Detroit syndrome. She charged that America, like Detroit, built obsolescence into all aspects of life. "Only the young person or the new model is desirable and marketable. The 'Detroit mentality' has taken us over as a society," she charges. "We are a wasteful society. We throw away people and before we throw them away, we warehouse them in institutions. We make them into vegetables, fit for nothing but scrap piles."

Like the Founding Fathers, Kuhn was blessed with vision—with the ability to see the future. She could see the important role seniors would come to play in society. She predicted that, by the year 2 000, one out of every five Americans will be over the age of 65 and nearly half will be over 50. "If we are going to continue to toss people on the scrap pile at the going rate, our society is going to be really sick—in fact it will be dying. We have got a few years' grace, we had better make the most of them," she warned.

Fortunately, Kuhn is also blessed with the gift of leadership, that is, the ability to galvanize public opinion and create an enthusiastic appetite for action. This translates as political power. She generates an amazing positive energy; call it charisma or something else, but people respond when she speaks. Her use of the language is simply wonderful, both in spoken and written form.

She has led a life rich in service to others. It has been a life of caring and compassion. Millions are better off today because Kuhn touched their lives. She is the personification of the best of Christian values. She is slow to anger, but she has no patience for those who place machinery and material things before the needs of people. She believes firmly that it is the God-given responsibility of all Americans to serve their country and their fellow human beings. As far as she is concerned, the ultimate sin is the waste of time and the waste of human potential.

Like the Founding Fathers, Maggie Kuhn is a revolutionary. Like Robert Kennedy, she sees things as they should be and asks "Why not?" Like Eleanor Roosevelt, she has been willing to devote herself totally in service to humanity. Her life and example serve to remind all of the validity of Robert Browning's reassurance: "Grow old along with me! The best of life is yet to be. / The last of life for which the first is made."

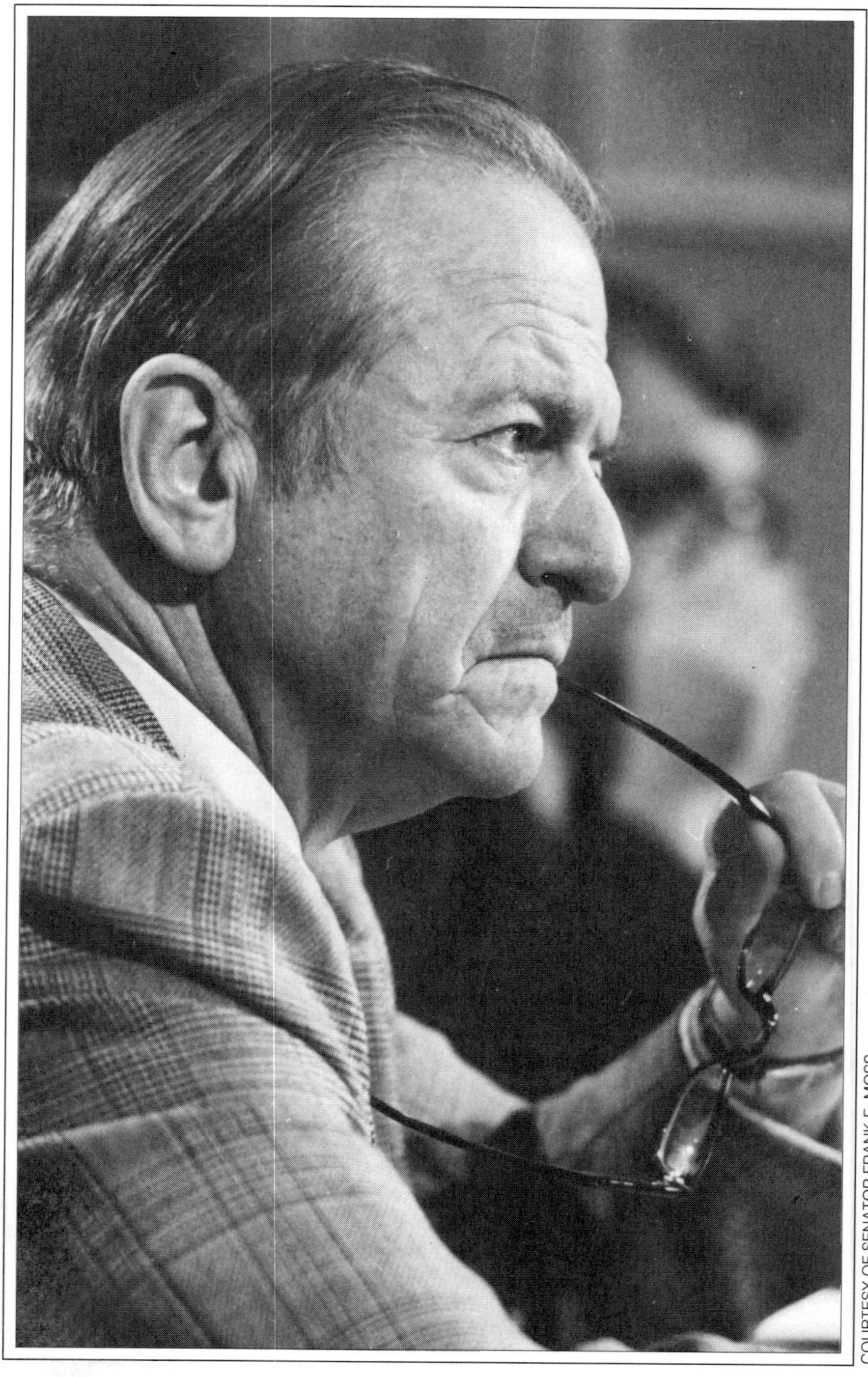

COURTESY OF SENATOR FRANK E. MOSS

FIVE

Frank E. Moss

To his colleagues, Frank E. Moss was known as "Mr. Integrity" or "The Senator's Senator." The media knew him as soft-spoken, effective, honest, and tough—a man of principle. His constituents knew him for his energy and his untiring work on their behalf. Insiders on the congressional staff remember him as likable, sincere, genuine, bright, and down-to-earth—the kind of man for whom everyone would love to work. His friends remember him for his hearty laugh, the twinkle in his eye, and the unbounded affection he heaped upon them. His neighbors remember him as a family man who lived the Ten Commandments and who remained totally unchanged by his successful climb to the top of the Senate ladder. To those who monitor the Washington scene, he became known as one of the three or four most powerful men in the nation; he was role model, teacher, inspiration, and friend.

Moss was, without doubt, one of the brightest stars to serve in the United States Senate. In his 18 years of service, he left a record of achievement to be celebrated by all. He established himself as an advocate of the people, not only of his home state of Utah, but of the United States of America.

He became, for example, the Senate's staunchest protector of the environment. He pushed through legislation protecting the air and water from pollution. He was also the nation's strongest advocate of conservation of natural resources. He single-handedly created more national parks than anyone. He worked hard to preserve the beauty of America as the birthright of Americans yet unborn.

He became the nation's foremost advocate of consumer rights. Virtually all the major consumer protection legislation enacted in the last quarter of a century bears his imprint.

Moss did as much as anyone to improve the health of the nation. He pushed for medical research and for the enactment of government housing programs for the elderly. He played a key role in the enactment of Medicare and Medicaid. One of his innovations was to take the U.S. Senate Committee on Aging on the road. He chaired dozens of hearings all across America. These hearings had the effect of galvanizing public support for Medicare and Medicaid. Against great odds, he turned the tide against smoking in America. He helped convert the technological breakthrough which came from research on the U.S. space program into diagnostic and therapeutic machinery to help in the fight against disease.

Certainly, no one has done more to protect the rights of minorities. Senator Moss was among the Senate's strongest advocates of civil rights. He spoke out against the inhumane policy of apartheid in 1962, a quarter of a century before it became fashionable.

Moss did as much or more than anyone to extend his personal integrity into government service. He believed that public service was both a high privilege and a public trust. He conducted more oversight hearings designed to ferret out fraud and abuse perpetrated against government programs than anyone in history. He succeeded where others had failed in bringing about the enactment of landmark legislation to establish the post of Inspector General in the Department of Health, Education and Welfare. He argued persuasively that every governmental department needed one official with extraordinary powers who would be responsible for the fiscal integrity of programs administered by that department. Thanks to Moss, every department and regulatory agency now has such an official, an Inspector General.

Nor will historians forget that he halted the decline of the U.S. space program and kept the nation committed to explore the last frontier. To those who argued that there was no value in such activity, he responded that the same arguments were made in the 18th century against pushing forth beyond the Ohio and Mississippi rivers.

Moss has many achievements; but among the jewels in his crown, none shines more brightly than his work on behalf of the poor, the disabled, and the aged. As is noted in this chapter, Moss was the preeminent voice for aging in the Senate. He conducted more hearings than anyone before him or since. His hearings had both substance and style. The reports he issued made sense and they also made news. Moss was responsible for putting aging on the front pages of major newspapers and as a result, the Senate Aging Committee became the most requested and most hotly contested committee assignment. The senator's success also proved to be the impetus for the creation of the House Select Committee on Aging. Never were the nation's seniors better served than when they had Claude Pepper fighting for their interests in the House of Representatives and Frank E. Moss as their prime advocate in the U.S. Senate.

It is also a testament to Moss's convictions that he has continued to contribute to society even after leaving the U.S. Senate. He has written books and articles, testified frequently before Congress, helped the Association of Former Members of Congress create traveling exchange programs with colleges and universities, helped create the Foundation for Hospice and Home Care and The Caring Institute.

Such are his contributions that a portrait of Senator Moss belongs in the Senate reception room alongside those of Clay, Webster, Taft, and LaFollette who were previously selected as among the most venerable to ever serve in the Senate chamber.

Early Years

Frank E. "Ted" Moss was born in Salt Lake City, Utah on September 23, 1911, and lived most of his life near Holladay in Salt Lake County. He was the son of James E. "Jimmie" Moss and Maud Nixon Moss. From the time he was old enough to remember, Ted worshipped his father—with good reason. Jimmie Moss was special and everyone knew it. He had blue eyes that sparkled in a way one could never forget. Jimmie was a teacher for over fifty years in Utah's high school system. For the same amount of time, he was everyone's favorite. He became known statewide as the father of high school athletics. Three generations in Utah still speak with reverence about Jimmie Moss and the values, the education, the love, and affection he poured into its people.

It is only natural that the great teacher would work even greater miracles with his son, Ted, than with those who graced his classroom for only a year. Young Ted Moss was a good student and played on the football team at Granite High School in Salt Lake City. He received his Bachelor's degree with high honors from the University of Utah in 1933. At his father's urging, he chose to follow a career in law at the George Washington University in Washington, D.C. He received his Juris Doctor degree with high honors in 1937.

From law school, Ted Moss went to work in the general counsel's office of the Securities and Exchange Commission. Those were exciting times. Franklin D. Roosevelt was in the White House and was doing his level best to bring the best minds into government to deal with the series of economic problems known as the Great Depression. Ted Moss was impressed with FDR, who reinforced many of the same values he had learned at his father's knee. He also made a number of lasting friends in Washington who would help him later in his life.

After two years, Ted Moss returned to Utah where he was selected as law clerk by the Utah Supreme Court. Thereafter, he opened a private practice in Salt Lake City and soon ran for elected office. He was one of the youngest persons ever elected to the post of City Judge in Salt Lake City. He was reelected and served a total of 10 years in that position.

Judge Moss settled into a quiet family life. He had married the beautiful Phyllis Hart, born in Logan, Utah, and they had a daughter and three sons. This idyllic life was interrupted by World War II. Judge Moss entered the U.S. Army Air Corps. He served in the Judge Advocate General's Department in the European Theatre and ultimately attained the rank of colonel.

Following World War II, Moss returned to Salt Lake City and continued his career on the bench. In 1950, he ran for and was elected Salt Lake County Attorney. As always, he performed so effectively that he was reelected easily. It was at this time that he came to the attention of the tiny regiment of Democratic party leaders in Utah, which has long been recognized as the most Republican and the most conservative of states. They told him that he should begin to set his eye on higher public office. Judge Moss began to think about running for governor.

In his role as Salt Lake County Attorney, Judge Moss handled one politically explosive case after another with a style and grace worthy of Louis Nizer or Clarence Darrow. One case is illustrative. His political advisors urged him not to personally prosecute the case of a man who openly flaunted the law by living with several wives. Polygamy was still a sensitive subject in Utah, having been condoned at one time, if not encouraged, by the predominant Church of Jesus Christ of Latter Day Saints until the federal government intervened. Utah had to outlaw polygamy as a price for admission to the Union; this was done, but it was done grudgingly. A tiny minority continued support for polygamy in response to what they considered the higher law of religion. Moss was told that it was at best a no-win proposition to prosecute the case and at worst it was political suicide to proceed. Characteristically, Moss never wavered. He said the law was the law and had to be enforced; he successfully prosecuted the case.

The Senate Race

In 1957, America was in a deep recession. Unemployment was high, production and sales were down. Dissatisfaction with the incumbent party grew widespread. It even reached the Republican oasis of Utah. President Dwight D. Eisenhower remained personally popular, but his party's policies were increasingly under attack. The Democratic party began to read signs that 1958 was going to be a banner Democratic year. The party in power traditionally loses seats in Congress during the off-year election, but the recession provided hope for a larger swing than usual.

Senator Arthur V. Watkins was running for reelection in 1958 and he looked unbeatable. Voters in Utah were 3 to 1 Republican and there was no one within Utah's Democratic party that seemed able to put together a challenge. Persuaded by Jimmie Moss and his attorney staff, Judge Moss threw his hat in the ring and won the Democratic nomination. Unexpectedly, Salt Lake City's controversial, ultraconservative mayor and former governor J. Bracken Lee announced he would run to oppose incumbent Republican Watkins and Democrat Moss, and run as an Independent candidate. Governor Lee had achieved nationwide fame of sorts for his refusal to pay income tax and for his outright defiance of the IRS and other authority vested in Washington. Governor Lee had a hard-core following, plenty of money, and soon launched a vitriolic attack at Senator Watkins and Judge Moss. He railed against Republican party officials who failed to support him, and was equally vitriolic about Judge Moss. The general election was held on November 4, 1958, and Frank E. Moss was declared the winner over both Lee and Watkins.

Some political pundits said the election of Moss was an accident. Some commentators said that he could not have won but for the fact that Governor Lee and Senator Watkins split the Republican vote. They asserted that Moss was much too liberal for the state; that his ideas were out of sync with the average voter and that he would be a one-term senator. Still others said that voters were casting their ballots for their beloved teacher Jimmie Moss, who stumped the state, and not so much for his son Ted. Phyllis Moss and James "Phil" Cowley, the senator's campaign manager, knew better. They knew Ted Moss was a man of destiny who would always rise to the top of the class because he is the personification of so many of the values that make America great.

Judge Moss was elected; he won it on his own, no thanks to the national Democratic party. As Senator Moss learned, his integrity would sometimes prove to be an impediment to his success in Washington. During that recent election, he had been desperate for funds. At the time, the Democratic Senatorial Campaign Committee was controlled by the Southern block. Lyndon B. Johnson was Majority Leader. Bobby Baker was his man on the Senate floor. As Senator Moss told it later, an emissary from the Democratic Senatorial Campaign Committee visited Utah and offered him a much needed $5,000 contribution, provided that he promise never to vote for repeal of the so-called oil depletion allowance, a special and lucrative tax break for oil companies. The senator refused to go along and did not receive the money. Moss protested and later received a $2,000 unrestricted grant from Senator George Smathers of Florida, Chairman of the Senate Campaign Committee.

Integrity proved an obstacle to Moss again in January of 1959 when the Senate was being organized for that session. The media had selected Moss as a rising star in the Senate. A cover story in *Look* magazine picked Senators Moss, Eugene McCarthy of Minnesota, Edward Muskie of Maine, and Phillip Hart of Michigan as the best and the brightest of the class of '59. Clearly, Moss had a few things going for himself. Then there was tradition: when a party elects a senator from a part of the country which it has historically been unable to carry, the party generally rewards the winner with as many choice committee assignments as possible to enable the senator and his party to hold onto the seat.

Senator Moss had asked for a seat on the powerful Appropriations Committee, the committee that decides how much money should be spent and what it should be spent on. He asked for a seat on the Armed Services Committee. He asked for a seat on the Aeronautics and Space Committee, then so prestigious that Lyndon Johnson, the Majority Leader, had chosen to chair it himself. It is to be recalled that this was the time of Sputnik and the very beginning of America's race into space. To his disappointment, Senator Moss was given what is generally considered the dregs of committee assignments, the Senate Interior and Public Works Committees.

Senator Paul Douglas, that great statesman from Illinois, once said that Moss's honesty and integrity had cost him his rightful place in the United States Senate. Speaker Sam Rayburn is said to have advised new congresspersons that one has to "go along to get along." The saying means that a senator has to close his or her eyes and assist others in their political deals if they expect reciprocity and, hence, advancement in Washington. Moss had established himself as someone who would think for himself and not simply go along with the crowd.

The same events occurred in 1963 when Moss again sought to get on the Appropriations and Aeronautics and Space Committees. Bobby Baker advised him to tell Senator Richard Russell of Georgia that he would never vote for changes that would make it easier to break a filibuster. The Southern block used the filibuster to block civil rights legislation from coming to the Senate vote and under Senate rules at the time, a 2/3 vote of the Senate was needed to shut off a filibuster. A change in this rule, making it easier to break a filibuster, could possibly lead to the enactment of civil rights legislation. Moss refused to go along, believing that it should be easier to cut off debate. Once again, Moss did not get the cherished committee assignments.

Making Lemonade

There is an old saying that goes, "If life gives you lemons, make lemonade." Senator Moss set out with his usual determination to make the best out of the committee assignments he had been given. It should be understood that committee assignments, in a very real way, shape what a senator can accomplish in Washington. It is hard to carve out a career in foreign affairs, for example, unless one is a member of the Foreign Affairs Committee. The same is true for Armed Services or Appropriations. Each committee handles specific kinds of legislation. By giving Senator Moss assignments on the Public Works and Interior Committees, the unfriendly senate leadership sought to sideline him. Through hard work and diligence, Moss had the last laugh.

The Public Works Committee is the committee that must approve the building of dams and roads—what are sometimes referred to as "pork barrel" projects. One by one, the members of the Senate, including the leadership, found that they needed Senator Moss's vote to win Senate approval for their pet projects back home. They also learned that Senator Moss was honest and fair. He would not automatically give approval to any project. He studied each one in detail. If the project was needed, and could be built at a reasonable cost, he gave his blessing—without asking for a quid pro quo in return.

Moss used his position on the Public Works and the Interior Committees to benefit Utah and the nation. As chairman of the Subcommittee on Mining, Minerals and Fuels, and vice-chairman of the Energy Subcommittee, he sought to alert the nation to the possible shortage of oil reserves. His legislation promoted research in alternative kinds of energy, from solar power to oil shale. His legislation created the Office of Coal Research to study ways of using coal more effectively. He was also the sponsor of coal mine safety legislation that established federal minimum standards and inspection of coal mines, authorized civil penalties for violations, and compensated miners who had developed black lung disease.

Senator Moss believed fervently that America should set aside some of its natural beauty to be enjoyed by future generations. He is more responsible for the creation or expansion of more federal parks and recreation areas than anyone. His legislation established the Canyonlands National Park, the Golden Spike Historic Site, extended the boundaries of Zion Park, created Arches National Park, Capital Reef National Park, Flaming Gorge Recreation Area, Glen Canyon Recreation Area (Lake Powell), and expanded the Park City and Brian Head Ski Resort areas, to cite only a few of his credits.

The senator became the nation's unchallenged expert on water resource management. He traveled to the Soviet Union as chairman of an American delegation to study the dimension of Soviet hydroelectric power. President John Kennedy said of him, "Senator Moss has preached the doctrine of the wise use of water with, I think, more vigor than any other member of the United States Senate." The Senator authored the authoritative book, *The Water Crisis*, and most of the major legislation relating to water management, research, and pollution control. The senator also had a similar interest in preventing air pollution. His overall interest in protecting the environment brought him awards and accolades from the Sierra Club, and a close friendship with actor and Utah resident, Robert Redford, who is devoting much of his energies to this important cause.

President Kennedy

Senator Moss had served two years with John F. Kennedy before Kennedy was elected president. The two shared interests in helping the elderly and the disadvantaged. Both were activists and both had a vision of the future. Moss had been the leader of the Utah delegation to the 1960 Democratic convention which nominated President Kennedy. Moss campaigned for him. During the years 1960–63, the president and senator Moss became quite close friends. The senator enjoyed easy access to the White House. It was a happy time for Moss. Being an insider at the White House allowed Moss to accomplish a great deal for his state. One of the happiest days in the Senator's life was his 52nd birthday. On September 23, 1963, President Kennedy came to Utah for the dedication of the Flaming Gorge Dam and made a ringing speech before a crowd of thousands crowded into the Mormon Tabernacle. The evening began with "Hail to the Chief" and a prayer and ended with the Mormon Tabernacle Choir singing "The Battle Hymn of the Republic." President Kennedy was at his best and the air was charged with electricity and indescribable enthusiasm.

Understandably, the president's death, barely one month later, was one of the real low points in the Senator's life.

Reelection: Consumer Affairs

In 1964, Moss answered all those pundits who had predicted he would be a one-term senator. He was reelected by the widest margin ever rolled up by a candidate for national office in Utah. The polls showed that Senator Moss was indeed perceived to be much more liberal than the average Utah voter. Moreover, the senator had to overcome the 3 to 1 Republican edge. Exit polls indicated that the people in Utah appreciated the hard work and constituent service that the senator had brought to them. They showed he was widely popular because of his engaging personality. The Utah voters were able to separate him from other elected officials, largely because of his work on the Interior and Public Works Committees. His work on these committees had an immediate effect on them—his efforts improved the quality of life and made jobs in Utah.

With his reelection, the senator was able to trade his seat on the Public Works Committee for the most prestigious Senate Commerce Committee. He soon became chairman of the Subcommittee on Consumer Affairs and his accomplishments were many.

Moss was responsible for the warning labels on cigarettes and for taking cigarette advertising off television. His legislation required federal inspection of fish processing plants and required the Food and

Drug Administration to take off the market drugs found by the National Academy of Sciences to be ineffective.

He is the author of the Poison Prevention Packaging bill that requires all household products which are potentially harmful to children come with child-proof caps. His legislation created similar child-proof caps for prescription medications.

The senator is also to be credited for the Toy Safety Act, which requires the Secretary of Health and Human Services to remove dangerous toys from the market. In the course of hearings, the Senator had found toy ovens that heated to 600 degrees, hotter than most kitchen ovens; non-insulated wires where water seepage could cause fatal shocks; cuddly stuffed animals whose ears could be pulled off to expose long sharp pins; and many other hazardous items. In other hearings, the senator documented that many breakfast cereals have limited nutritional value; the result was nutritional labeling.

Moss was one of the sponsors of the Truth in Lending legislation. A Moss bill called for open dating of perishable items and unit pricing in supermarkets. Another Moss bill standardized warranties so that no manufacturer could avoid the responsibility of standing behind a product. Still another bill upgraded the powers of the Federal Trade Commission so that it would be better able to deal with consumer problems.

Moss won praise from his colleagues for his work on behalf of consumers. Senator Warren Magnuson, Chairman of the Senate Commerce Committee, said: "Senator Moss has time and time again captained a strong consumer team that has scored heavily for the consumer—and for legitimate business. Consumers are fortunate to have a man like Ted Moss carrying the ball for them."

The Third Term: Top of the Senate Ladder

In November of 1970, Moss again overcame overwhelming odds and was reelected to his third term in the Senate. The Republican candidate, congressman Laurence Burton, had the advantage of voter registration and money. He spent thousands of dollars on a Madison Avenue advertising campaign that featured the congressman, a huge man, on horseback decked out in cowboy wear with the theme: "A man to match our mountains."

The primary factor in the election was image. Senator Moss was seen as likable, folksy, hardworking, and honest. The citizens liked his work on consumer affairs. Some orthodox Mormons voted for him for the first time because of his stand against smoking. The senator could point to 25 major proposals that had been enacted into law, whereas his opponent could not point to a single item that he had authored that had been enacted. The problems of the nation's elderly became a major issue in the campaign.

Congressman Burton had been an outspoken opponent of Medicare. He said it was unnecessary and merely a politically motivated gesture. "The Johnson Administration's medical care for the aged bill is either politically motivated or a deliberate plan to put the U.S. Government in the medical business one step at a time," he charged. By contrast, Senator Moss had cosponsored and supported the Medicare bill. As a member of the Senate Special Committee on Aging and Chairman of its Subcommittee on Long-Term Care, he had conducted numerous hearings which brought to light the health problems of older Americans. His hearings brought to light substandard conditions in the nation's nursing homes and his amendments created the home care benefit in both the Medicare and Medicaid programs. It was no contest; Moss won handily.

With his reelection to a third term, Moss advanced up the Senate seniority ladder. He acquired more power, more responsibility, and began to be recognized nationally as a leader. By now, Senator Moss was universally admired and respected by his colleagues for his intelligence, good judgment, hard work, and integrity. A reflection of this acceptance came early in his third term when he was elected as secretary to the Democratic Conference—the third-ranking Democratic leadership post after the Majority Leader and Majority Whip. This election also put Moss on the important Democratic Policy and Steering Committees, which decide legislative goals and committee appointments. As Phil Cowley had predicted in 1958, Senator Moss had made it to the top of the ladder.

Moss used some of his new power to help his friend Ed Muskie put together the Senate Budget Committee as a means of getting a handle on government spending. Moss served as the ranking Democrat on the committee and helped make it the powerful force that it is today. The committee sets budget ceilings and charts the parameters of government spending. Other Senate committees are bound by what the Budget Committee decides they can spend. The present move towards a balanced budget had its roots in the efforts of Senators Moss and Muskie in 1972.

It was in his third term that Moss finally realized his ambition to serve on the Senate Appropriations and Space Committees.

In 1974, the Democratic Steering Committee asked Moss to assume the chairmanship of the important Aeronautics and Space committee. The committee and the space program were in trouble. The Nixon-Ford Administrations had indicated their desire to stop the space program, to cancel the space shuttle, the Voyager project, the joint Soviet-U.S. space mission, and almost all other projects. Moss can be credited for keeping the space program alive. His hearings demonstrated the value of the program to the nation, not only in jobs but also in bringing about the creation of new technology that can be adapted to a multiplicity of uses.

As structured, the Space Committee was very powerful. It was tailored specifically by its first chairman, Lyndon Johnson. The enabling legislation authorized the chairman of the Space Committee also to sit as a member of the Appropriations Committee. As successor to Lyndon Johnson, Senator Moss sat in on Appropriations Committee hearings and meetings and thereby helped fund the American space program.

The Senate Aging Committee

During his third term, Senator Moss used his power as a senior member of the U.S. Senate Special Committee on Aging and chairman of the Subcommittee on Long-Term Care to expose all manner of fraud and abuse perpetrated against senior citizens. The work of the senator and this subcommittee can be credited with bringing the subject of aging to the attention of the American public.

Some 27 hearings were held on nursing home problems between 1971 and 1976 and a 12-volume report was issued that charged that 50 percent of the nursing homes in the United States were substandard, with one or more life-threatening conditions. Beginning in 1975, hearings were held on Medicare and Medicaid fraud. The committee held a dozen hearings on this subject between September 1975 and August 1976; 11 of the 12 hearings were front page news. Senator Moss and the committee's work made the cover of *Time*, *Newsweek*, *U.S. News and World Report*, and *Medical World News*, and repeatedly made the front pages of America's major newspapers. The volume of the publicity was so great that Senator and later Vice-President Walter F. Mondale wisecracked to staff, "Hey, can't you do something to get Senator Moss off the front page of the *New York Times*?"

The senator's investigations of Medicaid fraud in New York City were summarized on the evening news and carried live on educational television. One of the committee's investigations into fraud and abuse among clinical laboratories was covered by CBS's "Sixty Minutes." In that investigation, committee staff posing as physicians opened a medical clinic on the south side of Chicago. Salesmen representing 11 of the 12 clinical laboratories that received 90 percent of the money Medicaid paid for lab services entered the clinic and offered illegal kickbacks and rebates to the investigators. The episode was filmed by Mike Wallace who openly confronted the cheats.

In a related investigation, some members of the committee staff posed as Medicaid patients and sought treatment in the so-called Medicaid mills, which are found in abundance in America's major cities. It was learned firsthand that many of these clinics were billing for services they did not render at a scale few dared to imagine. Senator Moss decided to see things for himself. He put on old clothes, let his whiskers grow, and offered himself as a patient. On June 7, 1976, Moss made Senate history by going undercover to expose abuses and fraud in the Medicaid clinics of New York City.

In doing so, he took a very great risk. He was taken to the roughest areas of New York—East Harlem, Fort Apache in the Bronx, and into the den of the drug dealers on the Lower East Side. There was abundant evidence about the involvement of organized crime in the ownership of some of these facilities, which specialized in seeing as many Medicaid patients as possible in the shortest possible time and then billing Medicaid for the maximum amount possible. Thousands of dollars worth of phony claims were submitted by physicians who Senator Moss did not see and thousands more were billed in tests that were unnecessary or never performed.

The result of the investigation was a committee report documenting widespread fraud in the Medicaid program and the enactment of Moss's bills, which made Medicaid fraud a felony and created the Office of Inspector General in the Department of Health and Human Services to fight fraud. At the Senate hearings, Moss was able to give his firsthand account of how Medicaid fraud is perpetrated by some greedy providers. The investigation made headlines in every major paper in the country for four days running. The *New York Times* and most other major newspapers commended the work; the senator received kudos for his personal role in the investigation. When he made his appearance on the Senate floor following the hearings, his colleagues in the Senate gave Senator Moss a standing ovation.

The *New York Times* editorial said in part: "Senator Frank E. Moss and the members of his staff performed an extraordinary public service by personally posing as indigent patients as they sought to uncover Medicaid irregularities."

The *Macon Georgia Telegraph* was typical of other editorials: "With enterprise too seldom displayed by our elected officials, Senator Frank E. Moss has personally documented and publicized the blatant and long ignored fraudulent practices within the Medicaid program."

From 1962 through 1977, the Senate Aging Committee was featured on one or more of the three network television programs a total of 25 times, 22 of these related to the work of Senator Moss and the Subcommittee on Long-Term Care.

Views on Senior Issues

Senator Moss was in the forefront of most of the major issues in the field of aging from 1959 through January, 1977, when he retired from the Senate. With Claude Pepper, Robert Butler, Daphne Krause, and Maggie Kuhn, he led the battle against ageism. In an internationally quoted speech, he said in 1971:

> It is hell to be old in this country. It is a simple truth for most of our elderly. The pressures of living in the age of materialism and the pursuit of the good life has produced a youth cult in America. Our preoccupation with staying young virtually knows no boundary. We spend millions on elixirs and remedies all the way from pep pills to hair transplants and face liftings. Hang the expense. Drink Pepsi, drive a Ford, smoke Silva-Thins or do anything anybody insists will keep you looking young.
>
> Why this obsession with youth? Some blame the movies. Others blame advertising for the kind of images sold to the public. The real reason goes deeper. Most of us are afraid of getting old. This is true because we have made old age in this country a wasteland. It is T.S. Eliot's rats walking on broken glass. It is the nowhere in between this life and the great beyond. It is being robbed of your eyesight, your mobility and even your human dignity.

Senator Moss led the campaign to change the shabby way that elderly were treated in American society. He began with income and retirement practices.

> It is a national disgrace that millions of elderly find themselves living in poverty for no reason save the fact that they have chosen to retire. More than half have only their social security checks to rely upon. Many have become disabled and cannot work but the great majority can and want to do so. Unfortunately, we discriminate against them. We will not hire them. When we do, we pay them the minimum wage and penalize them by reducing their social security income by one dollar for each two dollars that they earn.

The senator introduced legislation to raise the amount of money seniors could earn without having to suffer offsetting deductions in their social security. He worked with Claude Pepper to help eliminate mandatory retirement.

Moss consistently fought to provide the nation's seniors with better and more affordable housing. "Fully 30 percent of all senior Americans live in substandard conditions without adequate plumbing or electricity. This fact is a blight on the American conscience," said the senator, who for a time chaired the Subcommittee on Housing for the

Elderly. In this capacity he helped enact legislation, which was known as the Section 202 program, that provided direct loans to churches and non-profit organizations at low interest to help build housing projects specifically designed to meet the special needs of seniors.

The senator championed the cause of national health insurance as the best solution to the health needs of all Americans. As an early co-sponsor of Medicare, he said:

> Older Americans are sick three times as often as the younger population. Their hospital stays on average are three times as long and their expenditures per capita are more than three times that of their younger counterparts. To add to this burden, most seniors cannot buy private health insurance coverage. They are considered an unacceptable risk. Even if such policies were available, seniors cannot afford them in their retirement years when they can count on less than half of the income they had prior to retirement. I believe that access to the highest quality health care is a right for all Americans—particularly the aged. Health care is a basic civil right which must not be abridged or limited to those who can afford to pay for what they need.

Moss wrote and said a great deal about nursing home care in the United States. He noted that he had been accused in turn of being the greatest friend and the greatest enemy of the nursing home industry. Indeed, his legislation helped nourish the industry and at the same time established tough federal minimum standards. On one occasion, he said in releasing a highly acclaimed report:

> The average older American regards nursing homes as a kind of purgatory, as the first step of an inevitable slide into oblivion. To seniors, nursing homes have become synonymous with death and the notion of protracted suffering before death. There are many wonderful nursing homes in America whose existence reinforces the fact that we need not tolerate substandard care and life-threatening conditions. The time for denials and mutual recriminations is long past and it is time nursing home owners and consumer advocates worked together to insure that all nursing home patients are given the highest quality services preserving their human dignity and sense of intrinsic worth.

In the course of conducting his 15 years of investigation of nursing home problems, Moss discovered home care, which he concluded was a better alternative for those needing long-term care than institutionalization.

> You have only to ask yourself which you would prefer, to be uprooted and placed in a nursing home or to remain at home with nursing and other medical, therapeutic and social services delivered to your door. Home care is much to be preferred from a social policy point of view. It is generally less expensive than institutionalization and it serves the important function of keeping families together.

Senator Moss was the sponsor of legislation creating the Medicare and Medicaid home care benefits in 1965 and 1967, respectively. He was also one of the first advocates of hospice care, as a participant in the first congressional hearings on this subject. In 1971 he said:

> Americans do not have a very enlightened view about death. It is after all, a part of life. In our society, there are far too many people who die friendless in hospitals and nursing homes when they could be at home. Hospice care, that is the provision of home care services to those who are terminally ill, can make a major difference in the lives of those who receive them and serve to support surviving family members in their hour of grief.

Awards and Recognition

Frank E. Moss has received awards too numerous to be listed here in their entirety. Here are but a few: George Washington University awarded him their Distinguished Alumni Award in 1963. The National District Attorneys Association gave him their Furtherance of Justice Award in 1961. The inscription on that award reads: "For his outstanding service as a prosecutor exemplifying his courage and humanity and the highest ideals of justice; and for his resourcefulness, initiative and continued interest in all federal legislation contributing to more effective law enforcement throughout our country." In 1969, he received the Bronze Medal for Distinguished Service to the Aging from the American Association of Homes for the Aging. This marked the first time the award had been given to a public official. He has received the Better Life Award from the American Health Care Association, "In recognition of outstanding service through unselfish and effective efforts that have resulted in lasting contributions to the improved health care of the aged in the community and the Nation." The Better Government Association of Chicago, Illinois honored the senator for his tireless efforts to root out abuse, waste, and fraud in government in March 1976. In June of 1976, he received the Award of Merit from the National Council of Senior Citizens. The citation for that award reads in part:

> Senator Frank E. Moss has served on the Senate Committee on Aging since 1963. He has distinguished himself as one of its most active members, chairing more hearings and introducing more legislation with respect to the needs of the elderly than any man in the history of Congress.
>
> He has consistently fought for increased social security or pension benefits to meet the income problems of the elderly and has sponsored legislation to help meet the housing needs of the elderly.
>
> Senator Moss has been an outstanding voice in the Senate and can be credited with greatly aiding health needs of seniors. He played an important role in the enactment of Medicare in 1965, and since that time has pressed for its expansion to provide eyeglasses, dental care, and out-of-hospital prescription drugs, as well as increased home health services.
>
> He has received national acclaim for his hearings on nursing home problems. Since 1969, he has conducted 38 hearings and issued a 12-volume report which the Department of Justice called the most comprehensive nursing home investigation ever undertaken. His hearings and reports have led to the enactment of new legislation to protect the infirm elderly and have served to bring criminals to the bar of justice.

On September 15, 1990, a federal courthouse in Salt Lake City was named in his honor pursuant to an act of Congress. A few days later, on September 27, 1990, he was named the second recipient of the Pepper Distinguished Service Award from the Mildred and Claude Pepper Foundation. The award is given to the person who has achieved outstanding results through the practice of the politics of compassion in the spirit of Claude Pepper.

Perspective

What makes Senator Moss so special? There are so many things that must go into the equation that any analysis will inevitably fall short of the mark.

One primary factor is the senator's values, his high moral character, his honesty, integrity, hard work, and love of his family and his country. Another element is the senator's personality. He is so warm and open, slow to anger and quick to forgive. He is sincere, genuine, and humble. He never confused the office with the man.

Another element relates to his veneration of the aged and his constant efforts to encourage young people. He is a strong advocate of education as the key to social mobility. He wrote thousands of letters to young people in high school encouraging them to go on to college. He said that one of his few regrets was that he did not have the opportunity to offer jobs to more young people from Utah so that they could be exposed to Washington and Capitol Hill.

He was also fair and treated everyone equally. He did not curry favor with the rich and powerful nor did he back off when his investigations implicated powerful political figures—even when they were members of his own political party.

He always aligned himself with the poor and the middle class—with the majority of the American public. He constantly asked himself what he could do that would improve the quality of their lives.

He was an activist in the Senate. He believed that government exists to help people solve their problems. If government is not being responsive, the answer is to make it work, not to do away with it. He had a great vision not only of things as they are, but as they will be and as they could be. He is a futurist who still believes government should attempt to find long-range solutions and not simply deal with the crises of the present.

Nor is he afraid of change. He often said the greatest challenge before America was to cope with the winds of change blowing fiercely throughout America and the world and still hold on to our democratic processes and our cherished freedoms. In a widely quoted speech delivered at Utah State University in Logan, Utah, on June 30, 1966, he said the following:

> What we need in America is more people who are not afraid to become involved in issues which are controversial. My experience is that where there is no controversy there is no progress. I do not want it said of our generation what T.S. Eliot wrote in his poem, "The Rock"—"And the wind shall say: These were decent people, their only monument—the asphalt road and a thousand golf balls." We can do better than that. We need a constant flow of new ideas. We also need respect from the people for such new ideas—a willingness to consider them fairly and without prejudice. Our nation has endured well into the Twentieth Century not because of our rhetoric and our wealth, not because we have the longest cars or the whitest iceboxes, or the first color TV, but because our ideas of individual initiative and individual freedom, and freedom of enterprise have proven to be more workable and more lasting.

He had the courage to follow his convictions wherever they led him. If that meant taking on the physicians, nursing homes, the broadcasters or the tobacco lobby, then so be it. He took on the fights and more often than not he won.

If only two words could be used to describe Moss, they would be joyous and judicious. The senator finds joy in whatever he does. He loves his law practice, his family, and his country. He takes great pleasure in helping others. Perhaps it is knowing that he had done everything he possibly could to help that gives him that sense of inner peace and that fuels his ready million-dollar grin. Above all he was and is judicious: fair, honest, and wise.

In 1988, Moss helped create the Caring Institute to promote the social values reflected in community service based on the belief that the solution to most human problems lies in the service of one human being to another. Among other things, the Institute every year seeks to identify the most caring men and women in America. When asked about this, Moss said:

> Society has reached a critical stage. We appear to have lost sight of our values; there has been a preoccupation with things material. The public record has been dominated of late by greed and selfishness. Somebody has to say, "Hey, we are off course." Whether we are talking about individuals or the nation, we are best served by

> transcending self. Someone has to nudge us back in the direction of being what we always were, the most caring nation in the history of the world.

In these times when some elected leaders rank in the public's favor somewhere below used car dealers, it is a pleasure to look back on the career of one of the greatest Americans. He left his mark in the U.S. Senate, opening new ground for others to follow. He anticipated problems before they became that and intervened with timely legislation. He became the voice of the voiceless, the friend of the friendless, and he brought hope to those without hope. He stands tall in his public service, having left a great legacy to all Americans. To his colleagues in the Senate, he provided an even greater service, he set the standard against which they will be judged in the future.

———— ❧ ————

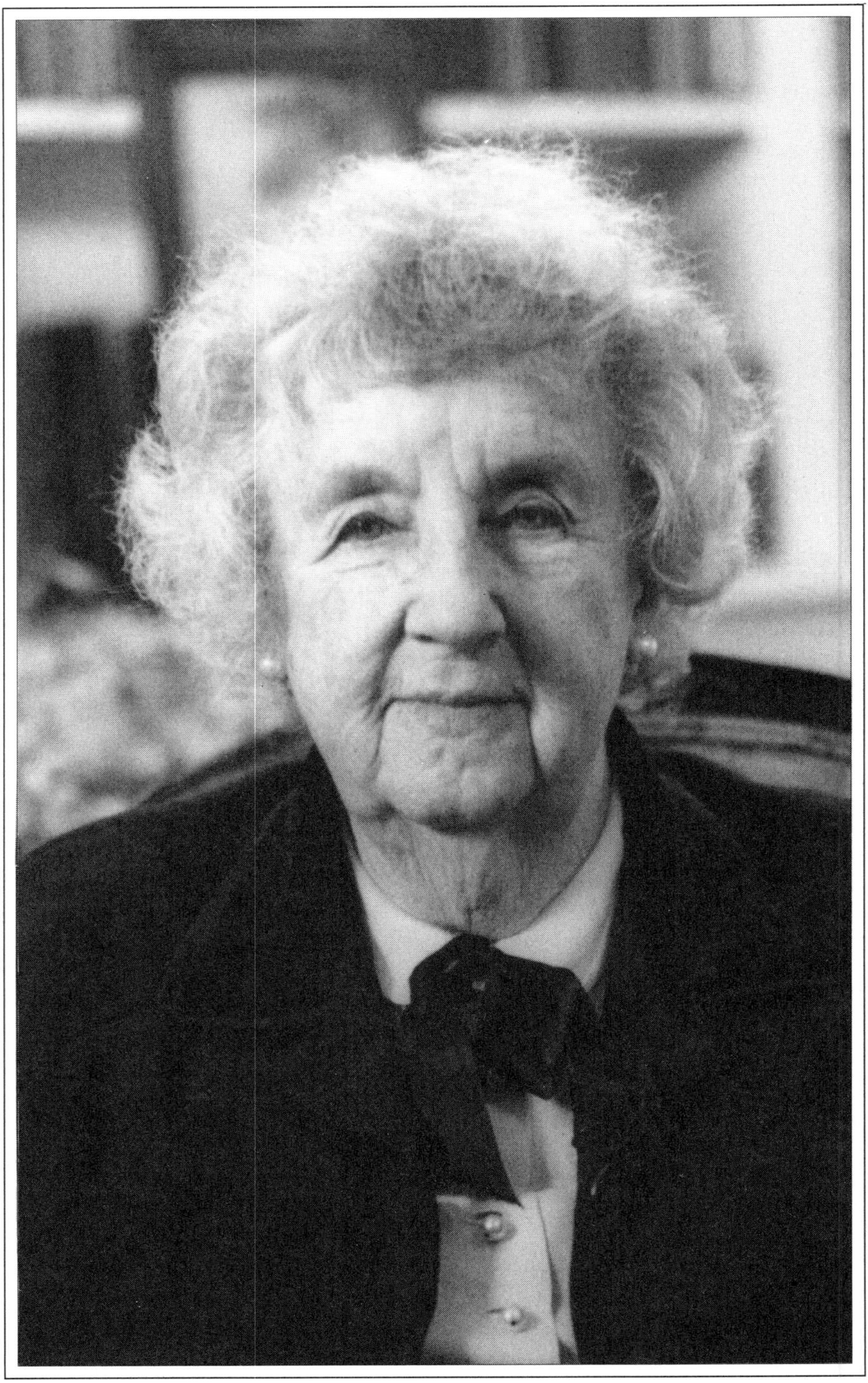

VAL J. HALAMANDARIS

SIX

Virginia Henderson

The field of nursing needs its own equivalent of Mt. Rushmore. There should be some place where all Americans can go to learn about those individuals who helped build what may be the noblest of all professions.

Certainly no other profession is so selfless. No other profession has contributed so much to humanity. No other profession has done so much good for so many millions of people.

Nurses have been legendary figures of mercy—mother substitutes, women of goodness and charity, going back to the very beginning of time. In some cases, they have been members of religious orders, and in other cases, they were simply Good Samaritans with empathy for other human beings.

What could be more noble than the prevention of illness or the treatment of illness and disease? What could be more humane than comforting those who are ill and in sorrow?

To be sure, physicians have played a similar role, but as anyone who has ever been in a hospital can attest, the quality of nursing and aide service determines the overall quality of care received by the patient.

Through all the years of goodness compounded by more goodness, four names have emerged to head the list of those who have contributed the most to the field of nursing. By consensus, the names to be chiseled on the shrine would be Clara Barton, Florence Nightingale, Annie W. Goodrich, and Virginia Henderson.

Virginia Henderson is a research associate emeritus from Yale University, best known as the author of the definitive textbook on nursing. Her ideas have shaped the field of nursing for several generations. She revolutionized teaching as it relates to the elderly, shattering myths and stereotypes and accenting the values of caring and concern.

Henderson is small in stature, but large in spirit. She has a heart as big as Texas, and at age 93 her mind remains razor sharp. She has blue eyes that sparkle with such intensity that they melt any thoughts of height or chronological age.

Virginia Henderson was born on the eve of the 20th century. She has witnessed a quantum leap in the extension of the human life span: during her lifetime, average life expectancy has increased by 66 percent. This miracle was made possible by modern science and the development of new medicine, technology, and medical procedures. However, this major advance could not have occurred without Henderson and the advances she helped pioneer in the field of nursing.

Henderson, more than any other person, helped transform nursing from an art to a science. She helped propel the profession out of the back wards of hospitals into the front line of American health care. Almost single-handedly, she pushed the nursing profession in the direction of research, statistics, and comparative analysis. It took her 11 years, but with the help of friends, she indexed all the known literature in the field of nursing. By this one act alone, she has left a legacy for future generations, the importance of which too few people realize. Henderson has given the nursing profession a gift that will become increasingly more valuable with time—the opportunity for perpetual growth and improvement.

Henderson was, and continues to be, one of the strongest advocates of the elderly and a leading proponent of home health care. On the completion of her studies, she chose to work as a visiting nurse, providing hands-on care to shut-ins, the disabled, and the aged. She still ranks this experience among her most satisfying career moves.

Virginia Henderson has guided nursing in the direction of personalized care and urges listening and learning from patients. By her life's example and her many achievements, she has brought dignity and respect to her profession and tremendous service to humanity.

Background

Virginia Henderson was born in Kansas City, Missouri, on November 30, 1897. She was the fifth child born to Daniel B. Henderson and Lucy Abbot Henderson. "It upsets my family when it is reported that I am a Missouri native," says Henderson. "My father's family is from Maryland and my mother's comes from Virginia. In fact, they named me after the state."

Henderson's paternal grandfather, Charles Henderson, was an industrialist with interests in real estate, mining, and transportation; he and his family resided in Hancock, Maryland. Her maternal grandfather was William Richardson Abbot, a soldier who upon returning from the Civil War began teaching school and ultimately became the principal of Bellview High School in Bedford County, Virginia. He held this post from 1870 until 1910 when the school was abolished.

Henderson remembers William Abbot as a stern man who also had a keen sense of humor. "Most people were afraid of him, but for some reason I was not. I never seemed to be afraid of anybody. Grandfather liked that and we became great friends." He was the "absolute king of the establishment. Grandfather influenced all of us because he was such a person of integrity and had such a wonderful mind."

Henderson says that her maternal grandmother was equally important in her formative years. "She was wonderful. She was the daughter of a physician and she was a pretty good doctor herself. The children in our family hardly ever had to consult a physician because Grandmother treated them. There were few laws and regulations in those days and Grandmother kept a whole little pharmacy, which she used to treat the boys. We had a country doctor, but he chewed tobacco and he would spit on his boot, sharpen a knife, and lance a boil. Grandmother knew enough to know that that wasn't a good idea."

Henderson's father was a lawyer by profession. He taught in Grandfather Henderson's school while he was studying law, which is where he met Lucy Abbot. They were married and moved to Kansas City, Missouri, where Daniel Henderson opened a law practice.

"My father was a quiet man, a small man with a delightful sense of humor. I think he was very handsome as a young man. He was also very idealistic. He devoted a great deal of his life to helping the underprivileged, particularly the Indians," says Henderson.

Daniel Henderson practiced law in Kansas City until 1902. By that time he had accumulated so much work on behalf of the Indians that he realized that he had to be near Washington, D.C. When Virginia was four, the family moved back to Bedford County near Lynchburg, Virginia. In this way, his wife, Lucy Abbot Henderson, and the children could be near her family, a comfort since his work required extensive travel to visit the Indian reservations out West.

> I think that some people thought that father should not have left the children to be raised by our mother. But he was home as often as he could be and mother was completely sympathetic with his devotion to do something for the Indians. Mother adored father. She used to say to me privately, "Your father is a hero."

Others shared this view, so much so that the portrait of Daniel Broshius Henderson hangs in tribute in the Smithsonian Museum in Washington, D.C.

Henderson says she learned many of her values from watching her father. "I remember on one occasion he said, 'I would like to think that my children could help people who did not have as many advantages as they have had.' I was very impressed with his taking that stand and thinking that this really was a very decent way to feel about things." Helping those who had fewer advantages became a lifelong commitment for Virginia Henderson.

Her father and grandfather were not the only figures who had a profound effect on shaping Henderson's character. Her mother, Lucy, was an equally strong personality. "She was very bright and had a wonderful sense of humor. She was supportive of everyone. She was bored with us as children. She loved us as babies, was crazy about us when we grew up, but as children she thought we were pretty silly. The trouble was that we did not entertain her. As somebody said about our family, 'The worst thing you can do to an Abbot is to bore them.' And she never corrected us so that when she did, it just burned into you. You never forgot it. She was a wonderful mother and a wonderful person."

Education

Henderson's education involved going to one of the two schools run by her family.

> I was educated by my family. It didn't amount to much. We seemed to have taught each other in those days. The aunts had school for us and when Grandfather's school was broken up, I went to my Uncle Charlie's school for neighborhood boys.
>
> There were 13 boys in the school. I was the only girl. One of the boys was very, very smart; in later years he made himself a fortune. I credit that boy for my education. We had a great rivalry, such as who would be the first to get the answers to problems in geometry. It was my effort to be as good as this boy, who really made me work and to use my head for the first time.

After she received the equivalent of a high school education, Henderson would have liked to have gone on to college.

> If I had had the money and I were a boy and worth educating, I would have been an architect. I loved building things—houses, furnishings, and so on. But that was out of the question. They didn't think I could be educated so I was having a grand time at home, doing things that I liked to do, making things for the family to wear and things for the house to wear.

World War I broke out and two of Henderson's brothers went into the service. This gave Henderson the idea that she, too, should try to help. She learned that there was a great need for nurses not only in the military, but also in civilian hospitals, so she enrolled at the age of 20 in the Army School of Nursing. The Army's program to train nurses had been the brainchild of Annie W. Goodrich, who suggested a training program comparable to West Point. "Miss Goodrich used to say, quietly, that it was the only constructive thing the Army has ever done," says Henderson.

Annie Goodrich

Annie Warburton Goodrich is Virginia Henderson's heroic figure—the person that she admires most in all the world. There is good reason for this. In most people's estimation, Goodrich is a towering figure in terms of her contribution to nursing and to humanity.

Henderson remembers Annie Goodrich as a diminutive and delicate person, yet as a person of great strength. "She had the air of a French countess, having come from an affluent family and having lived for a time in England."

Henderson met Goodrich through her sister Frances, who was working as a secretary in Washington, D.C., with the American Federation of Art and living in a friend's house. This was during World War I, and it was common for Washington families to open their homes, particularly to those involved in the war effort. As it happened, Goodrich was living in the same house as Frances Henderson.

> I used to see her just as an ordinary human being and Miss Goodrich and I were sort of friends before we had any reason to know each other as professional people. There were three generations living in that big old house in Georgetown. It was quite remarkable. The entire family was crazy about her.

Henderson reports that Goodrich saw old people being treated in an insensitive way and took an oath to do things better. "So she went to New York where she received her training at New York Hospital. Her talent was immediately recognized and she was installed as the director of the four biggest hospitals in New York City: New York Hospital, Roosevelt Hospital, St. Luke's, and Bellvue Hospital."

Thereafter, she set up the State Board of Nursing Examiners and went to the Henry Street Settlement, where she became director of nurses and then director of the Visiting Nurse Service of New York. Simultaneously, she taught public health nursing at Teacher's College, Columbia University.

Henderson reports that Goodrich fought a long battle to make the point that nursing should be based on education as well as experience. She led the battle to create schools of nursing and then to establish them as part of colleges and universities. She became the first dean of the Yale School of Nursing.

Goodrich set up training programs for nurses, which she ran out of the Army Surgeon General's Office. One such program was at Walter Reed Army Hospital in Washington, D.C., where Henderson received her training. The course consisted of a combination of academic instruction and supervised experience.

Ideas

When asked to describe the philosophy of Goodrich, Henderson says that her heroine and role model was far ahead of her time. "In the first place, she was a Jeffersonian Democrat and she was an egalitarian. She said that she would love to live in a world where the plumber read Plato."

> She thought the possibilities in our service were absolutely unlimited. She had learned how to cut through the red tape; she succeeded because she had such a beautiful sense of humor. She was really beloved in this most arbitrary medical world. I don't think she saw our work as so different and separate from what the doctor is doing now. She saw us working together as partners.
>
> She saw nurses as accepting this terrific responsibility of a 24-hour service, which the doctors have never done except as interns and residents. But she was not trying to say that what we did was greater than what they were doing. She admired the doctors' work.
>
> She was for national health insurance. I think that she would be disgusted to know that we remain the one developed country in the world that has no national health service. She would not have believed that it could have been postponed as long as this. I remember somewhere she wrote, "I see no hope for the poor, without national health insurance." And she was not any more afraid of tax-supported health care than she was of tax-supported education.

Goodrich was also a strong proponent of home care. "She wanted us to be able to move from the institution into the homes if this was possible in order that we might get the feeling of a continuum in health care. So, she put us into a visiting nurse uniform even as students, which essentially was a blue gingham dress with a black cravat."

Home care was an integral part of the training of nurses at the Yale School of Nursing under the direction of Goodrich. "Nurses followed patients back and forth from their homes to the hospital, and students kept careful records and were very much involved in people's lives," remembers Henderson.

During the course of her training, Henderson helped tend to wounded veterans at Walter Reed, worked in pediatric care on a floating hospital in Boston harbor, and worked in hospitals. In 1920, the year before she graduated, she developed a preference for home care over institution-based nursing.

> I developed the feeling that I would not like to nurse in hospitals. I was resentful of the hard-and-fast rules, which I thought were not desirable or in the best interests of the patients. I preferred to nurse where we had more control over the lives of patients. I thought that if we were not helping a patient, that they should be able to choose whether to open the door and let us in. Whereas, if you're in a hospital, you have a pretty hard time resisting anything anybody wants to do to you. You'd better behave yourself or you'll make it tough for yourself.

Predictably, Henderson's first position following graduation was with the Visiting Nurse Association of New York, also known as the Henry Street Settlement. Goodrich at that time was its director.

Employment

Henderson graduated in 1921 and spent two highly enjoyable years with the Visiting Nurse Association of New York and then another year with the VNA of Washington, D.C. Thereafter, she was recruited by her home state to help set up a program of nursing education and the State Board of Nursing Examiners. In 1924, she became instructor and educational director at the Norfolk Protestant Hospital School of Nursing, Norfolk, Virginia.

> They saw me perhaps as someone who could bring some of Miss Goodrich's ideas to the State of Virginia. I was the first full-time nursing instructor in the state. It was a wonderful five years. I succeeded in changing things in spite of the teetotal resistance to everything that I was doing.

She succeeded, she says, because she established an excellent relationship with the hospital physicians. To break the ice, she gave a party and turned the hospital's sun room into a cabaret.

> I invited the doctors to come and asked them to be the waiters. I told them to wear tuxedos and I put towels over their arms and they had a wonderful time. We had prizes for the best dancer and so on. From then on the doctors started giving the party for the nurses. It was a small thing but it made a difference because nurses and doctors began to see each other as human beings, not as master and slave.

Another key to her success, she says, is the fact that physicians soon realized that she was teaching the students to do far more for the patients than they had been taught in the past.

Henderson left her post in Norfolk in 1929 and became a clinical instructor in the outpatient department of Strong Memorial Hospital and School of Nursing at the University of Rochester, located in Rochester, New York.

She obtained her bachelor's and later her master's degree in nursing at Teachers College, Columbia University, and then joined the faculty, working closely with her friend and mentor, Annie Goodrich. She stayed at Teacher's College from 1934 through 1948.

> I was teaching an advanced course in medical-surgical nursing. It was a required course. I think it made a difference because we let the patients teach us. We taught the course around three questions. Every student had to conduct a clinic and was chairman of an interdisciplinary conference at which the patient, the family, and the physician were present. We asked the patient, "What have we done that's helped you?," "What have we done that hasn't helped you?," and "What do you wish that we had done that we didn't do?" The course was highly effective.

Henderson also stressed the importance of research and documentation.

> My nickname was "Little Three-by-Five," which was given to me because I would always ask students on what they based their conclusions and they had to produce these library slips which would show that they read such-and-such a thing in such-and-such a place. They knew that they did not get by without documenting everything for me.

Henderson joined the faculty of Yale University School of Nursing as a research associate in 1953. She stayed at that post through 1971. It was at Yale that she produced the books for which she will be most remembered.

Books

Virginia Henderson is the author of six books and articles too numerous to count. Among her work is the basic text on nursing, which has been used in schools of nursing for the past 50 years. The text, *Principles and Practice of Nursing*, has been translated into Spanish and Japanese. At the other end of her work is a biography on her heroine, Annie Warburton Goodrich, which was incorporated into the Dictionary of American Biography.

When asked about her textbook and how it came into being, Henderson noted that she was asked to write a text but refused, saying she could not write a better one than the current standard written by Bertha Harmer. "Then Bertha died and I was out of excuses." Henderson reworked the text, which was published under both names in its fourth and fifth edition. "It wasn't until the sixth edition that I found the time to do a complete rewrite and the book became my own," she says.

Having authored what is generally accepted as the best text in the field, Virginia Henderson became the dominant person in the field of nursing. Her thoughts and ideas have influenced several generations of caregivers.

Another Henderson accomplishment is even more prodigious. Together with staff at the Yale School of Nursing, Henderson produced the Nursing Studies Index, a compilation of annotations of all the reported studies; research in progress; research methods; and historical materials in periodicals, books, and pamphlets relating to nursing published in the English language. It took Henderson some eleven years to complete this project. The index is maintained and provides students with an invaluable tool to assist them with research on nursing topics. The index is also integrated with the catalogue of the National Library of Medicine and the Library of Congress. Henderson comments:

> The work was an outgrowth of my "Little Three-by-Five" nickname. I realized that our students did not know how to use the library and that the literature in the field of nursing was not indexed. I decided that such an index, a comprehensive guide to nursing literature, had to be created. I began pressuring for it so much that people got tired of me talking about it. One person even said that I ought to be renamed Virginia "Index" Henderson.

She began working with Leo Simmons of Yale, who obtained a small grant to fund the project. "I had a very fortunate experience because I did the field work. This meant that I traveled to most of the states asking people what research they had done or what research they would do if they had the money."

Creation of the index is, for Henderson, one of her proudest achievements. "Most people do not really know what was involved. It just took so much courage to keep the project from folding time after time when our money ran out and we had to find another grant. It also led to the creation of our ongoing International Nursing Index, which even now nurses do not appreciate."

Henderson wrote several other books as well, including *ICN Basic Principles of Nursing Care*, which was translated into 25 languages; *Nursing Research, A Survey and Assessment* (with Leo W. Simmons); *The Yearbook of Modern Nursing* (with Simmons); *Nursing Resources for the Information Age*; and *The Nature of Nursing*, which has been translated into Japanese and Hebrew.

The Nature of Nursing

In 1966, Henderson published a highly regarded book, *The Nature of Nursing*, which is really the story of her professional journey. She describes it as a personal memoir or a testament. "The journey which this book describes was very agreeable and fortunate for me. . . . But we are all travellers in what John Bunyan called the wilderness of the world and the best that we find in our travels is an honored friend. . . . We travel, indeed to find them. . . . Every book is, in an intimate sense, a circular letter to the friends of the author." In this book, Henderson makes many important points, among them are the following.

Henderson believes the proper definition of nursing practice is an unfinished and a dynamic process. She quotes Florence Nightingale, who said that the purpose of nursing is to "put the patient in the best condition for nature to act upon him."

She quotes Effie J. Taylor, who said, "The real depths of nursing can only be understood through ideals, love, sympathy, knowledge, and culture expressed through the practice of artistic procedures and relationships." She quotes with approval the 1962 definition fashioned by the American Nurses Association, which said that nursing "means the performance for compensation of any act in the observation, care, and counsel of the ill, injured, or infirm or the maintenance of health or prevention of illness."

She said there is some validity to the view of psychologists that a nurse is a mother substitute. In Henderson's view, the nurse is empowered to observe, care for, and counsel a patient and to supervise other health care personnel. The nurse, however, should refrain from diagnosing, prescribing, and correcting, since these skills are within the physician's domain. She notes that the quality of American medical care will never reach its zenith until physicians and nurses sort out their relative responsibility and begin working more closely together.

She adds a few general principles which should apply. First, a nurse must be a constructive force in society. Second, nursing care must be patient centered. Third, this care must be individualized. Fourth, nursing care at its best is an expression of love. Fifth, nursing care should be provided to individuals in their own homes as much as possible.

Given the chance, Henderson reiterates that her most rewarding work experience came as a visiting nurse. While in school, she learned that hospital care all too often means that a patient loses his or her privacy, freedom of movement, the choice of what to eat and what time to get up in the morning, and other prerogatives that are the very essence of human dignity. On a related point, Henderson notes that after following patients home from the hospital she learned that the institutional regimen often failed to change the patient's lifestyle, which was often what sent him or her to the hospital in the first place.

Henderson offers the following quotation from the text she wrote with Bertha Harmer, which best crystallizes her own ideas about the nature of nursing:

> The unique function of a nurse is to assist the individual, sick or well, in the performance of those activities contributing to health or its recovery (or the peaceful death) that he would perform unaided if he had the necessary strength, will, or knowledge. And to do this in such a way as to help him gain independence as rapidly as possible.

Henderson also emphasizes the importance of a nurse helping a person to face death with dignity and "even bring to it an awesome beauty." She adds that in American society we shrink from old age; we are afraid of death. "In this country when an aged person loses his independence, we are likely to tuck him away in a nursing home. It is a poor name for it as it has few of the characteristics of a home and there is little nursing there. Such custodial care as the average nursing home offers is a national disgrace."

She emphasizes the importance of nursing research; it is the obligation of all who practice. She believes the essence of good nursing education includes both tutorial and practical firsthand experience. In her view, there is no substitute for witnessing firsthand the provision of high-quality care.

She quotes L.M. Avery, an Australian nurse, who said, "To me nursing is like a seed planted in very arid soil, which by nourishment, constant love, and care and attention, grew into a sturdy tree with promise of future growth. We have been content to sit in the shade of its branches, forgetting that it is still a young tree requiring constant supervision in nourishment."

Henderson has spent more than fifty years of her working life helping to nourish the tree of nursing, with exceptional results.

Learned

When asked to explain her youthful appearance and vitality, Henderson says, "I attribute whatever vitality I have to the intense interest I have for health care and the work that I continue to do in it."

When asked what she would do if she were appointed by the president as Secretary of the Department of Health and Human Services, she says:

> I would get the best people I could find to work with me, and I would make enactment of a national health system my top priority. There are those who suggest that if you are for publicly funded health care that you are communist or at least a socialist. I say to them, "Did you go to the public school?" And they say, "Of course I did." I say, "Well, you're a socialist. You know, you got your education at the expense of the public." I don't see any difference myself.

When asked what is wrong with our current health care system, she says:

> I think the fee-for-service system corrupts the caregiver. I think it is sickening that *The Economist* of London can publish a study three years ago that showed that of the five countries (USA, West Germany, France, England, and Japan), the range that is spent for health care was from 12% of the U.S. gross national product to 5% spent by the Japanese. And they have got better statistics than we have by a long shot. In fact, the health statistics get worse as more money is spent. In my judgment, we are spending it wrong.

Asked how the money should be spent, Henderson says she believes that much greater emphasis should be placed on prevention, that there is an overemphasis on drugs, and that far too much money is spent on surgical procedures and other extraordinary measures performed at the end of life. "Under our fee-for-service system, the big fees go to health workers who have saved the lives of the critically ill. They don't go to those who care for children. They don't go for the promotion of health care for children or old people." Henderson says that ironically Cuba has a far better health system in some respects than does the United States. "I was told by a nurse who has been with the World Health Organization for more than 10 years that she thought the best health care system that she had ever seen was in Cuba."

When asked whether she would advise her niece to go into nursing or medicine, she responded:

> I don't give advice, but I would say to anybody who would ask me that I think the kind of satisfaction in nursing is a complete kind of satisfaction because you have the person's entire welfare in your hands; if you do it right you are in the position to do the most you can for that person. I feel sorry for doctors. If you read the statistics, they spend less than 10 minutes with a patient, and about all the poor devils can do is to order a drug. So they've got their whole world drugged—this whole world that we live in is drugged to death, and we are beginning to learn that it's no accident that all of our young people are taking dope. All the old people are taking dope, and it's prescribed for them by the doctor.

When asked why we undervalue nurses in America, she said:

> If you go back to the Sarah Gant time in history, you will see that they were uneducated people and probably didn't help people very much. It has taken us a long time to outgrow the impression that the public had. But there are other factors. Certainly one of them is that

> we undervalue women as workers, and nurses have largely been women. I also think we tend to value headwork more than handwork, and we see nursing as handwork rather than for what it is, a combination of your hand and your head and your personality, whatever goes into it. I think we have got to value the emotional, psychological, and philosophical aspects of health care much more than we do.

When asked about leadership, she quoted Goodrich, who said, "It shouldn't be the person that leads, it ought to be the idea."

> We have to understand that working with your hands, being a master of something you do, is a beautiful thing. I value the person who paints the picture much more than the art teacher. I get so irritated with my friends from the upper class who introduce me to a friend and I say, "I am a nurse." And my upper-class friend plunges in right away and says, "She is not really a nurse; she writes and she teaches." It just makes me so angry I can hardly stand it because the hero and heroine in nursing is the person who sticks with the ill patient day after day and never loses his or her desire to help that person.

Henderson says she worries about professionals in the health care field who are in it for the money.

> I do not believe that people should be working with their eye on the money they are going to earn from it. I feel sorry for them. I was impressed with the writing of Trevor Clay, who says that nursing at its best is an expression of love. I think America is in crisis because we are becoming so materialistic. It is sickening to me, but I think it is beginning to change.

She acknowledges that she is a crusader, fighting for the rights of the underprivileged.

> I am prejudiced in favor of the underprivileged. I am underprivileged myself. I have never had any money; I've never had any power, but I've had a fairly decent time and have led a very interesting life. I am a fighter, but I hope not a mean one. I am persistent in my beliefs and struggling to defend them.

When asked her views on the graying of America, she says:

> My reflection is that we have got to stop putting the elderly in institutions. We've got to visit these people at home. I think we've got to learn to make greater use of older people instead of making them feel useless. And I think there are plenty of things they can do that would be an asset to this country.

When asked what advice she would have for young people in future generations, she says:

> Be interested in what you are doing. Be so interested in what's happening that you haven't any time to feel sorry for yourself. I could have grown up feeling awfully sorry for myself because I feel sorry for everybody. I'm like my cousin, who once said to my sister, "Tell you the truth, I feel sorry for anybody if I think about them." And my sister Jane said, "I don't feel sorry for you." To which my cousin responded, "Well think about me!"
>
> I'm naturally a very compassionate person and I suffer a lot when I see people in trouble. I think I would suffer myself if I had the time to think about myself.

Honorary Degrees and Awards

Virginia Henderson has received honorary degrees from the University of Western Ontario, the University of Rochester, Rush University, Pace University, Catholic University, Old Dominion University, Boston College, Thomas Jefferson University, Emory University, St. Joseph's College, and Yale University.

She has been awarded honorary membership in the Royal College of Nursing in London, the Sigma Theta Tau Society of the Vanderbilt School of Nursing, the University of Barcelona in Spain, the Japanese Nursing Association, and the Registered Nurse Association of Ontario, Canada.

Among her many awards are a Citation for Achievement in Nursing Practice from Teacher's College of Columbia University; a distinguished service award from the American Nurses Association; the Presidential Bicentennial Award from the Boston College School of Nursing; the Mary Adelaide Nutting Award from the National League for Nursing; the Annie W. Goodrich Award from the Yale University School of Nursing; and a meritorious service award from the National Association of Nurses, Colombia, South America. She was also given an award from the University of Buffalo, School of Nursing, for promotion of research in nursing practices, and the Christine Reimann Prize presented by the International Council of Nurses. In October of 1985, Henderson was presented with the Excellence in Education

Award from the National Association for Home Care. The award was subsequently named the Virginia Henderson Award.

Remembered

"I think that I am normal, to the extent of wanting people to care about me," said Henderson in response to the question of how she would like to be remembered. "I'd like to feel that people believe that whereas I might be misguided, I was well intentioned."

> I would like to be thought of as a humanitarian, as someone who did not exclude other human beings from their sympathies. One of the young people I admire most is a man who works as a nurse with the criminally insane. I feel kinship with him because he is able to get the sympathy of those patients. I asked him what accounts for his ability and he said, "I don't know. I suppose it is because I like them. No, I love them."
>
> And I thought, "You are for me." And then he said something that pleased me; he said, "They're very much like you and me." I expect that we are all close kin to the criminally insane.

When asked about her plans for the future, Henderson answered by quoting Montaigne, who, she described as a great philosopher and writer:

> His advice to old people is "not to think about death but just concentrate on getting your cabbages hoed." And that is what I hope I can do. I don't dread death at all. I dread dying, especially in an institution, and yet I don't want anybody else to have to devote their life to taking care of me, because I don't think it is right. There are too many caretakers who are struggling to care for a loved one at the present time with no respite at all.
>
> I think some of the best things that we have done in health care in this nation is the work that we do in our hospices. I think what they are doing is quite beautiful. I hope I am lucky enough to get that kind of care. As a matter of fact, I have been invited by a young man named Steve Wright, who is from England and who does beautiful work in this area with the aged. He says that whenever I want I should get on a boat and come over there and he will see me through. Until then, I hope I can keep on hoeing my cabbages.

There appears to be little doubt that Virginia Henderson will be remembered for her contribution not only to nursing but to humanity in general. By her example, she has taught millions of caregivers that true meaning of caring. The nation's elderly in particular have been beneficiaries of her pioneering work in geriatric nursing, as well as her contribution to the fields of hospice and home care. Through her writing and research she has left a legacy to benefit generations yet unborn. Like those heroic individuals she most admires, she has made the very best possible use out of her head, her hands, and her heart.

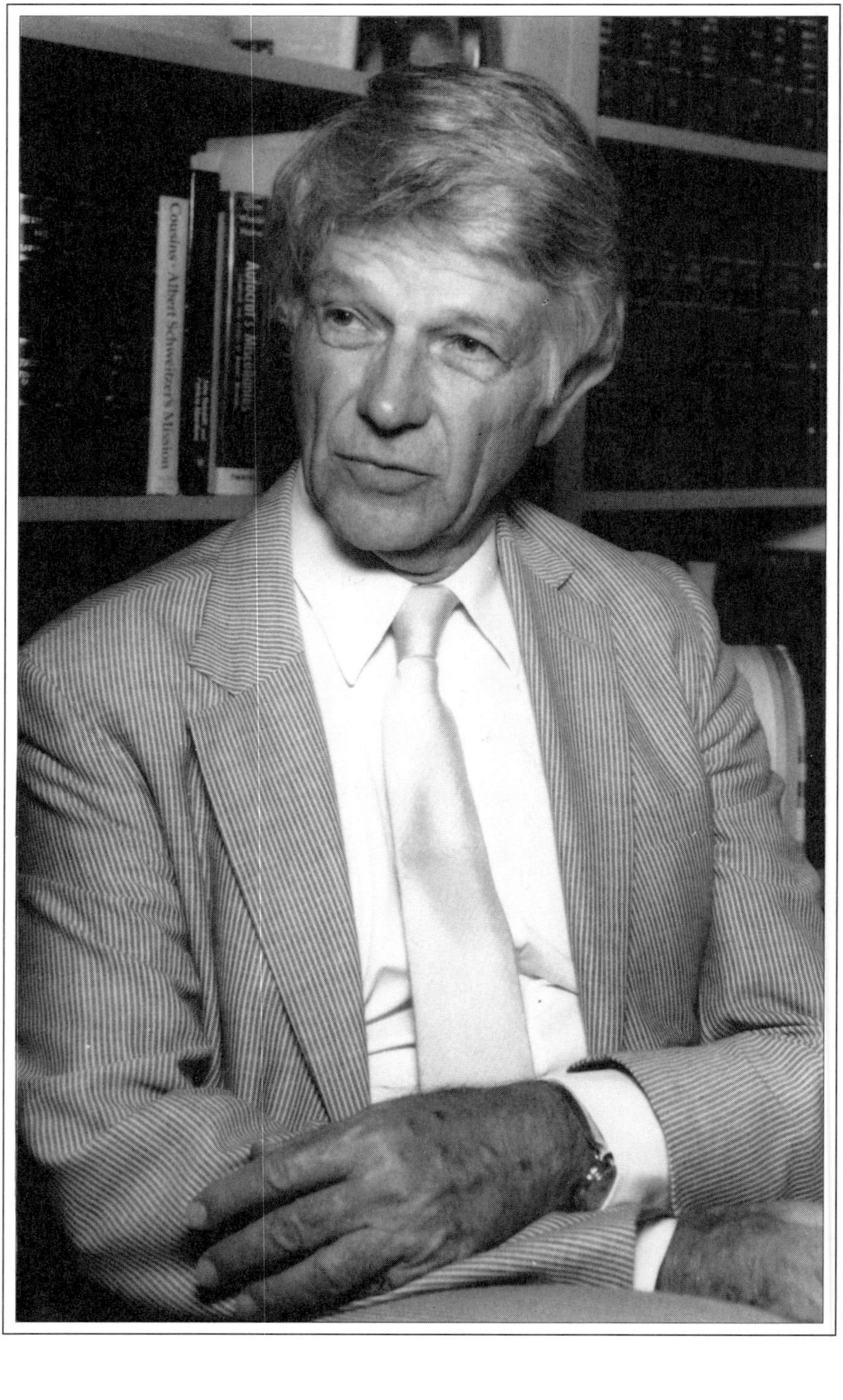

MARILU HALAMANDARIS

SEVEN

Robert N. Butler

James Michener once wrote that the care of the aged looms as the major problem facing America for the balance of the 20th century. There is no doubt that Michener was right; nor is there much doubt that Michener probably learned this truth by reading something written by Dr. Robert N. Butler. For years Butler's was a voice in the wilderness trying to alert the nation to the "graying of America." No one paid attention, of course, but he continued to shout his message. In the past few years, people have begun to listen when he talks about "an aging explosion" and when he predicts that the number of "elder people" is expected to increase 40 percent by the year 2010, at which time some 20 percent of the American public will be age 65 or over. A movement known as "Senior Power" has developed and is gathering steam. As their numbers increase, there is increasing concern about Social Security, adequate housing, health care, and other issues of importance to seniors—the fastest growing segment of the American population.

Butler is to the current revolution in geriatrics and aging what Thomas Payne was to the American Revolution. He has been the conscience of the public, crying out against the injustices perpetrated against those who are old. He helped popularize the term "ageism" to describe this most pernicious form of discrimination, which at one time or another will catch all Americans in its net. He has been researcher and scientist, looking for solutions to both medical and social problems with a tenacity that Sherlock Holmes would envy. He has been one of America's great healers. He has worked his magic not only on individuals, but on institutions and the body and soul of society as well. He is both a trail blazer and catalyst in awakening the American medical establishment to the special needs of the elderly.

Robert Butler is an authentic American hero. The fact that he has been propelled forward into public prominence at just this time proves the correctness of the belief that America has the uncanny ability to produce at just the right time the kind of person it needs to deal with its most pressing problems. Butler belongs in the company of great men such as Jonas Salk and James Watson; but in the end, his achievements will surpass them all. After many years of struggle and success, he has embarked on the greatest adventure of his life. Because of Butler, and the farsighted men and women of Mt. Sinai Hospital and Medical Center in New York City who believe in him, the life of future generations will be unalterably changed for the better. It may be that the next quantum leap in geriatric medicine will be developed at Mt. Sinai. If current preliminary findings are supported by clinical trials, scientists may find the key to Alzheimer's disease and thus extend the average life span to 85 or 90 by the end of this century.

When he visited the Soviet Union in 1978 to review Soviet research on aging-related diseases, Butler was treated like visiting royalty due to his staggering list of achievements. Recognition for what he has accomplished is increasing in the U.S., but still has far to go. Robert Butler has undoubtedly made a strong contribution and will do so for many years to come.

Early Years

Robert Butler was born in New York City in 1927. He never knew his father; he was raised by his grandfather, who passed away when he was seven. It has been said that Butler's concern with aging and medicine began at this time when all he knew was that his grandfather had disappeared. As he told one reporter, "There was no talk, no funeral—only a protective silence that was more confusing than the shared sorrow." Young Bob took an oath to become a doctor and help people live longer.

Butler spent his early years living in Vineland, New Jersey, with his stepfather, Fred Butler, who was a biochemist. He attended Vineland High, although following a move back to New York City, he graduated from Dewitt Clinton High School in 1944. He completed his undergraduate work at Columbia College, also in New York City, graduating in 1949, and moved on to Columbia University, where he graduated from medical school in 1953.

Butler completed his internship at St. Luke's Hospital in New York and performed his residency in 1954–55 at the University of California in San Francisco. Thereafter, he went to the National Institutes of Health, Chestnut Lodge, Rockville, Maryland, where he worked through 1963. During this time, he established an experimental unit on problems of the aged. In the years 1963–76, he was on the faculty of Howard University and George Washington University Schools of Medicine and served as an instructor at the Washington School of Psychiatry and the Washington Psychoanalytic Institute, all in Washington, D.C. He also had a lively private practice.

Butler's involvement with aging spans more than a quarter of a century. He remains today one of the most knowledgeable people in the country on this subject. In the early years of its history, Butler appeared before the Senate Committee on Aging with a regularity that was almost embarrassing. This was due to the fact that he was so far ahead of his time; he always had thoughts, papers, books, and reports to share with the interested solons.

In 1969 and 1970, Butler turned his energies toward helping the committee document abuses in nursing homes and enacting reform legislation. Butler outlined the essence of the problem—conclusions that were later documented by the committee; to wit:

1. that the U.S. has no policy with respect to treatment of the infirm elderly;
2. that the current system contains financial incentives that guarantee poor care;
3. that physicians have abdicated their responsibility for care of the aged;
4. that 90 percent of the care in nursing homes is given by aides who are largely untrained, and sometimes hired literally off the street;

5. that the system for enforcing nursing home regulations does not work.

At Butler's urging, the Committee on Aging sent a questionnaire to all the nation's medical schools in 1971 asking how many of them had a specialized program in geriatrics as part of their curriculum. No school said that it had established a Department of Geriatrics in its medical school, nor had anyone established this as a specialty. Only six of the 104 schools in existence at that time indicated they had electives that allowed credit to medical students who agreed to work with the aged in nursing homes.

The committee probed the reasons why physicians neglected the aged nursing home patients. It learned that Medicare and Medicaid regulations discourage physician visits; that physicians claimed they were too depressed by such visits; that they were deterred by the absence of trained nursing and supportive personnel; that they preferred to spend their time tending to the younger members of society because they felt that there was little they could do for the elderly. As still another excuse, the physicians said the kind of feedback that comes from seeing clients improve does not exist in nursing homes in the context of the infirm aged. Butler helped the committee shatter these myths. He pointed out that dramatic recovery is possible with respect to even the most debilitated nursing home patients, sometimes by doing nothing more than taking them off all the drugs being administered. Butler helped document the high incidence of adverse reactions that take place in nursing homes as the result of poor management of various drugs. For example, the committee documented that patients taking the heart stimulant digitalis and a diuretic at the same time can suffer adverse reactions owing to the fact that diuretics cause a loss of potassium, which increases the toxic effect of digitalis on the heart, sometimes leading to heart irregularities, which can result in death.

In 1975, the committee turned to Butler during one of its most sensitive and explosive investigations. A group of nurses had come forward, charging horrific and widespread abuses in the 2,200-bed nursing home run by Allegheny County in Pennsylvania. After numerous "undercover" visits by Senate investigators who documented that things were very bad indeed, Butler was asked to accompany

Senate staff on a tour of the facility. Even though a massive cleanup operation had preceded the visit, it could not disguise the multiple problems. Butler testified on what he had seen before a spellbound committee. The highlight of the hearing, however, came when the Catholic chaplain who served the facility and who was having great difficulty taking care of his aged and ill mother in her home was asked about the quality of care in the facility. The priest said, "I would rather see my mother dead than in [this facility]."

The Pulitzer Prize

In 1963, Butler authored the first of many books on the subject of aging. This book, entitled *Human Aging*, was written along with Myrna Lewis, the highly intelligent woman he later married. They wrote another book in 1973 entitled, *Aging and Mental Health.* One of the most telling points of that book is the connection it draws between early forms of research on aging, and the negative attitudes that are particularly intense for the institutionalized elderly. He said:

> Until 1960, most of the medical psychological, psychiatric, and social work literature on the aged was based on experience with the sick and institutionalized, even though only five percent of the elderly were confined to institutions. A few research studies that have concentrated on the healthy aged give indications of positive potential for the entire age group.
>
> But, the general, almost phobic, dislike of aging remains the norm, with healthy old people being ignored and the chronically ill receiving half-geared custodial care. Only those elderly who happen to have exotic or "interesting" diseases or emotional problems or substantial resources ordinarily receive the research and treatment attentions of the medical and psychotherapeutic professions.

A few years later, Butler produced a book entitled *Sex after 60*, long before this subject hit the "Phil Donohue Show." In addition, Lewis and he published a flurry of scientific papers, each one more impressive than the last. One of the most impressive was "Age-ism: Another Form of Bigotry," which appeared in *The Gerontologist.* In a later writing, Butler probed the possible causes of ageism, saying:

> In the West, death is considered as outside of the self. To be a self (a person) one must be alive, in control, and aware of what is happening. The greater and more narcissistic Western emphasis on individuality and control makes death an outrage, a tremendous affront to man, rather than the logical and necessary process of old life for new. The Western predilection for "progress," conquest over nature and personal self-realization, has produced difficult problems for the elderly and for those preparing for old age. This is particularly so when the national spirit of the country and the spirit of this period in time have emphasized and expanded the notion of measuring human worth in terms of individual productivity and power. Old people are led to see themselves as beginning to fail as they age, a phrase that refers as much to self-worth as it does to physical strength.

In 1975, Harper and Row published another of Butler's works entitled, *Why Survive? Growing Old in America*. Butler summarized the book for reports in one line: "We have shaped a society which is extremely harsh to live in for the old." This stunning and insightful exposition of growing old in America won the Pulitzer Prize for non-fiction. Butler received notice that he had won the award on May 1, 1976, the same day he learned that he had been nominated to be the first director of the National Institute on Aging.

The National Institute on Aging

From his earlier tenure in the late 1950s when he had established an experimental unit on aging, Butler had felt there needed to be greater emphasis on problems of the aged at the National Institutes of Health (NIH). Others had latched on to the idea, including Senators Frank E. Moss and Thomas Eagleton. Legislation introduced by both senators and by Claude Pepper in the House to establish a separate National Institute on Aging (NIA) was enacted in 1974. The purpose of the Institute was to conduct biomedical and behavioral research on the aging process and diseases affecting the elderly. In fiscal year 1976, the first year of operation, the Institute had a budget of $19 million. In large part thanks to the careful management of Butler, Congress increased the budget to $84.5 million in fiscal year 1983. Butler noted that he was grateful for this increase in funds, but pointed out that this amount was only 2.5 percent of the *total funding* for NIH, which at that time was something like $3.4 billion a year. He added that, at the time, the elderly accounted for about 60 percent of all health spending.

As NIA director, Butler spearheaded a number of impressive programs and conferences that will pay ongoing dividends for years to come. For example, the National Conference on Mental Health and Aging, also supported by then-First Lady Rosalynn Carter, was widely heralded for sensitizing the public to the need to improve mental health services for older Americans. Several conference resolutions have been acted on, including one that called for expanding mental health benefits covered under Medicare.

Butler had a major role in planning the 1981 White House Conference on Aging, although his role was diminished following the 1980 election of Ronald Reagan. Still, the resolutions calling for greater emphasis on research and establishment of a national policy on long-term care bear his imprint.

In 1980, Butler teamed up with Congressman Claude Pepper in sponsoring the first of an ongoing series of International Conferences on Cancer and Aging. This conference brought together the best minds of the world, including numerous Nobel Prize winners, to share and discuss their research findings. Chairman Pepper termed it, "The Manhattan Project of Medicine."

The Institute can count numerous other successes. One of these came when Butler persuaded the National Cancer Institute to change a rule that had prohibited cancer research on individuals over age 65, even though 55 percent of all cancer occurs after that age. Another success came with Butler's trip to the Soviet Union, where he and other Americans obtained permission to work with physicians from the U.S.S.R. to study the long-lived people who inhabit Abkhazia, that small mountainous republic that lies between the Caucasus Mountains and the Black Sea. This research may help unlock the secret of why these people routinely live to remarkable old age.

Another major success of the Institute has been to help break the myth that senility is a normal part of the aging process. Butler told a reporter recently, "We've learned first that it is not a given, second that it's not arteriosclerosis, third that it's in fact predominantly due to a disease called Alzheimer's disease. And there are now some major leads for potential interventions in the next decade. We may soon be able to treat what is probably the number four or five cause of death among the aged."

Butler told Carol Krucoff of *The Washington Post* that, "Another good thing that is happening is the beginning of the development of geriatric medicine in the United States so that older persons can feel that their doctors and nurses will be taught in medical schools by people who have made their life's work out of understanding the particularities of aging and the disease and disabilities associated with it."

Butler pointed out that as of 1989, 50 of the nation's 127 medical schools have "something going on in geriatrics." Obviously, this is a far cry from what the Committee on Aging learned in its 1971 questionnaire. But the most exciting development in the field of aging has been the creation of a full-scale Department of Geriatrics at Mt. Sinai Hospital and Medical School and the fact that Robert Butler was named to head it.

Mount Sinai Department of Geriatrics and Human Development

Under the able direction of Alfred Stern, former chairman of the board, and Frederick Klingenstein, the current chairman, the Mt. Sinai Hospital and Medical School has made a commitment to become the major force for the study of problems of the aged in the United States. In 1984, that institution took the bold step of being the first medical school in the nation to establish a full-scale Department of Geriatrics within its medical school. Specifically, the new unit includes a diagnosis referral unit, a demonstration unit in clinical geriatrics, an aggressive research program, and an in-depth orientation of all medical students to geriatric practice in both inpatient and outpatient settings.

Butler planned the program to reach maturity in 1990. Based on past performance, it is likely that it will continue to attract top-flight scientists and physicians from all parts of the nation and the world.

Butler points out that one benefit of the department has been to force the hospital to avoid unnecessary institutional admissions. The plan allows for patients to move back home, where they prefer to be, as soon as possible. Moreover, the curriculum includes an ambitious program whereby physicians, students, and interns make house calls. Another major element in Butler's plan is the linkage with the Jewish Home and Hospital, a well-respected long-term care facility.

Butler believes that with the proper research he can document that the sociomedical needs of geriatric patients can be identified and assessed and met effectively and efficiently in the home or by community resources. He is betting that he can get the established disciplines to cooperate and incorporate greater attention to geriatrics in every aspect of the medical school curriculum. He is betting that significant new techniques in preventive medicine can be established that will help seniors avoid health problems. Moreover, he is betting that with the proper help there will be significant discoveries in medical research.

Officials at the institution have given Butler a broad grant of authority and the financial support he needs to assemble an incredible team of professionals to execute his plan, which is clearly unparalleled in American medicine. Still, demands are so great that he spends much of his time raising funds.

Butler was given the opportunity to serve on the curriculum committee. By the committee's agreement, the first two years of school now include 20 hours of instruction in the general aspects of aging. In addition, all medical students in their fourth year are required to complete a four-week clerkship in the school's clinical geriatric program, and geriatric medicine is offered as an elective for fourth year students. The basic goal of the medical school curriculum is to disseminate knowledge among the specialities concerning appropriate geriatric practice.

The school also offers a fellowship program leading toward a combined M.D./Ph.D. program to train physician/scientists for a career in academic gerontology.

The master plan contemplated the creation of a new hospital, the first in the nation to be designed specifically with the aged in mind.

The plan is for the hospital to include a geriatrics assessment and referral unit which will receive cases for diagnosis and consultation and conduct preadmission screening. A clinical demonstrations unit will be established at the hospital. It will handle referrals from other Mt. Sinai departments, mostly complicated and unusual cases.

As noted, medical students and residents receive part of their professional educations in several nursing homes, which also cooperate in research on such questions as how to prevent the misuse of medications and how to prevent bedsores. One nursing home agreed to provide a newly endowed geriatrics professorship in the department, with responsibilities both at the home and at Mt. Sinai.

The new geriatrics department also coordinates research and educational activities underway at other Mt. Sinai-related facilities, such as Beth Israel Hospice, Elmhurst Hospital, Hunter College Brookdale Center on Aging, the Hospital for Joint Disease, and the Bronx Veterans Administration Hospital.

The department plans to establish hospice services as part of its curriculum. A Geriatric Demonstrations Home Care Service will be established in which all medical students will be required to participate. A wellness clinic will also be established to do low-cost health screening. A mobile unit now enables physicians and nurses to visit shut-ins to provide them with medical care and advice on self-help and counseling. Also underway are in-service and pre-service training programs for nurses aides and a model curriculum in geriatric medicine.

Views

Due to his longstanding work in and commitment to the field of aging, Butler has a keen insight into the problems facing senior citizens today. He feels that some progress has been made "in that there is a greater awareness of the problems of the aged, and greater attention paid to the problem of long-term care." More progress is represented in the form of new regulations that have been put into effect with the hope of improving the quality of nursing home care. He points out that at least 10 of the current 127 medical schools now offer significant training programs in geriatrics. "Finally," he says, "there has been a virtual end to mandatory retirement in our society, thanks to Claude Pepper."

Butler, however, thinks that we still have a long way to go in improving the quality of life for America's aged, saying retirement income is inadequate:

> Some one-third of our elderly now live at or near the poverty level, and this is just unacceptable. Widows are especially hard hit. In fact, they are one of the twin shames of our society: Impoverished widows and impoverished children. About 20 percent of our widows and children live in poverty.

He also mentioned housing problems:

> Some 30 percent of our seniors still live in substandard housing. Then there is the misconception based on the misuse of statistics that 70 percent of the elderly own their own homes. This ignores the fact that many of these homes are old and badly in need of repairs, which the seniors either cannot make themselves or cannot afford. This means there is little market for the family home if they were to try to sell it, and finding adequate replacement or rental housing can be a major problem. Escalating real estate taxes and high rents continue to plague the elderly, forcing them to choose between a roof over their heads and such essentials as food and medicine.

Butler also feels that, in some instances, America has regressed with respect to the health problems of seniors:

> We have clearly lost ground with respect to the health care needs of the elderly. People pay more out-of-pocket proportionately than they did before Medicare was enacted. The problem is that Medicare was designed as if old people were young people. We need a massive transfusion. We need a Part C of Medicare to cover long-term care, particularly noninstitutional home care, day care, and nursing home care. And I frankly think we can do this without adding massive new expenditures to the federal budget.

When asked if some future president were to appoint him the Secretary of the Department of Health and Human Services, Butler said that his first task would be to broaden the health agenda.

> Our health agenda must be broadened. We must broaden our research beyond AIDS and currently recognizable diseases. Actually, AIDS taught us a valuable lesson, which is that we must invest

> the necessary funds to isolate and understand new viruses in the continuing struggle between microorganisms and human beings. On a related point, we need better integration between the National Institutes of Health and the rest of the health establishment. Second, we must do something about the growing problem of long-term care. Third, we need to tackle the environment. We can't just warn people to be careful about their health habits. We have some responsibility to stop the pollution of our air and water, and this can't be done without developing a conceptional framework that is broader than any one government department.

Butler is an advocate of home care as the best solution to meeting the long-term care needs of the nation. "The data suggests that home care can save health dollars," he asserts. "Home care should be brought to the chronically ill recuperating from hospitalization, to those who may be acutely ill but can be treated outside the hospital and to those who need help from time to time to fill the gaps left by declining functions and the loss of friends and relatives."

As Chairman of the Commission on Elderly People Living Alone, of the Commonwealth Fund, Butler released a report in 1989 that proposed broadening the scope of Medicare to provide a long-term care home care benefit to assist the 1.6 million elderly living alone and suffering from serious disabilities. He talked about the proposal:

> It really is a rather modest proposal. We sought to provide help for a group about which there can be no debate. They are severely impaired. They need help, there is no doubt about it. This group has enormous impairments and they in turn create enormous burdens, particularly to the women of our society. Our proposal would authorize day care and home care services under Medicare for this most vulnerable population.

To Butler, research is of preeminent importance to the health of America.

> Research is the ultimate service because you can prevent people from having a particular disease. It is also the ultimate in cost containment in that you do not have to spend money for treatment. In the past few years we have discovered that there is no such thing as senility. Mental deterioration is not an inevitable part of growing older. What we used to call senility is in fact a host of diseases, many of them treatable. We have learned, for example, that Alzheimer's

disease is a consequence of multiple deficiencies in the neurochemicals found in the brain.

He feels that through research we can hopefully reduce the need for nursing homes. He commented that "nursing homes are the iron lung of geriatrics." When asked to explain this, he said:

> I was trying to demonstrate to Congress the value of research. I offered the example of the polio epidemics of the past. Polio was a terrible virus for which we found a cure when the children of the nation led the way through the March of Dimes. I said that nursing homes were the iron lung of geriatrics in the sense that it is a halfway technology. Nursing homes at present are needed and we cannot just dismiss them. On the other hand, if we can recognize that Alzheimer's disease is the polio of geriatrics, and if we can find the cure for it, we will reduce the need for nursing homes.

Butler feels that while progress has been made, more needs to be done to insure that doctors of the future are trained in the special needs of seniors:

> We have made some progress but not enough. While 10 of the 127 medical schools have a program in geriatrics, only one has a full-scale department of geriatrics within its medical school. At the same time, there is not enough being done to sensitize students to the problems of death and dying. Ageism still takes root in our medical schools. Students are all too likely to continue referring to the elderly in disparaging terms such as "crocks," "old biddies," and "gomers." There has been some improvement in overall attitudes because of people like Claude Pepper, George Burns, and Arthur Flemming, who prove that it is possible to be fantastically productive for our entire lifetime.

Butler is quick to point out and reemphasize that many of the problems of the elderly are social in nature. In fact, negative mental attitudes, a feeling of hopelessness and uselessness, he says, often leads to the manifestation of physical symptoms. In this connection, he says many of the problems of the elderly stem from the fact that they feel lonely and unloved:

> We really do not have a philosophy of growing old. We do not have canons that offer guidance on how we should conduct ourselves. As a result, many older people feel lonely and abandoned. The answer must be found through love and developing effective com-

> municative relationships between people. We must find ways to build more caring and love into our society and its institutions. Our leaders must show imagination in calling for this kind of spirit, and I do not think that we can excuse our leaders for any failure they may have in addressing this important issue.

When asked for other root causes of the problems facing America's seniors, he pointed to the discrimination against women that exists in contemporary American society:

> In many ways the problem of age in our society is the problem of women. Women make up about 75 percent of those who reside in nursing homes. It is the women of our society who generally live the longest, suffer from multiple disabilities, and become dependent on others for help. At the same time, the burden of caring for an older relative generally falls on younger women, who often must leave their jobs in order to care for parents or in-laws. Women's organizations need to be more attentive to the rights of older women. Aging must be put on the political agenda now and in the future.

Butler feels that America should strive to be a fully integrated society—one in which races, cultures, and ages live together and learn from each other. "We have the chance to be the world's first successful multiracial, multicultural, age-integrated society. Why should we fritter this away by having age-segregated housing? At the same time, I favor free choice, but I feel we are better off with age integration."

Through years of research, Butler has ratified his early beliefs that seniors can play a vital role in society if they are allowed to do so. He is heartened that mandatory retirement has been eliminated in law, if not in fact, and he sees greater appreciation for the talents of older workers in the coming years, particularly as the shortage of employees becomes more acute. He also believes there is a natural alliance between the young and the old in society:

> Older persons have a lot they can contribute. But more than that, corporate leaders are discovering that retirement benefits can be a heavy load to carry. They are finding that providing older persons with meaningful work pays dividends to both the individual and the corporation. . . . I believe that older persons are uniquely suited to playing roles as teachers, counselors, conserving our heritage and natural resources. In other societies it has been proven that they do well in judicial and administrative roles. I also think that there is a

> great affinity between the old and the young, and as much as possible we should have older persons work with and encourage our young people.

When asked for the secret to effective aging and whether he favors the "engagement" or the "disengagement" theory of aging, he said that the secret lies in service to others:

> I believe that seniors should be activists; one has to keep on growing, working, and learning right to the end of life. In our studies at NIH we learned that those people who had goals in their lives, some purpose and structure to their everyday life, were the ones who lived the longest. The lesson from these scientific studies is clear: one must have a goal, and continue to work towards it. It is all the better if the goal is something beyond one's self and has social good associated with it.

Remembered

When asked how he would like to be remembered, Butler had this to say:

> As someone who tried to improve the quality of life not only for older people but for all people, because there is after all a continuity in life—today's older people were once kids and today's children will one day be old.

Carl Sandburg wrote that nothing happens but first a dream. It is evident that Dr. Robert Butler has come a long way since he took an oath as a seven-year-old to help people live longer and with more meaning in their lives. Butler has already seen many of his dreams come true. To the extent that the elderly of America and across the world have seen progress, he has been a major part of it. To the extent that they will have the benefit of scientific and social policy breakthroughs in the future, this too, will be because he has acted on his dreams and has inspired others to share them. Fortunately for everyone, Dr. Robert Butler is still a youngster; he will not reach his 65th birthday until 1992. Even then, age should not be a barrier to his achievements. Like those he admires most, he promises to remain "fantastically productive" for his entire lifetime.

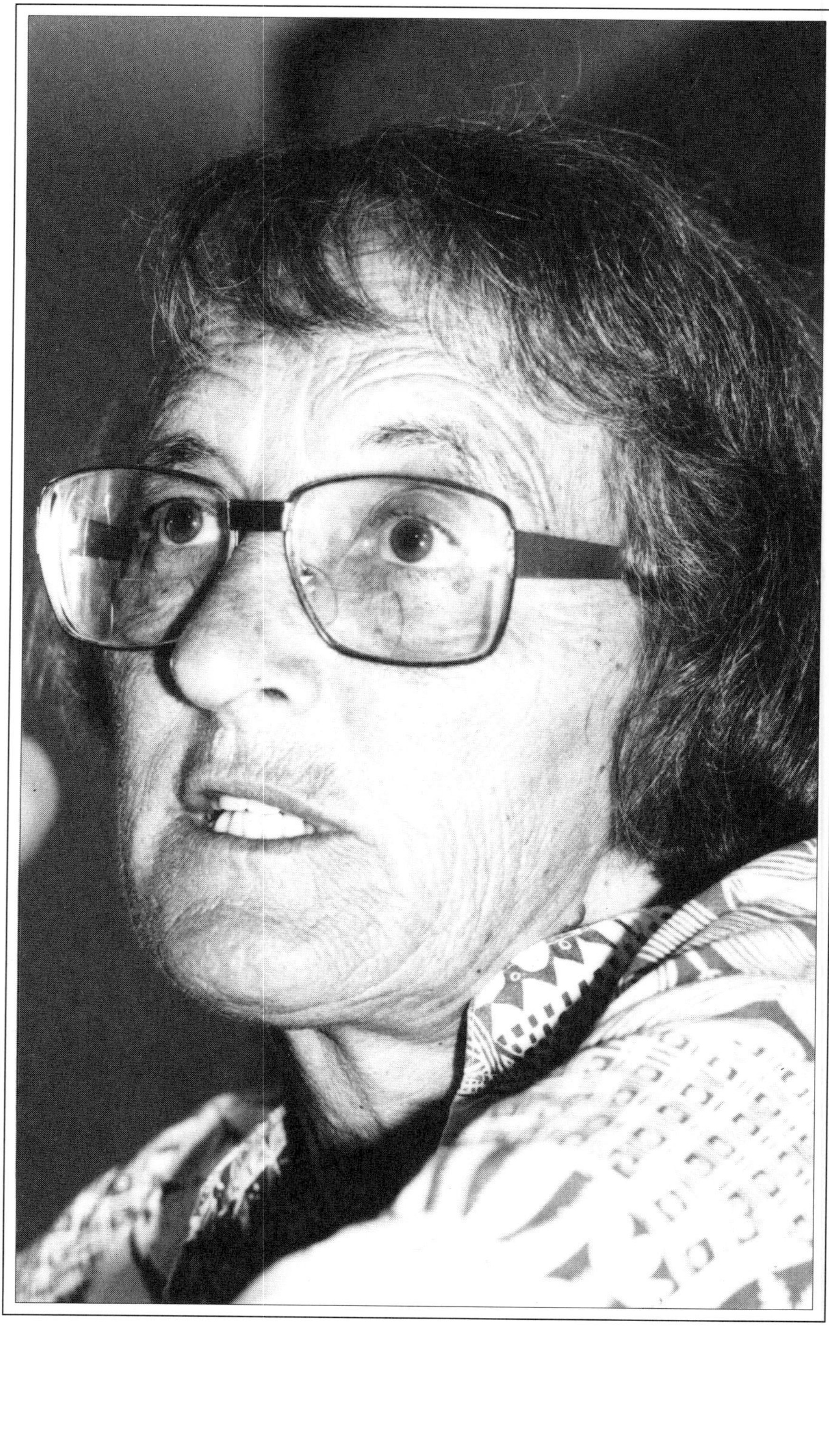
MARILU HALAMANDARIS

EIGHT

Elisabeth Kübler-Ross

Dr. Elisabeth Kübler-Ross is one of the towering figures of the 20th century. She is a pioneer who, more than a quarter of a century ago, dared lift the social taboo and open the door to discussion of issues related to death and dying. She authored the classic book, *On Death and Dying*, and identified the five stages (denial, anger, bargaining, depression, and acceptance) that mark the transition through the final days of life. She has been a prime mover in the field of hospice and home care, helping millions of people to see death as the final stages of growth and encouraging them "to live to the end of their days."

She is something of an anomaly: she is a physician who makes house calls and who does not charge for her services; her primary surgical instrument is the power of love. She is a modern-day Gandhi whose long-range goal is to bring about human maturity. All ages have benefited from her contributions, not only the aged, sick, and dying. "What do dying people teach us? They teach us how to live. Death is the key to life," she once said.

She has authored some 14 books in an effort to get her message of unconditional love across to the public. She sees herself as "catalyst and translator," helping people to rid themselves of their fears and guilt so that they can live fully and not be afraid of either living or dying. She has tried to help people understand what it means "to love thy neighbor as thyself" and that "death as an end to things does not exist."

While her goal is to change society, to do away with the evils of war and racism and injustice, she is a strong proponent of individual responsibility. Societal changes, she believes, will be brought about only as a by-product of changes in the lives of individuals who free themselves of their own negativity and devote themselves in unconditional love to others.

Few people have done more for the nation's senior citizens than she. She challenged western notions that success is defined in terms of acquisition of material possessions and that casts death as the ultimate defeat. Rather, she believes that people should be valued by what they do for others and that the opportunities for caring only multiply with advancing age. Death, she believes, far from being a defeat, or consequence of either original or individual sin, is like birth—a natural part of life.

"Both birth and death involve great changes and adjustment, often inconveniences and pain but also joy, reunion, and a new beginning," she wrote. "If it were not for our inner knowledge that we are on this earth plane for a relatively short period of time, then why should we strive for perfection, for love and peace, if it were not for the desire to leave this place a little bit better, a little bit more human than when we entered it?"

Through her prodigious work, Kübler-Ross has made an invaluable contribution to improving the quality of life for its most vulnerable members, and in the process, she has helped liberate future generations from self-imposed fears and burdens based on the notion that death is somehow punitive, unnatural, and inhuman. Kübler-Ross is one of the world's great humanitarians, a practitioner of preventive psychiatry, and a healer of the human heart.

Background

Elisabeth Kübler-Ross was born on July 8, 1926, in Zurich, Switzerland. She was the first of triplets and weighed barely two pounds at birth. This precarious introduction to life may have had something to do with her eventual work with the dying. "I was not expected to live and if it had not been for the determination of my mother, I might have not survived," said Kübler-Ross. She adds that her mother believed firmly that the life of a weak infant depended on its closeness to the parent in a home environment and not in a hospital.

At the age of five, Elisabeth became critically ill with pneumonia. It was another experience that would have a great effect on her. She was taken to a children's hospital and kept in isolation for weeks, able to see her parents only through a window. She has described this room as "a cage," saying, "There was no familiar voice, touch, odor, not even a familiar toy. . . . If it had not been for my vivid dreams and fantasies, I am sure that I would not have survived the sterile place."

During World War II, she helped out at Zurich's largest hospital, helping refugees who had fled Nazi Germany. At the end of the war, she hitchhiked through the war-torn countries of Europe. She worked for a time in a small clinic and helped open first aid stations and even traveled with a gypsy caravan. She worked as a cook, mason, and roofer and visited one of the concentration camps. At this point, she made her decision to take up medicine. "It was there in the midst of suffering that I found my goal."

The visit to the concentration camp at Majdanek changed her life forever.

> It was a place where 960,000 children were killed. I saw train-loads of baby shoes of the murdered innocent children and carloads of women's hair taken from the victims, to be sent back to Germany to make cloth. At this camp, I met a young Jewish girl whose grand-parents, parents, brothers, and sisters had all died in the gas chamber. She was saved only because there was no room in the gas chamber to squeeze in another person. She said that she was determined to survive in order to tell the world of the atrocities committed in Hitler's Germany. Yet, she said when the liberating armies arrived, she realized that if she had done what she intended that she would have been no better than Hitler himself—because she, too, would be spreading hate and negativity. This young girl touched my life more than anyone ever has by teaching me that there's a "Hitler" in every human being.

The experience of caring for others helped Kübler-Ross temper her soul. She remembers that her parents taught her good values and that she lived in an affluent home. However, her parents did not give her much affection. Being a triplet, she also felt as if she had no real identity. The visit to Majdanek changed all of this. She enrolled in medical school in order that she might provide even more help to those who were suffering and in need. Even at this young age, Kübler-Ross was an advocate of doing good work and not just talking about it. She reports, for example, being disillusioned with religion because of the contrast that she saw between the preachers' incredible oratory in the pulpit and their lifestyles. She found ministers to be judgmental and critical instead of caring and loving; therefore, she rejected formal religion for a time and looked elsewhere for heroes.

She received her medical degree from the University of Zurich in 1957. A year later, she married a fellow medical student, Emanual Robert Ross, a neuropathologist with a practice in Illinois. Elisabeth Kübler-Ross came to the United States in 1958 and took her internship at Community Hospital in Glen Cove, Long Island, New York. She also took psychiatric training at Manhattan State Hospital and Montefiore Hospital, both in New York City, and in 1962 at the Psychopathic Hospital at the University of Colorado in Denver. In Colorado, she became an assistant professor in psychiatry and psychophysiology and achieved some success in treating chronic schizophrenics. It is reported she used a technique that she later used with dying patients: asking patients what they thought would be most helpful to them.

The Book

In 1965, Kübler-Ross became an assistant professor of psychiatry at the University of Chicago Medical School. A group of theological seminary students came to her to ask for her help in a study of death. Kübler-Ross suggested a series of interviews with dying patients to see if they would talk about their feelings and thereby help instruct the professionals. The sessions were organized at Chicago University's Billings Hospital and involved doctors, nurses, and social workers in addition to theology students. She soon learned that dying patients were anxious to talk about their feelings and experiences. The result of this work was the internationally known best seller, *On Death and Dying*. In the book, Kübler-Ross wrote as follows:

> Surprisingly, perhaps, most dying patients are anxious to talk about death. They welcome a breakthrough of their defenses. They welcome a frank, unemotional, honest discussion and a sharing of their feelings. Other factors contributing to their willingness may include a break in the lonely monotony of waiting, a feeling of being useful or worthwhile for something, and for a few perhaps, a gratification of exhibitionist needs, to show "how strong" they are, or some may just be unable to say no to the chance to gratify some dependency needs.

The book is a collection of anecdotes taken from the more than 500 interviews with dying patients, augmented by some generalizations reached by comparing what was common to each. In the book, Kübler-Ross advanced the notion that patients have to go through five stages of denial before they can cope with their death. The first is the "No, not me" stage; then the "Why me?" stage; the bargaining "Yes me, but" stage; depression; and finally acceptance.

Kübler-Ross noted that those people who lose their eyesight or suffer other kinds of losses (whether physical or emotional) experience these same psychological stages to one degree or another.

On Death and Dying became a standard reference text on counseling the terminally ill. In her book, Kübler-Ross made the case for including a course in the art of counseling the dying in medical, nursing, and theology schools, as well as in schools of social work. It is an eloquent plea for home care as opposed to treatment in an institutional setting, and it makes the case for choice. She argues there comes a point when heroic measures only serve to prolong suffering and therefore should be withheld. She suggested that patients should have a voice in determining their own destiny.

Kübler-Ross commented:

> The fear of death is the most inescapable fear of human beings and the most unavoidable one. . . . Dying is still a distasteful but inevitable happening which is rarely spoken about. One might think that the scientific man of the twentieth century would have learned to deal with this uniform fear as successfully as he has been able to add years to his life span, or to replace human organs, or to produce children through artificial insemination. Yet, when we compare dying in less civilized and less sophisticated countries, we cannot

> help but see that we, in the so-called advanced civilization, die less easily. Advancement of science has not contributed to, but rather detracted from, man's ability to accept death with dignity.

The U.S. Senate Hearings

In 1972, the U.S. Senate Committee on Aging conducted the first national hearings on the subject of death with dignity. These hearings were without doubt one of the most important events in the death awareness and hospice movements. They generated a great deal of publicity both for Kübler-Ross and the causes she espoused.

In her testimony, Kübler-Ross said she preferred to talk about living with dignity—living until the end of life—instead of dying with dignity. She made the case that many dying patients are neglected. She said that when she came to the United States, she was surprised to see that 80 percent of all death took place in an institution rather than at home. This was true despite the fact that most people want very badly to die at home.

She said there are many reasons why this has happened. She cited changes in demographics, the disappearance of the three-generation family, and the enactment of Medicare and Medicaid, which provide financial incentives to institutionalize people. She said some people feel there is something morally wrong or sinful in keeping a person at home where the latest devices of science are not available to prolong life. She said that family members do not realize that with a little training they could help the terminally ill person care for her- himself and remain at home.

Kübler-Ross noted that she was surprised that children are not encouraged to visit nursing homes in the United States and concluded that they are sheltered from death, rather than educated that it is one of life's experiences. She said that research established that family members believe it is best not to tell a loved one he or she is going to die. She said the opposite is true. Only with this knowledge, she believes, can the dying person make the journey through the five stages she identified in her book.

Kübler-Ross said, "We live in a very peculiar death-denying society. We isolate both the dying and the old, and it serves a purpose. They are reminders of our own mortality."

Kübler-Ross said things used to be simpler in this country and abroad when death was part of life. She said that when she was a child, people were born at home and died at home. Dying patients were not institutionalized very often. While this did not always make dying easier for the patient, it helped the children and grandchildren learn that dying is a part of life.

She said that dying patients need essentially two things. The first is hope; but hope is not always associated with cure, the treatment for prolongation of life. Hope may be expressed in terms of a third party. A dying mother may hope that her children grow to fulfill their destiny and lead a happy life, for example. The second need is for reassurance that they will not be deserted. "And yet most of our patients who are beyond medical help feel deserted."

Kübler-Ross had several recommendations. She said that more emphasis should be placed on teaching children and others that death is part of life. Second, she said, "We should not institutionalize people. We can give families more help with home care, visiting nurses, giving the families and the patients the spiritual, emotional, and financial help in order to facilitate the final care at home." She said, "We need more physicians who make house calls." Nursing homes, she said, should also incorporate a day care center for children. Greater emphasis should be placed on thanatology in schools of medicine, nursing, and social work. She said that nurses who work with the terminally ill should not be required to work more than four-hour shifts because the work is extremely exhausting. To do otherwise requires the depersonalization of the patient.

Under questioning from Senators Frank Church and Frank E. Moss, she reemphasized the importance of shifting dollars from hospitals and nursing homes into home care and hospice. She specifically rejected the notion that a new kind of facility be erected for the terminally ill.

"I would be very leery if the care of the dying patient would become institutionalized. I would be opposed if we have modern death houses which are just institutions for the dying." She mentioned the positive example of St. Christopher's Hospice in England, but said, "We really cannot duplicate it in the United States." The primary reason, she said, was the British national health system which supports clients and which "does not cost the patient a penny." Rather than new facilities for the dying, she said that we need to train doctors, nurses, and social workers who love to work with the old and dying patient. "Then you will not need special institutions for the care of the dying patient and the majority would be allowed, at least for final care, to be at home."

One of the results of these hearings was the first legislation to be introduced in the U.S. Congress by the above-named senators to provide federal funds to support hospice programs. Some 11 years later, in 1983, legislation was finally enacted in the form of an amendment to Medicare that provides hospice coverage for clients certified to be in the last six months of their lives. Medicaid hospice coverage was added as an optional benefit as late as 1988, and there are now 31 states which offer the benefit.

Shanti Nilaya and the Elisabeth Kübler-Ross Center

Kübler-Ross continued her research and her writing. Additional books included, *Questions and Answers on Death and Dying* (1974), followed by, *Death: The Final Stage of Growth* (1975), *To Live until We Say Good-bye* (1978), *The Dougy Letter* (1979), *Living with Death and Dying* (1981), *Working It Through* (1982), *Remember the Secret* (1982), *On Children and Death* (1983), and *AIDS: The Ultimate Challenge* (1987). Her fourth book, published in 1978, includes a description of a Shanti Nilaya, which means "Home of Peace" in Sanskrit. Kübler-Ross built a retreat or "healing center" on 42 acres overlooking a lake not far from San Diego, California. At this "home," Kübler-Ross conducted five-day live-in workshops on the subject of "Life, Death, and Transition." Fees to attend were modest; still, no one was turned away for lack of ability to pay.

This non-profit operation, which has assisted thousands of people, is subsidized in large part by the fees that Kübler-Ross earns from lectures. She travels more than 200,000 miles a year and is very much in demand as a public speaker. She remarked to one interviewer that this is a "lonely life." "People don't treat you like you are human. You virtually live in airports and motel rooms. You are adored and put on a pedestal, but you have dinner and breakfast alone."

There are many reasons why people are drawn to the Elisabeth Kübler-Ross Center. About one-third of each workshop's attendees are made up of people diagnosed as having a terminal illness. Family members who are having difficulty coping make up another sizable segment. The remainder is made up of those who are going through what Kübler-Ross calls "little deaths," such as the breakup of a marriage or disfiguring surgery. They come for catharsis, to purge themselves of the heavy emotional baggage that they have been carrying. Kübler-Ross calls the sessions "preventive psychiatry."

In early 1984, Kübler-Ross began work on the East Coast complement located on the Virginia-West Virginia border. The Elisabeth Kübler-Ross Center was established as a children's resource center to enable disadvantaged children to share the feeling of unconditional love, thus giving them an understanding of what it means to have "a loving and positive attitude to all that life has to offer." On July 8, 1990, Kübler-Ross closed the San Diego center and held a dedication ceremony at the new center in Virginia.

In her 1987 book on the subject of AIDS, Dr. Kübler-Ross explained her early plans for the center and how they changed:

> When I bought a lovely farm in Virginia it was with the intention of having a place of rest and recuperation, to raise animals, and grow vegetables, to offer my lovely land during the summer to needy inner-city children, and hopefully to build a center for my own workshops. I had the fantasy that this would become my own healing place, where I could rest between my travels and recharge my batteries so as to be better able to give to others. But this was obviously not to be. It appeared that my work had already been cut out for me in a different direction. I had always listened to my inner guidance and I felt that I had no choice. I had no idea what fate had in store for me—in Headwaters, Virginia, no less! But I—as I have done many times in my life—would bury my private dreams and follow my destiny.

Her plans to open the center to a dozen babies infected with AIDS caused a firestorm of protest in Highland County, Virginia, which has a total population of less than 3,000. Despite all the assurances of the best medical professionals, residents could not be persuaded that AIDS is not an infectious disease. The new center continues to host workshops, but at least for now, plans to create a hospice for AIDS babies has been put on the back burner.

Children's Hospice International

Kübler-Ross has made it a point to spend a good portion of her time helping chronically and terminally ill children. In 1983, she helped found Children's Hospice International (CHI) along with Ann A. Dailey, an impressive woman in her own right.

CHI was founded to promote hospice support through pediatric care facilities, to encourage the inclusion of children in existing and developing hospices and home care programs, and to include the hospice perspective in all areas of pediatric care, education, and the public arena.

Kübler-Ross participated in a press conference and gave a lecture at Ford's Theater in Washington, D.C., to help launch CHI, a cause still very close to her heart. She was introduced on both occasions as "a great teacher and leader who ranks with Mother Teresa of Calcutta for her humanitarianism and her work on behalf of mankind."

Kübler-Ross began her speech by confessing that in her work with the dying, she had avoided children for many years. She said that she was not mentally prepared to deal with them. She said she was surprised to find out how open they were and that working with sick children can be "the most wonderful thing in the world." She said that sick children intuitively know when they are dying. They may not learn this fact intellectually for some time but somehow, they know. She said that children communicate this in a symbolic language, in which they say obliquely what grown-ups will not allow them to express openly.

One role of the caregiver is to serve as translator and show the parents what the child is trying to say through this symbolic language.

One key to the symbolism is to ask the child to paint a picture. Such pictures are revealing, Kübler-Ross said. She talked about the law of compensation. When children are dying, "their spiritual quadrant increases so that parents inevitably say the child was the most special person they ever met."

Kübler-Ross said our goal should be to educate the next generation so that books on death and dying are unnecessary. "We should keep kids at home within the family structure. We must get beyond our uneasiness and discomfort in dealing with the dying children," she said. Caregivers cannot afford to be negative, "Negativity feeds on negativity; you must be positive."

Kübler-Ross said she was disappointed that so few hospices are willing to deal with terminally ill youngsters at the present time. She said that this comes from misunderstanding and uneasiness because of "our own unfinished business and concerns about our own mortality." She added that dying children are very open and honest: "They are not afraid of death. They pick up this fear later as they grow older. They are not afraid because they know better than any of us that death is not an end to life but just a new beginning."

She emphasized that in the education of children, nothing is more important than the example set by parents. "You have to serve as a healthy example of the best values and ideals. The parents' greatest gift to their child is to work out his or her own unfinished business. If you want to raise healthy children, you first have to heal the child inside of you." She said parents should love children unconditionally, but that they should still be firm. Children should always know that they are loved although at times parents may not love their behavior. "Don't go overboard in shielding children from the hardships of life," she cautions, "they have to be tempered by life's experiences if they are to survive and prosper later on. Should you shield the canyons from the windstorms, you would never see the beauty of their carvings," she said.

"You can change the world with love," advises Kübler-Ross. "Children need this kind of support. If unconditional love is combined with firm discipline, the result is healthy and happy children. We must learn how to love without expectations, without applying strings," she stressed.

She said that all too often children are not allowed to die with dignity. Young dying patients suffer from heroic efforts to prolong life, which often results in the prolongation of suffering. She added that she was not advocating euthanasia or mercy killing, but that she was opposed to "the artificial prolongation of life when it becomes meaningless." Kübler-Ross added, "We must learn to accept the things that we cannot change."

Kübler-Ross said that we should give children a role in deciding what is to be done with and for them. "We must learn to listen to our inner voice and that we cannot assume that children are not mature enough to make intelligent decisions about their wellbeing," she said.

Kübler-Ross continues to serve on the board of directors of CHI, which also directs attention to the problem of abused children. She noted that perhaps 25 percent of all children have been abused in one way or another prior to reaching the age of consent. There are about 1 million runaway children in the United States each year, an indication that something is wrong. She added that suicide prevention is another important cause, as suicide is the third leading cause of death among the 6-16-year-old age group.

In large part thanks to her efforts, hospice programs for children are being created across America. In addition, significant progress has been made in preventing child abuse and in increasing public awareness of this devastating problem.

Perspectives and New Challenges: AIDS

When asked to look back on more than 25 years of work in the field of death and dying, Kübler-Ross said she was pleased with the progress that had been made, although a great deal more remains to be accomplished:

> Life was tough in the early days. There was much resistance, so much fear and reluctance. Many thought it "odd" or at least unworthy of a physician to spend so much time with dying patients.
>
> Two decades later, laws and attitudes have changed. Thousands of books and papers written on the subject of terminal illness have led to another subspecialty, thanatology. Patients and families now talk more about impending death, and thousands prepare their own

funerals. By accepting their deaths, patients are more willing to finalize their Last Will and Testament to ensure that their wishes are known and the family taken care of. There is rarely a medical or nursing school or a seminary or social work institution where courses are not given on the needs of terminal patients. The clergy have also come a long way in their counseling. Hospices have sprung up in every major area and palliative care units are available. Dying patients and their families now have several alternatives to dying in a regular hospital. Patients now have the option of signing themselves into a hospice where quality of life is emphasized and not the prolongation (at all cost) of dying.

As is typical of life in general, new problems have a way of appearing even as major progress is made with respect to old ones. Kübler-Ross believes that AIDS is now the major problem that confronts humankind. She writes:

> AIDS has become the largest social political issue, a dividing line for religious groups, a battleground for ambitious medical researchers, and the biggest demonstration of man's inhumanity to man—even far exceeding the leprosy in Father Damien's day.

She says that Americans have become known as a death-denying people, so that in a way it would be consistent to pretend that AIDS does not exist. The only thing worse than denial to Kübler-Ross is hypocrisy. "We hear weekly from thousands of pulpits, 'Love thy neighbor' but when it comes to putting that into practice we quickly add a few conditions. And it is those who preach the loudest who have shown the poorest records in their care and compassion."

> We still live with the illusion that it shall happen to thee and not to me. How many more wars and epidemics, famines, or other tragedies do we humans need before we open our minds, hearts, and ears and finally believe that whatever happens to our fellow man happens to us? We were taught that we are our brother's keeper but we quickly add all sorts of conditions before we even consider such a possibility.
>
> I believe that in view of man's horrible history of destructiveness toward the world of nature, man against man, we have been given many chances to learn our lessons. And there have been many great teachers sent to prepare us. But we in our own ignorant, grandiose ways, thought we knew better—for ourselves and/or our country. We gradually replaced the old inner knowledge of our spiritual origins

with the "god of material wealth and power, politics, and conditional love. We have learned little from past wars. One war escalating into another, one religion fought against the other—in the name of God! We were always able to turn off our radio set or our television if it started to get to us and so we needed a reminder that we could not continue our destructiveness against nature and against our fellow man any longer—or else there would be no planet Earth left.

Is it possible that our AIDS patients, children and adults alike, chose to contribute their short life spans on planet Earth to open our eyes, to raise our consciousness, to open our hearts, and minds and finally to see the light?

We can make our choices based on love and begin to heal, to serve those with AIDS and other diseases, to show compassion and understanding, and finally before it is too late, to learn the final lesson, the lesson of unconditional love.

Since we can no longer deny that AIDS is a life-threatening illness which will eventually involve millions of people and decimate large portions of our human population, it is our choice to grow and learn from it, to either help the people with this dread disease or to abandon them. It is our choice, to live up to this ultimate challenge or to perish.

If we are not careful, the emergence of the AIDS epidemic will continue to polarize the population: a split between those who offer help and those who judge, label, and denigrate those afflicted. If we choose not to help persons with AIDS we will find ourselves with no hope for the future and no hope for mankind.

Awards and Honorary Degrees

Dr. Elisabeth Kübler-Ross has won more than her share of awards. In 1977, *Ladies Home Journal* selected her as Woman of the Year. Later, they selected her as one of the eleven Women of the Decade. She has received the Tielhard Prize from the Tielhard Foundation, the Golden Plate Award from the American Academy of Achievement, and the Modern Samaritan Award from that society in Elk Grove, Illinois.

She has received honorary Doctor of Science or Doctor of Letters degrees from the following universities: Albany Medical College, Smith College, Malloy College, Regis College, Farleigh Dickinson College, University of Notre Dame, Hamline University, Medical

College of Pennsylvania, Anna Maria College, St. Mary's College, Amherst College, Loyola University, Bard College, Union College, D'Youville College, Rosary College, and the University of Miami.

The Foundation for Hospice and Homecare, established in 1983, presented Dr. Elisabeth Kübler-Ross with its first annual award, given each year to the person in the world who does the most to advance the cause of hospice and home. The award is now known as the Elisabeth Kübler-Ross Award. Kübler-Ross has graciously agreed to serve as one of the members of the Foundation's prestigious Board of Trustees.

Perhaps the greatest awards come in the form of recognition and respect from her peers. Even the most conservative critics in traditional organized medicine cannot argue with her results. *Medical Economic* in August 1980 carried a series of quotes that illustrate this point. Some of them are repeated below:

"The technique that Elisabeth teaches," said Charles J. Filipi, a general surgeon in Walla Walla, Washington, "is effective to the point that I know she will be making another major contribution in the field of psychiatry. But far more important, she is effectively demonstrating that society's emotional ills are mainly based on a lack of love. We need to listen to this woman!"

Internist Joseph Fennelly said: "It had to be a little foreign woman with gut feelings and a guttural language who embarrassed us male chauvinist physicians in America. We don't understand what change is in the medical profession. We still want to deny death and dying. Elisabeth is out there in the front line, and every front-liner gets into a little trouble."

Dr. Ira Sapan of San Francisco, who does volunteer work at a hospice, described the workshop he attended as a tremendous personal experience. "A lot depends on the trust that builds between people there," he said. "There were individuals who had seen their children die violently being freed, and I developed a tremendous faith in humanity from what people individually and humanity in general could go through and yet survive."

Dr. Sapan followed up on some of the participants to see if the beneficial effects of the workshop were lasting. He reported: "One woman who recently lost a daughter had been catatonic in an institution many years earlier after the loss of a son. At the workshop she was able to say good-bye to the daughter and let go. Two years later, she's still feeling free and feeling good about herself. Another woman I talked with recently has had multiple sclerosis for about 30 years. She had actually planned her own suicide. Then she attend the workshop in 1978. I saw what I can only call 'Obstetrics of the soul'—this woman being reborn with a tremendous lust for life. She now leads counseling sessions at UCLA for MS patients."

Dr. Sapan's description of Kübler-Ross as a "tremendously caring, considerate lady" is typical of several reactions—in fact, the word "caring" is most common in descriptions of her.

Beliefs

The thoughts and beliefs of Kübler-Ross are well chronicled in her 14 books. Asked what was the most important thing that she learned in life, she said it was that all religions basically teach the same thing: "Respect thy neighbor, and love them as you love yourself." She adds:

> After half a century, my understanding of the human being in this world is simply that we are all children of the same God. We are in the most literal sense of the word brothers and sisters. The ultimate lesson all of us have to learn is UNCONDITIONAL LOVE, which includes not only others but ourselves as well. As long as we judge, label, criticize ourselves or others, as long as we fight and kill our fellow man, no matter who he is, we have not learned our lessons, and we should not consider ourselves religious men and women.
>
> I believe that it is in the most literal sense true that we reap what we sow. Generosity, compassion, understanding, love will plant seeds of the same kind and will, in times of need, return to us. On the other hand, seeds of intolerance, criticism, hate, and discrimination will equally return. All true benefits have to be earned and they are always mutual.

She believes that free choice is the "Greatest gift that God gave to his children" and that the journey of the soul is everlastingly determined by our choices. "It begins with us and it ends with us," she said.

She believes in action rather than passivity. "Healthy people don't react, they are in control of their lives. But if you spend your entire life reacting to others, you never live your own life. You become a cripple," she said in an interview with *Mother Jones* magazine.

She also believes in leading a life of limited regrets:

> AIDS poses its own threat to mankind but unlike war, it is a battle from within, knowing no borders or national boundaries. Are we going to choose hate and discrimination or will we have the courage to choose love and service. Choose wisely. Take the highest road so that you will have no regrets at the end.

She believes that there are five natural emotions: fear, grief, anger, jealousy, and love, each one of which is capable of being corrupted into unnatural emotions that drain energy and lead to ill health. Fears can become phobias, grief can be transformed into guilt, anger to revenge, jealousy to competitiveness, and love may be compromised when harnessed to other conditions. "Most of us are raised with 'I love you ifs.' We try to buy people's love with compliance. That is not love, that is prostitution. Real love has no claims or expectations. It doesn't judge. It listens and respects the individual as he or she is. Real love is unconditional."

She has identified five basic fears that haunt all people—the fears of rejection, failure, illness, getting old, and death. She cites love, honesty, and action as the attributes to help people ride out these rough seas. She has a different view of pain than most people. She sees it as a gift. "When you look back on times of anguish, suffering, and trauma, you'll see that these are the periods of greatest growth. Looking back you will see that positive things—togetherness in the family, faith, or whatever came out of pain."

When asked to define strength, she said it is being honest:

> We make progress in our society only if we stop cursing and complaining about its shortcomings and we have the courage to do something about them. It is painful to admit our own fears, sense of guilt or shame, inadequacy or low self-esteem; however, it is the brave one who will admit these things, the strong one who will fight his own negativity, and the trusting and faithful one who will see the light at the end of the tunnel.

Kübler-Ross is an advocate of individual responsibility. "Because the world is so violent and so nasty, you can be a little island of love, peace, and light. The only way to heal this world is to heal yourself."

She believes that within each of us there is a Hitler and also a Mother Teresa. The important goal is to look within ourselves, identify the negative elements, and eliminate them. "If you become honest, like children, you can get rid of your Hitler and truly become a Mother Teresa or Gandhi, or whoever is your private saint."

When asked what advice she has for others, she stressed the importance of learning to be open and honest with others. "You should never judge your fellow man unless you have walked a mile in his moccasins." Kübler-Ross also stressed the importance of being consistent in thought, word, and deed:

> The pattern of your essential self is woven by the threads of all that you have desired and loved, of all that you have done, believed, thought, felt, and willed since you were born. As long as you breath, those threads continue to weave and reweave the patterns of the person you are. There is no escape from the process. It goes on whether you recognize or deny it. Most of the process remains hidden in the depths of the unconscious. At the core of this process there is the essential you that is continuously evolving in response to the impact of daily experience. We in religion call that developing essential person, the soul.
>
> Guilt, fear, and shame are the only enemies of man. And if you look at your own bookkeeping and you can truly say, and mean it, that you have no fears, no shame, no guilt, then you most likely will have no unfinished business. If you get mad at somebody for more than fifteen seconds, look to your own Hitler, and you know that you have work to do on yourself. If you have to go see "ET" to cry, then you have a lot of unfinished business and a great deal of unshed tears.

Kübler-Ross also stressed the importance of religion, saying that the people who most easily faced death were those with strong religious convictions. Asked about her perception of God, she said, in essence, that God is love:

> It's my contention that God is *all* love, made up of so much love you cannot even conceive of it.
>
> Yet many so-called Christians judge other people. And many churches use fear and guilt to fill their pews. Why? Christianity

> teaches us to love our neighbors as ourselves. It does not discriminate or condemn. Christ, by his example, was the best teacher of unconditional love *imaginable*. He accepted and loved and healed and worked . . . everywhere he went. He didn't ask people whether they attended such and such a church before helping them!

When asked about her views on life after death, she said: "I have always felt that something significant happens a minute or so after clinical death. Most of my patients have fantastically peaceful expressions, even those who had struggled terribly with death." She also referred to several cases where patients were declared legally dead only to spontaneously come back to life sometimes after several hours. These patients, she said, were able to describe in minute detail what was done for them by the resuscitation team. The frequency of such out-of-body experiences led her to believe that there was life after death. It also caused her to come under criticism and lose credibility with some quarters of the scientific community.

"Medical science is still wearing baby shoes," she said, noting that all major scientific advances were greeted with skepticism in the beginning. "Let people believe what they are ready to believe. It is not my place to tell them what to think. I have a practical mission in life, which is to love my neighbor as I do myself and by my example, and I try to teach that."

She continues to be a strong supporter of hospice and home care, saying, "Home care is our primary goal." She advises people to volunteer to work with hospices and home care agencies:

> We have moved from institutional care of the dying to a new healthier way of caring for them in their own environment; at home they are surrounded by their families and in control of their own needs and wishes which is almost impossible to achieve in the best of hospitals.

When asked what she expects for the future, she told *Mother Jones*:

> Primarily I see growth in human awareness . . . including our finally learning who we really are, and I also see us beginning to put our energy into constructive projects—growing vegetables, trees, and flowers, say—instead of creating military machines. I think we're approaching a time when the world is going to be much, much more fair. I truly believe that, within four or five generations, we'll ultimately outgrow war and hate and weapons.

Asked how she would like to be remembered, she said, "As a

person who tried hard to love my fellow human beings as I love myself and who tried to help people to settle their unfinished business and become positive practitioners of unconditional love."

There is a poem by Richard Allen which may capture the essence of her teachings. She often recites these lines:

> . . . as you face your death,
> it is only the love
> you have given
> and received
> which will count . . .
> if you have loved well
> then it will have been worth it . . .
> but if you have not
> death will always come too soon
> and be too terrible to face.

Elisabeth Kübler-Ross will be remembered and her positive contribution will influence generations to come. She has helped people overcome their fears and prejudices. She taught millions of people how to cope with terminal illness and that death is a natural part of life. Through her life, she has proved the healing power of positive thinking. In helping to correct the truly abominable treatment of the aged, ill, and dying that she has helped heal the body and soul of America.

❧

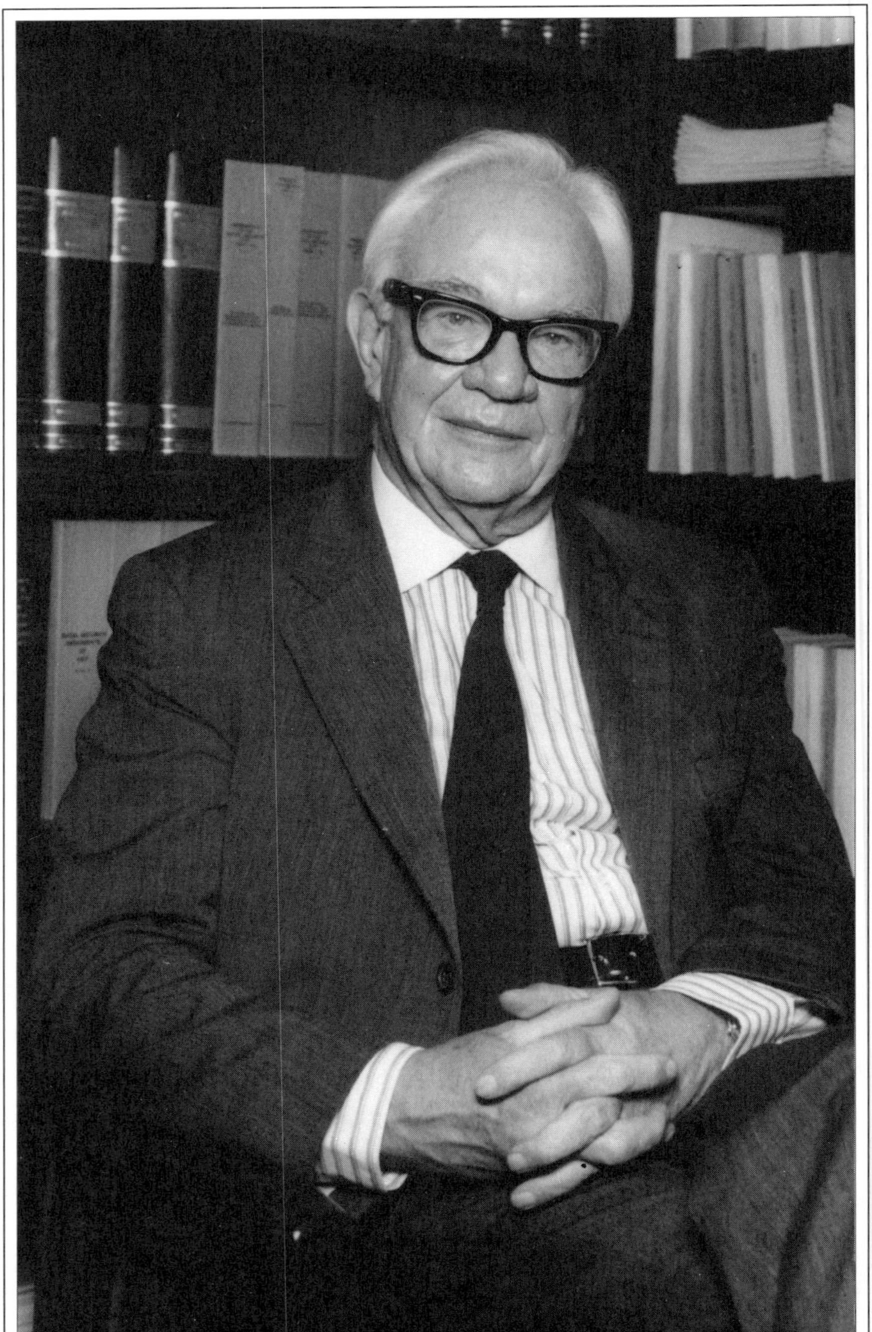

MARILU HALAMANDARIS

NINE

Robert M. Ball

Robert Ball is a tall, cerebral man who moves with ease among the power elite in Washington, D.C. He has been counselor and confidant to four presidents and a key advisor to scores of senators and congressional representatives. He is a man with a reputation for having the facts and telling it straight; a man with high principles and great integrity.

He is the kind of man that people such as Congressman Claude Pepper pointed to when they wanted to illustrate the personification of the best in public service. He is a man who has devoted his life to helping others, and he has done so with amazing effectiveness.

A philosopher once wrote that an institution is the lengthening shadow of one man. If the institution in question is the Social Security Administration, the man casting the shadow is Robert Ball. Modesty would not allow him to take the credit, but the fact is the Social Security Administration will forever bear his imprint. He, more than any other American, made it what it is today—the most efficient and most respected of government agencies administering two of America's most popular programs, which together represent almost one-fifth of the federal budget.

Few people can claim that they have done as much for the nation's elderly and disabled. In a career that has spanned almost fifty years, Ball has guided the extension of the Social Security programs, helped bring about the enactment of Medicare, established the administrative structure for Medicare, and brought millions of older Americans out of poverty by indexing Social Security payments to the cost of living.

He has served as architect and chief defender of the Social Security programs. In 1981, for example, a serious effort was made to make Social Security into a voluntary program and/or to involve the private sector in its administration. Still other efforts were made to reduce the number of individuals eligible for service and the amounts paid out under the program by 25 percent. It was Robert Ball who stepped into the breach and who did more than anyone to save Social Security.

Saving Social Security once would be achievement enough for any lifetime, but Robert Ball has helped do this at least three times in his career. At the age of 75, he remains active and involved; he continues to be one of the most energetic and articulate spokesman for seniors and disabled Americans. Ball's current crusade is long-term care. He has long believed that the failure to provide coverage for long-term care is the greatest gap in America's system of health care. He knows firsthand the devastating problems facing those with severe functional disability and the hardship this causes their families. He believes that things have reached the crisis stage and that government must now act to deal with the problem. He has authored a plan that has received widespread acclaim within the Congress. It is a plan that is based on home health care and that integrates nursing home care only to the extent that home care, respite care, and day care have been found to be inappropriate to meet the long-term care needs of the individual.

Background

Robert Ball was born in New York City in 1915. His father, Archey Decatur Ball, was a Methodist minister, which meant that the family moved frequently from parish to parish. When Robert was two years old, the family moved to Walden, Massachusetts; by the time he was ready for the first grade the family was living in Ridgewood, New Jersey, a suburb of New York City. It was here that young Ball spent most of his formative years.

Robert Ball has always had a special feeling for the elderly. It began, perhaps, out of the affection he had for his paternal grandfather, who lived with the family when Ball was seven or eight years old. His grandfather had worked as a traveling salesman and came to live with the family at the age of eighty-five. Ball remembers that his grandfather paid him what seemed like a very high sum of three dollars a week to perform certain small chores. "I had the room next to his and I would try to take care of him the best I could. I was very fond of him. He died in our home and I remember his death well."

When asked about his strongest childhood memories, he said, "I had a lot of fun. I was the third child in the family, and I think that all the hard part of being parents was pretty much absorbed by my brother and my sister. By the time I came along, my parents were much more relaxed and we had a very easy, friendly relationship throughout my early life." Ball says that being a minister's son carried its share of privileges, but also obligations. "We lived right next door to a large church in Ridgewood, New Jersey, and my father was the head man. This made me something of a special person. I also remember that I had to do things I wouldn't have had to do had father been a lay member of the church."

He says that his parents were clearly the most influential figures in his life. He remembers his father as being a very positive role model. Reverend Ball had a broad social conscience and was very involved in public affairs, but he always found time to discuss philosophy with his son. "My father and I used to stay up until two and three in the morning arguing every question, from the meaning of life to the future of the world. He accepted me as if I were a grown-up and would argue with and treat me accordingly from my teens through my college years." The Reverend Ball helped his son fashion his value system, based in large part on the Golden Rule and care and concern for others.

"He also passed down, without words, enjoyment of life. He was a very social person who, regardless of the seriousness of his goals, enjoyed almost every minute of every day as he went. He was full of laughter and full of humanness, and through the years I've tried to learn from his example," said Ball. He remembers his mother, Laura Elizabeth, as a very dignified and somewhat reserved person, at least in public. She was, after all, the minister's wife and she had certain responsibilities, such as running the Sunday school and coordinating fundraising to assist foreign missions. To her own family, however, she was not at all reserved, but playful and warm. "I was just terribly lucky to have such wonderful parents and to be associated with the Methodist Church, which emphasized what they call the social gospel, that is, trying to improve the lot of people here on earth," says Ball.

Robert Ball graduated from Ridgewood High School in 1931 and enrolled in Wesleyan University, located in Middletown, Connecticut. He majored in English literature and graduated Phi Beta Kappa in 1935 with a master's degree in economics. He has vivid memories of his college years and believes that the college had a wonderful influence on his life. "It was then and is now a college that has very small classes and prides itself on interaction between the professors and students. It was a somewhat protected environment, but obviously we were all touched by the events associated with the Great Depression. I was the president of a fraternity that was primarily known for its social activities, but even so it was perfectly possible to get half the fraternity to travel to Hartford to join the picket line in support of higher wages for coal miners."

Early Employment

Ball's first job was with Wesleyan University. He was given a fellowship, the opportunity to further study economics, and to do some teaching. "This allowed me to live better than if I had obtained a job on the outside. Frankly, there were just no jobs in existence at that time. This was also the year when I got married. My wife, Doris, and I spent a two-month honeymoon camping in the Adirondacks living in a borrowed boy scout tent. It was really quite romantic; we lived there on about $50 in this beautiful setting. Then I obtained a job at the handsome salary of $16 a week at the Stern Brothers Department Store in New York City, where I had the impressive title of Assistant to the Assistant Comptroller. What I did was balance hundreds of hundreds of items in about five checking accounts. I can still do a pretty decent job of balancing my checkbook."

At the age of 27, Ball got his next job, with the Social Security Administration. "I think one thing I learned both from my parents and from Wesleyan was the importance of public service. Government jobs at that time were held in high esteem. The New Deal had attracted the best and the brightest to Washington. I took a civil service exam which resulted in an offer to work for the Social Security Administration for the princely sum of $1,620 a year. This was early in 1939. The Act had been passed in 1935, but very little had been done in the way of administration until 1937 when they started issuing numbers to people. So I came in very early on the ground floor."

Ball began work in a district office in Bayonne, New Jersey. He visited employers to inform them about Social Security and to try to get them to improve their reporting practices. He also would visit the homes of people who were too ill to come to the office and would help them fill out forms in order to claim their benefits. Through hard work and dedication he was promoted to the post of assistant manager in the Newark, New Jersey, Social Security office.

In 1942, he was promoted to the central office of Social Security in Washington, D.C., where he worked in the training office. "I used to tell classes that I taught that they were the nucleus of what was going to be a huge organization and that they had a great responsibility and great opportunities. As the number-two person in this office, I frequently had the opportunity to substitute for the top person in executive staff meetings, which meant that very soon I became acquainted with all of the division directors within the organization. At a very young age, I developed a wide acquaintance of the top people in the organization. The head of the training office had a sink-or-swim philosophy and he would say to me go teach this or that subject when I had really no opportunity for preparation on the subject. This meant that I had quite a lot of opportunity for public speaking. I was very nervous about doing this when I was in high school, but through repetition it came easier and easier for me."

Bob Ball remembers the war years in Washington. For one thing, the building that had been built for the Social Security Administration on Independence Avenue was quickly taken over by the War Manpower Commission. It had specially designed floors to bear the weight of the huge Social Security printing and mailing equipment, but it was adapted to another purpose, which meant that the headquarters of Social Security was moved to makeshift facilities in Baltimore. From World War II to the present, the Social Security headquarters has always been split between Washington, D.C., where the commissioner retains an office, and Baltimore, where most of the employees work.

"I believed in Social Security with all my heart. I saw this program as making a major contribution to the solution of the problem of poverty in the United States. Its emphasis on self-help, with rights based upon work and contributions, was very important to me. I considered social insurance to be a practical method of accomplishing a great social goal in a way that protected freedom of the individual," remembers Ball. Any effort to give Robert Ball credit for the success of Social Security is quietly deflected. He credits the work of the "giants" who came before him, such as Professor Edwin Witte, who headed the committee that drafted the Social Security law, Arthur Altmeyer, who served with distinction as the Commissioner of Social Security, and Wilbur Cohen, a protégé of Professor Witte, who later became Secretary of the Department of Health and Human Services.

After the war ended, Bob Ball left Social Security to work with the American Council on Education as its assistant director. It was an opportunity to work with a good friend and mentor, Karl de Schweinitz, who had been the head of public assistance programs in Pennsylvania and director of the School of Social Work at the University of Pennsylvania.

> What we did, among other things, was to run short-term seminars for different groups of people. By short-term I mean 10 days to two weeks. One group that we taught was the top administrators of the Social Security programs from across the country; another group was the professors who were teaching social security at universities as part of their larger responsibilities. We held most of these seminars in Washington, although not all of them. This proved to be very successful and stimulating. I met a lot of important people and learned a great deal. We would discuss such topics as, "Is a contributory social insurance program the right way to go?," "What's wrong with relying entirely on a means-tested program?," "Why not let everybody save for their own retirement?" Obviously these questions are still around today.

Advisory Committee on Social Security

Ball stayed in the position at the American Council on Education until the Senate Finance Committee established an Advisory Committee on Social Security in 1948. The Republicans were in control of the Senate at this time and Eugene Milliken of Colorado was chairman of the Finance Committee. The senator was certainly no New Dealer, but he had strong views on the importance of Social Security. He established a bipartisan Advisory Committee on Social Security and gave them the responsibility of fashioning a report that would guide the committee with respect to future legislation. Professor Sumner Slichter, the Harvard economist, was selected to chair the committee and Robert Ball was its staff director. The result was a very substantial report that resulted in the 1950 amendments to the Social Security Act. It is no exaggeration to say that these amendments had the effect of saving the concept of contributory social insurance in America. The Social Security program had really been stalled since 1939. There had been no significant amendments for some ten years and inflation had reduced what were really very small benefits to the point where they were fairly meaningless. Only about 15 percent of the elderly in the U.S. were eligible for Social Security benefits in 1950. "I don't want to denigrate the 1935 and 1939 accomplishments, they were the great framework upon which everything else was hung. But the program had stalled, and the 1950 amendments really got it going again. They greatly increased the benefits, raising them something like 72 percent immediately. The eligibility requirements were greatly liberalized," said Ball. "Our report made recommendations not only on old-age survivor's insurance, it recommended a program of disability insurance; we issued a separate report recommending public assistance improvements and a separate report on unemployment insurance. It was a comprehensive job of which I am still very proud." Thanks to Robert Ball, Social Security was broadened in scope to include self-employed farmers, business and professional people, farm workers, employees of nonprofit institutions, members of the Armed Forces, and employees of state and local government, all of whom had been previously excluded from coverage.

Return to Social Security: Medicare and Beyond

Ball returned to the Social Security Administration in 1949, this time as its assistant director. He was put in charge of the Bureau of Old

Age and Survivor's Insurance programs. His responsibilities included research and helping to coordinate the flow of legislation through the Congress. Following the election in 1952, Arthur Altmeyer, the dominant figure in charge of the development of Social Security from 1938 up to the election of President Eisenhower, turned more and more responsibility over to Bob Ball. Ball served as acting director of the bureau and then deputy director for the better part of ten years. When President John F. Kennedy was elected in 1960, he appointed Robert Ball to be Commissioner of Social Security. Ball was the first commissioner to be chosen from the civil service ranks. Ball held the post from 1962 through 1973. Such were his accomplishments that he was continued in this position by three presidents—Kennedy, Johnson, and Nixon. In the early 1960s, Robert Ball played a pivotal role in Congress's decision to enact the Medicare program, which took place in 1965. It was his responsibility to help set up and to administer the Medicare program. Bob Ball remembers President Lyndon Johnson calling this the biggest federal undertaking since D-Day.

> I appointed a committee to help establish Medicare and I'll never cease to be impressed with how people with such diverse views could really come together and work cooperatively to put the program into effect. It was an amazingly successful job. Kermit Gordon, who was at that time president of the Brookings Institution, served as chairman of our advisory council, but we had representatives from organized labor, from the American Medical Association [AMA], the American Hospital Association [AHA], and virtually every other health care organization. We accepted a large number of the recommendations of this advisory council and built them into the Medicare program. The straight administrative task in launching Medicare was enormous. While all senior citizens were entitled to participate in Part A, participation in Part B of Medicare was optional. We were not sure how many senior citizens would elect to come under the physician's part of Medicare. We were successful beyond our expectations. Some 95 percent of the older Americans signed up for Part B. I didn't think you could get 95 percent of Americans to agree even on the premise that Columbus discovered America, but somehow it worked. We had cooperation from everybody. We even had the Forest Service looking for hermits in the woods. The Post Office had big signs on the sides of their trucks

> notifying the public that they had until March 31st to sign up. We had the General Services Administration turning itself inside out to find a space for several hundred offices. We had everybody quickly and easily behind this job. There was no bureaucratic infighting, and no attempts to second guess what we were doing. It was all quite amazing.

In 1972, Robert Ball helped bring about another significant expansion of the Social Security program. In that year, Congress enacted Public Law 92-603, otherwise known as the Social Security Amendments of 1972. Among other things, these amendments made the disabled eligible for both Social Security and Medicare. They increased Social Security payments by 20 percent and, in one stroke of the president's pen, lifted several million of the nation's elderly above the established poverty line. These amendments also indexed Social Security payments to the cost of living, which had the effect of protecting seniors and their fixed incomes from the erosion caused by inflation and ever-escalating costs.

In recognition of his achievements, Robert Ball has been given numerous awards. One of the most impressive of these is the Distinguished Service Award, given to him in 1954 by the Department of Health, Education and Welfare. He was the first recipient of this award. Some people say that he was the inspiration for the award and that there was support to select him as the recipient every year thereafter until he retired from government in 1974. Ball also received the Distinguished Service Award of the National Civil Service League in 1958 and was selected by Princeton University to receive the prestigious Rockefeller Public Service Award in 1961. In 1968, he received the Arthur J. Altmeyer Award. Ball received the Clarence A. Kulp Award in 1980 and the Presidential Award from the American Society on Aging in 1988.

Ball left the Social Security Administration in 1973, but his influence continued. His counsel continued to be heard at the highest levels of government. For example, he served as the chief policy advisor to President Jimmy Carter in the late 1970s and, with his good friend Wilbur Cohen, he helped found Save Our Security (SOS), a coalition of organizations of the aging and disabled, labor unions, and social welfare groups.

Save Our Security

In 1980, Ronald Reagan was elected president, bringing with him what he thought was a broad mandate to cut government entitlement programs, including Social Security. The Reagan Administration proposed legislation that would have turned Social Security over to the private sector, significantly reducing benefits as well as eligibility. Robert Ball, Arthur Flemming, and Wilbur Cohen formed Save Our Security and worked with Congressman Claude Pepper to head off this most serious threat to Social Security.

But there remained a shortfall in Social Security revenues; there was a cash flow problem and clearly something had to be done. There were differing views on what could be done, ranging from doing nothing to scrapping the program entirely. The Reagan Administration decided to attack this program entirely on the side of benefit cuts. President Reagan had strong reservations against raising taxes for any reason, but certainly would not do so in order to continue or expand entitlement benefits. The Administration came up with a recommendation that would have decreased Social Security protection over the long run by about 25 percent. It was to be done by a series of seven or eight different proposals which, when added up, would amount to a massive reduction. The proposals were couched in technical language which went over the public's head. But as Bob Ball remembers, they made one serious tactical mistake: they failed to understand what a serious backlash would be created by their proposal to scale back the retirement benefits for people who become eligible for early retirement at age 62. They underestimated the number of people who were counting on retiring at 62 instead of 65. This choice of early retirement already has the effect of reducing benefits by as much as 42 percent, but the Reagan Administration's effort to eliminate this option met with fiery resistance. This resistance was already so strong that the Senate passed a resolution disapproving of the entire package of Reagan cuts.

The result was the creation of a Social Security Commission made up of 10 people, five appointed by the Republicans and five appointed by the Democrats. The president appointed five members and agreed to appoint two Democrats within the five. The Speaker of the House also appointed five—three Democrats and two Republicans. Ball and the other members of the commission spent the better part of a year looking at various means of insuring the solvency of Social Security well into the next century.

There were serious public policy and political disagreements about what should be done. Bob Ball credits the commission chairman, Alan Greenspan, for doing an excellent job of keeping the group focused. "It was clear that he was not going to let the commission break down on any perceived unfairness or procedural difficulties. He let us participate in the selection of staff that would be more or less responsible to us." The staff director was Robert J. Meyers, who had been the chief actuary of Social Security and had served as deputy commissioner of Social Security in the early days of the Reagan Administration. Meyers, a longtime friend and colleague of Bob Ball, credits Ball with coming up with a compromise that brought together the Reagan White House and the Congress. The proposal, which sailed through the Congress, solved the short-term cash flow problems for Social Security and insured its long-term viability. The Social Security trust fund is now showing a healthy surplus. The idea was to build up reserves that would be left inviolate in the trust fund to protect against the day when the "baby boom" generation begins to retire. At that time, such reserves may be needed as it is projected that there will be fewer people in the work force and that they will be paying taxes to support growing numbers of retired individuals.

"Bob Ball made a wonderful contribution and insured the continuation of the Social Security program," said Congressman Claude Pepper to a reporter at that time.

Long-Term Care

Robert Ball has set as his next major objective the enactment of a new program to provide coverage for long-term care within the context of the Medicare program. He believes that long-term care is and will continue to be one of the most pressing needs of the nation. He has proposed a plan that is based on home health care. He outlined his plan at a 1989 meeting of the Brookings Institution and at his May 27,

1988, appearance before the Senate Finance Committee. Certainly no one has more credibility to speak for what is needed by the nation's elderly and disabled than Robert Ball. In his testimony, he said the following:

> The most important public purpose long-term care needs are (1) providing help to family members who have taken on the responsibility of caring for the seriously disabled at home; (2) protecting the income and assets of nursing home patients who may return to private or semi-private living arrangements and thus have a continuing personal need for their income and assets; (3) the protection of family income and assets for use by spouses of nursing home patients.

By way of solutions, he said:

> These high priority public purposes can be largely met by a universal public program that provides (1) a universal home care benefit of indefinite duration; (2) a respite care benefit to relieve the primary family caregivers; (3) a six-month nursing home benefit; and (4) an extended nursing home benefit for as long as there is a spouse living in the community.

Robert Ball told the committee that he firmly believes that home care is the best and most important choice in the provision of long-term care and that the funding of any long-term care program should be done be increasing Social Security payroll taxes by a small percentage. He argued for a universal federal program that could be supplemented by private insurance. He said that private insurance would be in the advantageous position to provide protection of assets in the case of long-term stays in the nursing home. Many of Robert Ball's ideas have been incorporated into Senator Kennedy's long-term care proposal, known as Lifecare.

Keys to Success

When asked what are the keys to his success and what advice would he give future generations, Robert Ball advises the nation's young people not to be afraid to take risks: "I guess that one thing I got from growing up a Methodist minister's son was security at a low level of economic wellbeing. I think that bred in me the feeling that I could take chances."

Inevitably, his thoughts turn to Social Security.

> I have no doubt that Social Security will be around as a permanent institution and that young people should have every confidence. To be sure there will be changes. But changes, whether they increase benefits or decrease them, need to be made only after very careful consideration. Too much is at stake here. People cannot continue to have confidence in the system if it is up for grabs in every budget negotiation in every year. Social Security is separately financed by dedicated taxes to be used only to support Social Security and they ought to be treated that way. I believe that young people should have no fear of contributing to Social Security. I am confident it will be there when they retire.

Robert Ball was asked about his extraordinary administrative skills. For example, the federal cash benefit Social Security program sends 99 cents out of every Social Security dollar to beneficiaries; only one cent is paid out in administrative costs. Medicare returns in excess of 93 cents on the dollar to beneficiaries in the form of claims, meaning that administrative expenses are limited to 7 percent or less. This contrasts with private health insurance companies, which struggle to keep their administrative expenses as low as 25 cents on the dollar. His response was that you need to find highly motivated people at every level of the organization. It cannot be limited to the leaders in the head office. You have to have motivated people with the right values and clear goals and you have to give them the right kind of training. When asked how to go about creating high morale, Robert Ball stressed the importance of encouraging people to participate in the decision-making process.

> I think in those days when we set up Medicare, no one was intimidated by knowing that their opinions were going against the dominant leadership. We wanted disagreement. You have to have people who are willing to tell you you are wrong. You have to have people who are willing to stand up and say, "I don't think you should do it this way" and then you can argue it out. Now that doesn't mean that in the end the leadership won't make the decision. A government department or an agency like Social Security isn't a democracy, but you want to have everybody's views and opinions.
>
> Now that leads me to a somewhat different point. I really do think that leaders make a difference and I have felt sometimes that in

> the last several years we have not made the most of the resources we have. I think that people at the top-level jobs have to be willing to quit, to resign, or to be fired. You don't do very well if your objective becomes to hang onto your job. The spirit of innovation and willingness to disagree is very important.

In the end, it all comes down to caring for others, says Ball. You must treat employees with the same respect and consideration that you would like were you in their place. You must be willing to give credit for the work and ideas of others. You must promote your common values and keep them constantly in the forefront. "We really strove for an understanding on the part of all employees as to our mission at Social Security. I personally wrote a set of objectives. They became the Social Security Administration objectives, which laid out for every employee what we were trying to accomplish in broad public service in each one of twenty categories. This document is used in orientation; it was used as a basis for work planning; and it was used to bring everybody together in a common approach." Former Secretary of Health, Education and Welfare, Arthur Flemming, said of Ball's document, "This is the finest statement of its kind by a government agency that it has been my privilege to read."

The statement of principles begins by listing four points of responsibility, which reflect Robert Ball's personal philosophy. He told employees they were responsible:

1. To the public: To safeguard and insure the rights of the public under the program, to provide the full measure of service to which the public is entitled, and to promote economical administration.

2. For the program: To improve the program so that it will more completely achieve its purpose and play its optimum role in providing economic security to the nation's workers and their families.

3. To the government as a whole: For the contributions we can make to government-wide policy and programs.

4. To the employees of the bureau: For the establishment and maintenance of an administrative climate and working conditions that will foster an effective career service.

Summary

In the past few years, it has become fashionable to make fun of those who elect to work for government. The assumption seems to be that it is the repository of those who could not find gainful employment in private industry. This attitude is in sharp contrast with the clarion call to government of President John F. Kennedy and the philosophy of President Franklin Roosevelt, who believed that there was no more noble or important calling than public service. Kennedy and Roosevelt believed that government was much too important to be left to amateurs. It was a place for professionals, meaning by that the best and most talented people available. The problems that currently confront the nation are testimony to the need to attract good people to government. The American public is sick and tired of reading about mismanagement and waste in government programs at the same time that people are going without the services they need. Some conservatives conveniently read the public's reaction as a call to cut back in government entitlement programs. But the polls continue to show strong public support for programs that help people, such as Social Security and Medicare. What this says in tones both loud and clear is that the real argument in America has never been the question of whether the public wants more government or less government. What the public wants is better government, which is to say more efficient government. Robert Ball put it in these terms:

> The business of the United States is the most important, challenging, and exciting business in the world, and we must be able to attract to it the best minds and skills of the next generation. We who are in government owe it to the country to set an example of government business that will compare favorably with the very best in private industry.

Neither Social Security nor Medicare are perfect, but despite efforts to water them down and to place barriers in the path of beneficiaries, they remain highly efficient in relative terms. They remain so because the Social Security Administration, which manages both programs, has been blessed with excellent leadership and excellent management. It is paradoxical that the two skills are not often found in the same person.

Robert M. Ball is the exception that proves the rule. He is both a charismatic leader and a highly effective manager. The nation owes a great debt of gratitude to Robert Ball for what he has done and for the continuing role model that he provides for all Americans. It is to describe such men as Robert Ball that the poet invented the phrase, "a true gentleman and a scholar."

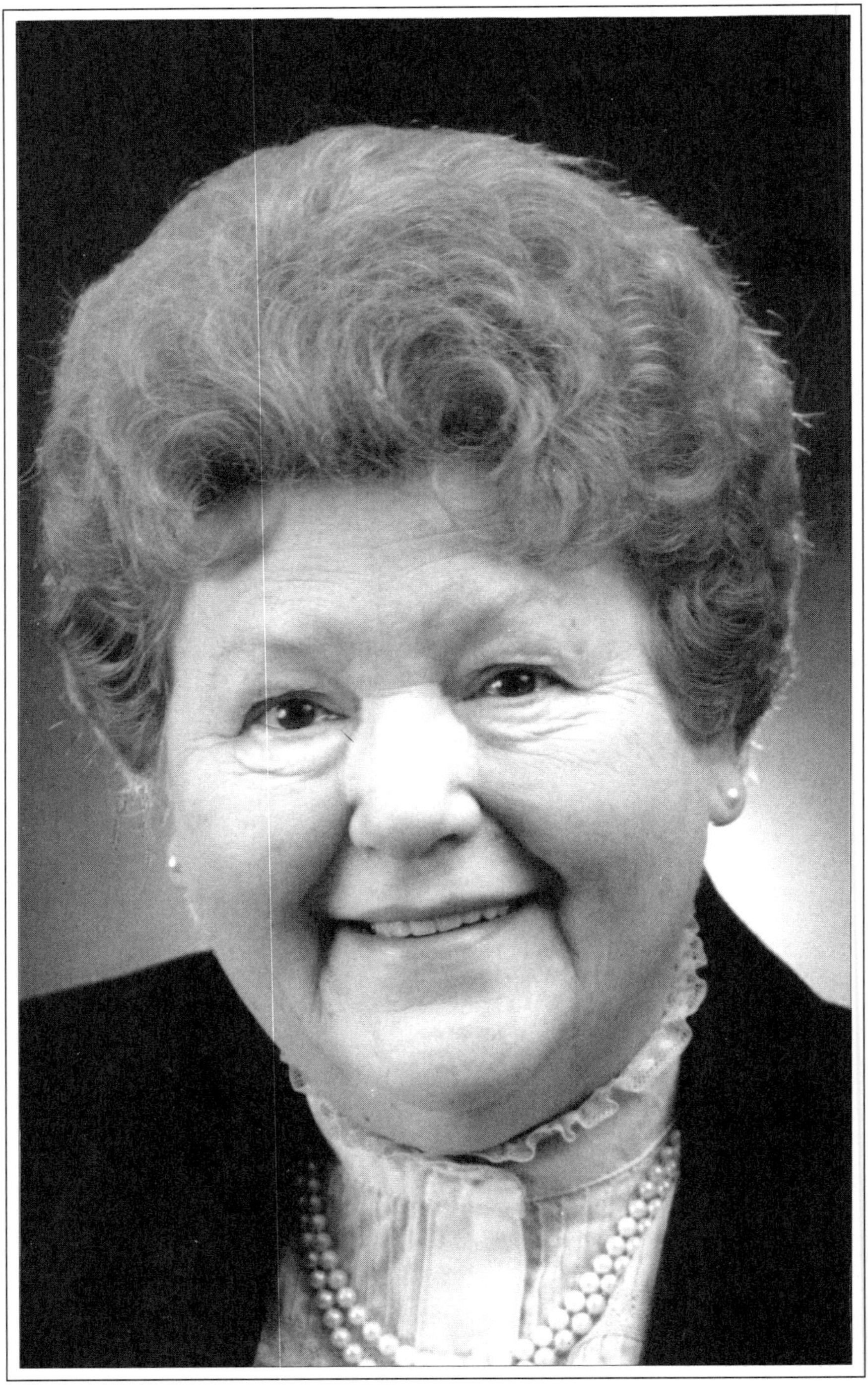

COURTESY OF DAPHNE KRAUSE

TEN

Daphne H. Krause

Daphne Krause tries to avoid the spotlight. Whenever possible, she credits others and minimizes her own contribution; but the truth is her efforts and achievements are extraordinary. Such are her achievements that she has been inducted into the Senior Citizens Hall of Fame; several state legislatures have passed resolutions commending her; and newspapers, magazines, and television stations by the hundreds have chronicled her success. She has made a national reputation by simply doing everything she can to help others. It is a classic case of doing well by doing good.

She has amassed an impressive record fighting injustice and fighting discrimination on the basis of race, creed, color, and sex. She has put most of her energies into fighting ageism—which she describes as the most pervasive form of discrimination in America.

Her battle against ageism led her to create the Minneapolis Age and Opportunity Center (MAO), which stands as a model of health and social service delivery programs not only in America but throughout the world.

In the dedication of the first building owned by MAO, Senator Frank E. Moss said:

> I see in the Minneapolis Age and Opportunity Center much more than just another lovely building. It is more than an innovative program. I believe MAO may be the first tangible evidence of an important shift in this country's values. MAO may mark the decline of the American youth cult and the growing acceptance of the graying of America.

> The effects of MAO can be seen on the faces of the elderly of the Twin Cities area. They look forward to the future with anticipation and not with dread. They approach life with a certain serenity born out of security in the knowledge that MAO will be there if they ever need help. MAO is a tribute to the courage, patience, and perseverance of Daphne Krause and the seniors of Minneapolis who, like Eleanor Roosevelt, would rather "light a candle than curse the darkness."

Senator Moss said it best, "Daphne Krause is a wonderful person; her life is an adventure in caring."

Background

Daphne Krause was born in Gloucester, England in the comfortable days before World War II to a family that was on the upper crust of British society. She grew up in a world of high propriety, "stiff upper lip," and stiffly enforced rules of behavior because certain things "just weren't done."

The family had at least three homes. A town house in Knightsbridge, London, full of antiques and servants, a palatial estate in the country in Buckinghamshire, and a seaside resort at Suffolk near Chestershire.

Krause remembers an idealistic world. "It was extremely peaceful and quiet. I took the way of life for granted. I was never spoiled but I was heavily protected as a child. I didn't see anything ugly or cruel, and it never occurred to me that people could be cruel."

This idealistic world was shattered by the death of Krause's father when she was three years old and not too long thereafter by the shower of Nazi bombs, which interrupted her education at St. Mary's Abbey and the Royal Academy.

> I grew up during the bombing of London. I remember seeing half of London on fire. I remember laying on my back in the garden with my father's binoculars and watching the dogfights. My family was horrified, worried that I might be hurt or killed by a stray bullet or from the falling shrapnel.

Krause remembers her mother opening the family home to take in refugees. She came home from school one day to find a child who had horrible ridges on her back from being beaten. "It looked like something out of a nightmare. I remember how shocked I was when mother told me that this beating had been administered simply because the child was Jewish."

Daphne went to stay with her great-uncle and guardian, Lionel D. Lewis, who was the founder and managing director of one of the largest engineering and construction firms in the world. Lewis built most of the American air bases, the British freeway system, and some of the largest dams anywhere in the world. Because of the war, the family retreated to the country estate in Buckinghamshire. The town house had been bombed and the seaside resort taken over by the armed forces to guard against the Nazi's landing on the beach via submarines and under the cover of darkness.

Daphne adored her uncle, whom she came to regard as her father. "He was a remarkable man. It wasn't just that I loved him; I respected him and he liked me. We used to go riding together and I used to caddy for him. He was a man of strong principles."

As a youngster, Krause was raised to be seen and not heard, but this didn't keep her from listening. A parade of the most famous men and women of the world passed through the family home. For example, she remembers a church bazaar held on the back lawn where she set out to win a stuffed tiger. She came up short in her efforts to throw rings onto well-spaced pegs. Second place got her a bar of soap. She remembers a tall man, who, on taking note of her sad face, insisted on exchanging the the bar of soap for the coveted stuffed tiger. The man was Joseph Kennedy, U.S. Ambassador to the Court of St. James and father of the future president. "I thought he was nice, but not too swift," remembers Krause.

She remembers that the Prime Minister Lloyd George was around the house from time to time, but he and her father never seemed to agree. Her father got along better with another prime minister named Winston Churchill.

> I remember the first time I saw Churchill. He was really quite short, but you didn't realize it; his presence was so tremendous that his height didn't matter. He reminded me of my father: Proud, determined. You just didn't say no to him.

General Dwight Eisenhower was a frequent guest, often staying at the home on weekends. "I would like to remember him saying something erudite or witty. What I actually remember is that he gave me a package of gum. I had never had chewing gum before and I remember him fondly for that."

In a sense, Krause was given a unique opportunity to be an eyewitness to history, to eavesdrop on the conversations of important people who gathered in her drawing room. She poured them tea and absorbed much, if not always realizing it at the time.

Coming to America

Following the end of World War II, Krause married a quiet man from Minnesota who had been working in the American Embassy. This meant new responsibilities, a move to the U.S.A., and it soon meant children and the difficult problem of trying to learn the peculiarities of the language and customs of her new homeland.

> Coming over here made me feel disconnected. It was an entirely different way of life. I was so busy trying to learn how to be an American wife and mother. I had never before heard of the PTA. I remember receiving a call from a teacher asking me to be a homeroom mother. I was horrified. I didn't know what that meant. It was the school nurse who called me and she had a voice like an old sergeant major so I dutifully trotted down there. I don't know why but she took one look at me and decided that I was manna from heaven.
>
> She used to tell me that the students needed milk or their brains would not properly develop and order me to find some milk for the kids. This was before school lunches were common. Somehow I managed to do it. What I found out is that if you properly describe the problem there is somebody in this country who will help you solve it. All you have to do is ask. Nothing has ever been easier.

Krause helped raise money and created scholarships for children from poor families. She set up a rummage sale in the church basement and helped bring clothes to the poor. In addition, she set up an exchange system of boy and girl scout uniforms. Her reward for each success was a new title and more responsibility.

When a small child was abducted and sexually abused one Halloween night, she offered the solution of a Halloween party in city hall. The mayor and city fathers loved it. So did the children and their parents. Krause got merchants to donate candy, and the city police patrolled the neighborhood. The city hall Halloween party has since become a tradition in Minneapolis.

She became known as a sort of Mrs. Fixit; if you had a problem in the Twin Cities the word was that you take it to Daphne Krause. For example, one woman bought a used car and was defrauded into paying more interest than the contract demanded. The woman brought this case to Krause, who brought in a legal aid attorney to handle the case. A woman on welfare wanted to learn how to be a secretary in order to earn a living. Krause helped her find a group that would instruct her. A friend complained that the ballot counting in Hennepin County needed improving, so Krause organized a group of women to do it. She organized a group of women into an organization that she called "Wise Wives." It was her effort to reach out not only to children but also to adults.

> On the surface these women kept busy; they did crafts, played cards and brought up their children, but their lives were still pretty empty. I helped them to learn how to care for each other. We started with a small group, but they brought in more and more volunteers. The few soon became an army.

Krause learned that you never turn anything away. "One man's discard is another's treasure. You have to know where it is going and also how to give it away. It is terribly important that it never come across as charity. For example, someone donated six tons of licorice. The weight of it nearly broke my porch. What do you do with six tons of licorice? We gave it to senior citizens. They went around to all the high-rises, organized senior volunteers, and gave the licorice to the other seniors, suggesting that they might give it to their grandchildren."

In the Twin Cities people began to learn that if you had six tons of licorice or 500 dinners left over from a political fundraiser that you could call Daphne Krause at any hour of the day or night and she would know what to do with whatever it was. Wherever possible, she made the recipients of the gifts responsible for their distribution to others, thereby avoiding the stigma of charity.

MAO

As Daphne Krause puts it, "One thing leads to another." In her case, all of her work with the community led to the establishment of the MAO.

Krause noticed that a large number of the people who came to her with needs and problems to resolve were senior citizens. She diagnosed the cause as a not-so-subtle discrimination against older Americans. This was in the 1960s when America was mired in Vietnam. She first used the term "ageism" to describe this invidious form of prejudice.

> I kept asking myself, "Why should there be ageism in this great nation?" That is when I became aware of the first death of the mind, which is the fear of death itself. I coined the term "thanatophobia" to describe the phenomenon. I am proud to see the word broadly accepted today and I believe it is the most fundamental fear that we have. Many things that happen to us are as a result of our fear of growing older, because death waits for us at the end and we simply don't want to face it.

Krause said that at this time she became aware of the sharp differences between the healthy older people and the sick and frail elderly. She learned that people with functional disabilities need help to remain independent in their own homes. She also learned that the alternative was deterioration, neglect, and death. She learned that not only did the quality of nursing home care in America leave a great deal to be desired, but also that the only federal program to help with long-term care carried the double insult of first requiring people to impoverish themselves by "spending down" all their income and assetts, and then only offering help through nursing home placement. It was to assist seniors struggling with the problems of functional disability and long-term care that Krause helped to found MAO, which has come to be accepted as the nation's best example of a comprehensive health and social service delivery program. MAO is a home care program, with an image that many hospitals and home care programs now try to replicate.

Senator Frank E. Moss, then chairman of the Senate Subcommittee on Long-Term Care, described MAO in these glowing words:

> I have tried to analyze what makes MAO so special—what makes it tick, so to speak. One thing that stands out is that it is built on one basic concept: It is planned by seniors, for seniors. It is what they want and what they need most. The seniors serve on the MAO board and control the destiny and direction of the program. It is a bootstrap operation, which has been put together with hard work and love.
>
> Next, I was struck by what I call the MAO approach. MAO has managed to take the elements of hope, service, dignity, and care and roll them into one. Each client is seen as a special individual and treated accordingly. Each is a valued member of society with hopes, aspirations, human desires and lifted by love and self-dignity.

When a senior walks into MAO, a counselor meets with that person in an intimate, comfortable setting. The counselor asks about personal problems and assesses the full range of the client's needs—social, emotional, and medical. Then a personalized, comprehensive "prescription" is written, tailored to meet those special needs. MAO takes into account the whole person and tries to help, using community resources. Only as a last resort does MAO provide services directly.

For example, if a person is malnourished and eligible for food stamps, the person is enrolled. If the person needs health care and qualifies for Medicaid, the person is made eligible. If the person is homebound, meals-on-wheels are arranged. If home health care is necessary, a nurse or an aide will call. If the person needs legal help, MAO has legal services attorneys who help the senior at no cost. If the senior is lonely and wants to work, he or she is put to work at MAO helping others. If the person needs minor repairs to allow her or him to stay at home, then MAO provides these improvements by way of retired carpenters who want to keep busy. If the person needs telephone reassurance, that is arranged. If what the person needs is employment, MAO has people to help the senior find a job.

As implied above, MAO keeps one chart that integrates both the social and the medical information concerning its clients. MAO offers homemaker services, it is a certified home health agency, and it has a unique free clinic in cooperation with Abbott-Northwestern Hospital in Minneapolis. When the counselor completes his or her work, the client is referred to the clinic for medical evaluation.

The MAO clinic has received national attention. Senior citizens with incomes below $10,000 a year are eligible to receive free care at the clinic. This is to say their Medicare coverage is accepted as full and final payment. The clinic absorbs coinsurance and deductibles. The doctors who provide care at the clinic have agreed to accept Medicare as full payment. In addition, free transportation to and from the clinic is provided and drugs can be purchased from the MAO pharmacy at cost.

If the patient needs hospitalization, Abbott-Northwestern admits him or her for whatever period is necessary and accepts Medicare as full payment. The doctors who provide medical attention in the hospital also accept what Medicare pays. MAO even pays for the first three pints of blood that might be used, an item not covered by Medicare. What is most encouraging is that the clinic has been in operation for several years now. It has proven that it is possible to provide unlimited care and still survive, even prosper, financially.

It is most significant to note that this innovative program has proven itself economically feasible from the hospital's point of view as well. In the past, Abbott-Northwestern has been plagued by a less-than-desirable occupancy rate. Since its venture with MAO, its occupancy rates have been in excess of 90 percent, which means the hospital is in a stronger financial position as a consequence of this program.

Although it is embellished by other programs, MAO is, at its heart, a home health agency. It is dedicated to the principle that intervention in time can prevent unnecessary and costly stays in the hospital or the nursing home. MAO's president, Daphne Krause, has made the point of the cost effectiveness of home care more eloquently than anyone. She has kept meticulous records of the services offered to MAO's clients, and she has contrasted these costs with the cost of equivalent nursing home placement.

In one case, MAO delivered services to a retired man for three years. He received counseling about once a month, three housekeeping (chore) services a month, occasional nursing services, and two home-delivered meals a day, seven days a week. The total cost of MAO services was about $10,000 over the three years. By contrast, the cost of placement in a nursing home for the same period would have been about $80,000.

But cost savings is only one benefit of MAO; more to the point, it has had a profound effect on the people whose lives it has touched. Said Senator Moss at a U.S. Senate hearing:

> I have talked to seniors who say they literally owe their lives to MAO I have heard they have willed half of their meager estate to MAO and half to their children. Clearly the availability of free health care has extended the lives of many needy older Americans.
>
> Once again, it is important to realize that MAO services go far beyond medical care. For the man who wrote me about losing his estate, MAO would provide free legal services. For the sick woman who must walk a long way to the hospital, MAO would provide free transportation. For the homebound elderly, MAO provides meals-on-wheels, nursing care, and homemaker/chore services. For the lonely widow who used to look forward to my newsletter, MAO provides telephone reassurance. For the senior who wants to work, MAO provides employment. For the families faced with the unpleasant task of placing a loved one in a nursing home, MAO offers an efficient, less expensive, and preferable alternative.

In counting the reasons for MAO's success, one cannot leave out the contributions of the community. Thousands of citizens in the Twin Cities area give of themselves and their time to make MAO a reality. The only government funding available to MAO has been Medicare, which pays for costs in its home health agency and clinic, along with small amounts from the Older Americans Act and from Title XX to pay for homemaker and chore services. The remainder of the money comes from contributions, bequests, and grants.

Policy Research

Yet another service of the MAO is to gather the facts on various problems confronting seniors. This documentation, compiled by MAO volunteer and legal aid attorneys, is sometimes fashioned into a report that is presented to the State Legislature or to the Congress. In 1971, MAO and Daphne Krause prepared a report on the conditions of nursing homes in the Twin Cities area and presented it to Senator Moss and the U.S. Senate Committee on Aging. Nurses, working "undercover" at the facilities, had been compiling data from more than a year. It was the most damning indictment of nursing homes ever made. The evidence was both compelling and deep. The hundreds of sworn affidavits from the nurses were entered in the record of the Senate hearing. In 1980, Krause presented the results of a similar investigation to the House Committee on Aging, chaired by Congressman Claude Pepper. The result in both cases was a number of prosecutions and convictions; sweeping reform laws were enacted both in Minnesota and in the nation's capital.

The success of the Minneapolis Age and Opportunity Center since its humble beginning in 1968 has been heralded far and wide in America and overseas. Both the U.S. Senate and House of Representative Committees on Aging have praised it and lauded its leader, Daphne Krause. Representatives from more than 50 foreign nations have journeyed to Minneapolis to study the unique program. Among those to send delegations were Great Britain, France, Canada, Japan, Norway, and Sweden—some of the most advanced nations in the world in terms of treatment of the elderly.

MAO has been lauded in countless newspapers and magazines. All three national television networks have featured its work. In July of 1974, CBS's "Sixty Minutes" featured a special segment on the work of MAO entitled, "Old Folks at Home." The program was an extremely positive endorsement of the concept of home care, as well as a tribute to MAO.

It hasn't all been easy. Every year, Krause faces the ongoing battle of how to come up with the funding to support the good works of MAO. Like every other administrator of a home care agency, she has had to contend with the Medicare program's bureaucratic red tape, tardiness, and refusal to pay for services rendered.

For example, in 1974 thousands of bills were rejected by Blue Cross of Minnesota (the administrator of the Medicare program in that state) which originated in the free clinic operated jointly with Abbott-Northwestern Hospital. The clinic was free in the sense that the clinic and the physicians who worked there accepted Medicare as full and final payment.

Krause tried to reason with Blue Cross, but to no avail. After several months of non-payment threatened the very life of the organization, Krause took her case to Washington. The result was a highly publicized hearing chaired by Senator Edmund S. Muskie on behalf of the U.S. Senate Special Committee on Aging. Nine U.S. senators listened to testimony from Blue Cross that they were paying all appropriate claims and that they had nothing against Krause or MAO. The facts showed otherwise. The committee counsel had uncovered and entered in evidence a "smoking gun" memorandum written by a high-level staff member of the Blue Cross organization.

The memorandum said, in simple terms, that Blue Cross had set out on a conscious effort to deny claims in an effort to force the free clinic out of business. Further evidence disclosed examples of identical claims, one paid by Blue Cross and the other rejected. Still other claims were introduced which had been submitted and paid to other doctors for treatments that Blue Cross had ruled inappropriate when delivered by MAO clinic physicians. The result was that both the Blue Cross representative and the representative of the Medicare program were royally barbequed by the senators present. The clinic was left alone for a time.

In 1980, a similar series of events took place that again threatened the life of the clinic. This time Congressman Claude Pepper intervened, asking the U.S. General Accounting Office for an investigation and personally making a tour of MAO.

The battle for funding continues to this very day. It is a battle to find donations, to find volunteers, and to obtain payment from the government for services that it has promised to pay under the Medicare program. All of this can be wearing, but Krause is known for her stamina and grit. She will avoid a fight wherever she can, but when the vital interests of MAO and the seniors are concerned, she can be a tiger.

The Enemy of Injustice

When asked to describe the greatest problems facing the world, Daphne Krause answers, "ignorance and injustice."

> I have really only met one person in my life who is evil, that is she truly enjoys hurting other people. I have, however, met a good number of people who are ignorant. I think that is the problem with President Reagan. I sometimes wish that he could come into the homes of some of the people that we serve and see the effect of DRGs—the new payment system he put into place for Medicare hospitals. I am thinking of the man sent home from the hospital whose cancer had progressed in his tongue and throat to the point where he could not swallow, much less take care of himself, and yet they sent him home. We were not allowed to serve him for more than a few weeks because someone decided that he was terminal and therefore not covered by Medicare.

Krause is the enemy of injustice. She says she learned from her father that all that was needed for evil to thrive is for good men and women to sit by and do nothing. "You must be outraged and you must challenge evil and injustice wherever you find it," she asserts.

Few things make Daphne Krause more angry than to tell her that this nation cannot afford good health care or cannot afford to care for the elderly. She contends that this is sheer nonsense, pointing out the tremendous waste in some government defense contracts. She has sharp words for some health maintenance organizations that cut corners in order to save money, depriving seniors of their Medicare health care entitlement.

Krause has few worries about the graying of America. She sees it as a natural progression. She believes that America can handle this problem in style. She contends that the seniors of tomorrow will be in better health and have relatively more resources than those of the present. She believes that it is very positive to allow the elderly the opportunity to continue to work. She believes that it is activity and purpose that keep people vital and alive. She advises seniors who can no longer work in their garden to grow a few things in pots. Those who can no longer do this should move to window boxes. It is a matter of adaptation to the environment and to disability, she says. She reminds people that relatively few of the elderly will ever become disabled. A little less than 10 percent of the U.S. population under age 65 is disabled, while slightly more than 10 percent of the over 65 population falls into this category, she notes. "This fact should punch holes in the old stereotypes of the elderly who are portrayed as frail and inactive."

Krause believes the failure to cover long-term care is the nation's number one problem. While she is an advocate for the elderly, she is also an advocate for children. She believes that functional disability and not age should be the key determinant in measuring eligibility for any federal entitlement program. She believes that home care is the best solution to the nation's long-term care dilemma:

> I think home care is becoming as much a respected partner in the health scene as are hospitals and physicians. When we started years ago, I coined the term a "viable alternative," meaning that it was the preferable alternative to nursing home care. But it isn't just an alternative anymore. It is and should be the standard and preferred method of providing care to frail seniors. After all, they want nothing so much as to remain in their own homes. I am glad to see home care being recognized as a full partner in the medical continuum.

Asked if she worries about anything at all, she cites the deterioration of our environment:

> I worry about the growing number of genetic disorders that are due primarily to pollution in the environment. I don't think we have even begun to understand the mess that is there waiting like a bomb to explode. We will see problems not only with infants and young people; more seniors will live longer and these environmental hazards are going to be manifested in them. Since we have poisoned them, the least that we can do is to take care of them.

Lessons Learned

When asked what she has learned, Krause responded:

> The most important thing I have learned is that it is a privilege to serve people. In my youth sometimes I was denied this honor. One time I remember I was caught by the nuns as I was swinging on the bars of the cubicle which surrounded my bed when I should have been asleep. The Mother Superior came in and caught me; she gave me demerits and I was not allowed to feed the poor who used to gather outside the convent gates. I learned that you had to be good in order to serve; that it definitely was a privilege.

She also stressed the importance of facing unpleasant situations.

> It is a fundamental belief of mine that you can't turn your back on situations that are unpleasant with the hope that they will go away. They will not go away. They have to be confronted and challenged. We must never forget that all kinds of barbarous things are going on and that we must fight to prevent these injustices from occurring.

She emphasizes the importance of religious faith. "The only people that I have ever seen who can face death with calm, and I envy them, are those of tremendous, unshakeable faith. I have to struggle with my faith all the time, I think that many of us do."

When asked to name her favorite poem, she says Longfellow's "Psalm of Life" which contains a great truth in the stanza: "Lives of great men all remind us / We can make our lives sublime, / And, departing, leave behind us / Footprints on the sand of time."

From her experience as the "Mrs. Fixit" of Minnesota, she says she learned about how wasteful we are and that the solution to human problems is often under our noses if we but choose to see, to ask, and to act. "There is nothing more wonderful than being able to put something discarded to good use," she says.

From Vice-President Walter Mondale she says she learned that you are known by the enemies that you make. "I don't like making enemies but sometimes if you believe that something must be done, that is the result. There are times when you must stand up for principle. You cannot turn your back and walk away, at least not and continue to live with yourself."

From Vice-President Hubert H. Humphrey she learned the importance of retaining the child-like innocence and curiosity that all of us are born with and which all too quickly fades into cynicism.

When asked specifically what advice she would offer to younger generations, she responded as follows:

> The bankers tell you to save your money for old age and that is good advice, but the wisest thing you can do is to learn how to stay healthy. Learn how to be flexible and adapt; learn what resources are available to you. It isn't how much you know as a person; nobody can possibly know enough, but the idea is that you must know how to find what you need.
>
> Moreover, you must never be so cynical or hurt by loving that you stop caring and build a wall around yourself. It is better to be

hurt, pick yourself up, and go on loving. Hatred turns in on you and it negates you. I believe that more illnesses are caused by hatred and stress than can possibly be imagined. And you must have faith in yourself. Never forget, every time you give of yourself, you get it back one hundred fold; it is sort of a shot of adrenalin to your mind and spirit.

Finally, it is never too late to try. I believe in picking yourself up and going on. It is not defeat that is the measure of a human being. It is the ability to get up and go on that is the measure of a human being.

Honors and Remembrances

In recognition of her many years of service, Daphne Krause has received a great many awards. Because of her work with the elderly, she was inducted into the Senior Citizens Hall of Fame in 1976. Her work in civil rights brought her an award from Minnesota's governor in 1975. She was named Woman of the Year in Minnesota in 1978 and 1979. The Minneapolis mayor and city council have passed a resolution saluting her work with the elderly, and she received the Sara M. Boyd Award from the Visiting Nurse Service of Milwaukee in 1986. She is in demand as a public speaker, having been asked to give guest lectures at Harvard, Yale, U.S.C., the University of Texas, and the University of Minnesota. She was selected to represent the United States at the International Anglo-American Conference on Aging in 1976. In 1978, the Senate and the Assembly of the state of California passed a joint resolution commending her for her "illustrious contribution to senior citizens of the United States and throughout the world." In 1987, she received the National Association for Home Care Special Award.

In 1978, a special awards dinner was held in Minneapolis honoring Daphne Krause and her work with MAO Among the guests present to pay their respects were Edgar Bergen, Jimmy Breslin, Joan Fontaine, Ellen Goodman, Ruth Gordon, Garson Kanin, Maggie Kuhn, Senator Frank E. Moss, Maureen O'Sullivan, Jesse Owens, and Studs Terkel.

When asked how she would like to be remembered, she replied:

I don't know that it really matters if they remember Daphne Krause. What really matters far more to me is whether I

> have made a difference. I have been so fortunate to be able to touch so many lives. I have been benefited in this even more than those whose lives I have touched. What matters to me is being able to do it. And you know, the terrible thing is that as soon as I say those words, I hear a voice, probably my father saying, "It isn't enough. You must do more."

Summary

This short profile cannot do justice to the career and work of Daphne Krause. It can only offer suggestions as to why she is an heroic figure. It is likely that no one will ever know the half of what she has done to help others. This is because, like the ancient Greeks, she believes that the only higher calling than service for another is service for another that is rendered anonymously. But somehow those who have been the beneficiaries of her kindness know from where it comes. To walk with her on the streets of Minneapolis is to walk with the saints. She is revered wherever she goes and properly so. By anyone's judgment, what she has done with her life is more than enough. No doubt her father would swell his chest with pride if he knew of her achievements. The good news is that she is still a comparative youngster and full of ideas, energy—and outrage. This means America can look for still greater achievements in the years to come and in departing many years from now, she will indeed leave behind her footprints on the sands of time.

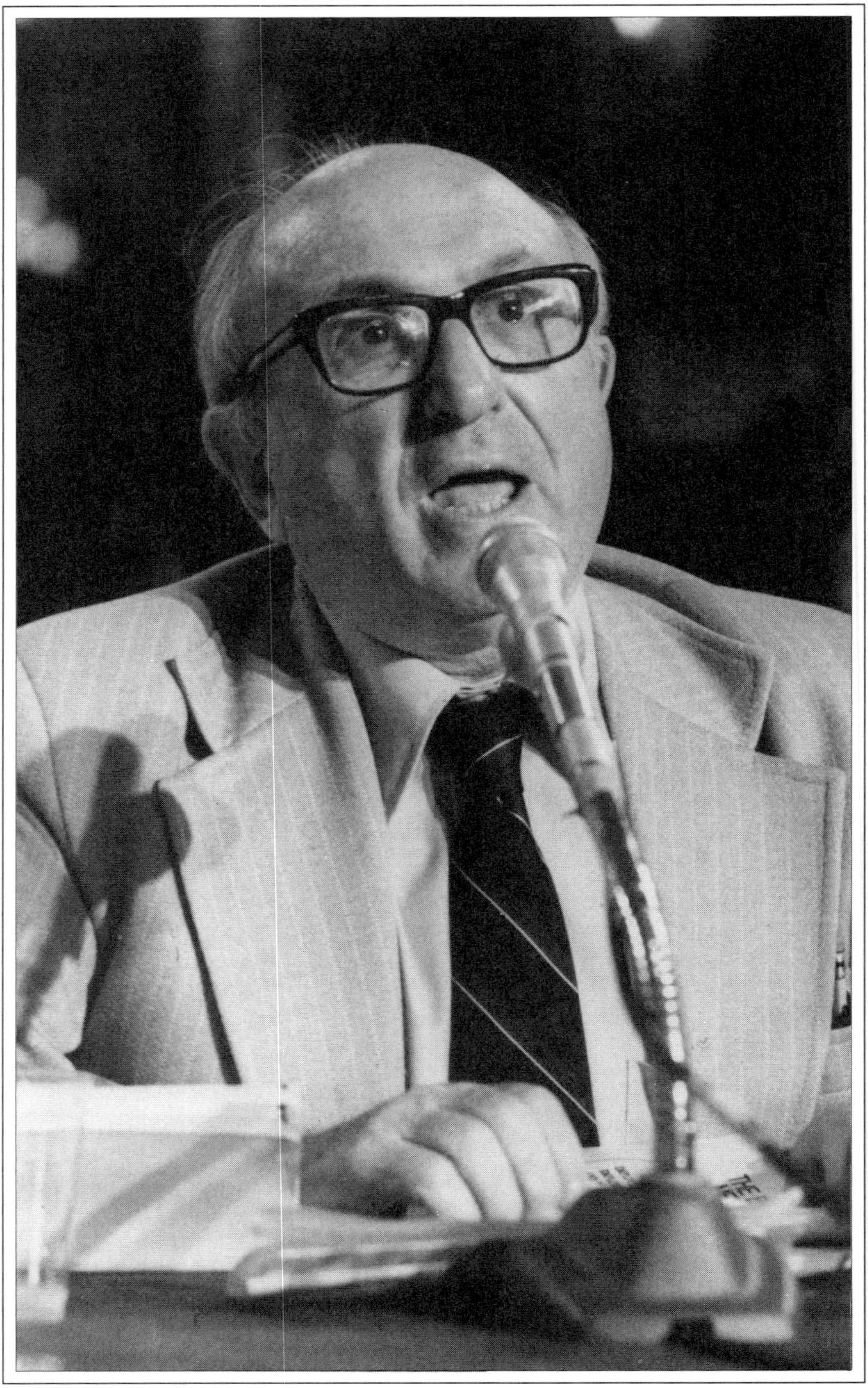

MARILU HALAMANDARIS

ELEVEN

Wilbur Cohen

He stood five feet six inches tall and weighed 160 pounds. His lively face, framed with wisps of grey hair on a balding head, gave him an ordinary appearance, which put people who met him instantly at ease. His blue eyes sparkled through thick glasses.

He was renowned for his amiable nature, always upbeat and positive. He was also driven by a profound sense of right and wrong, with a fierce determination to make life better, not only for the present, but especially for future generations.

He had witnessed the Great Depression and watched as good people through little fault of their own lost farms, houses, and jobs. He looked to mutual dependence and cooperation both within and without government as the best solution to prevent similar economic catastrophes.

He dreamed of a better world, not only for vulnerable Americans such as children, seniors, and the poor, but for everyone. He never lost sight of these dreams in his battle for economic, racial, and social justice.

Many historians refer to him as "Mr. Social Security," while his friends remember him simply and with deep affection as "Wilbur." By any measure, he stood tall on the American landscape and his contributions were anything but ordinary. For example, *Current Biography* wrote of him in these glowing terms:

> Since beginning his government career as a research assistant in 1934, Cohen played a key role in the formulation of virtually every important piece of social legislation in the United States, including the original Social Security Act of 1935 and the Medicare Act of 1965.

Shortly after he died on May 19, 1987, *The Washington Post* carried a eulogy, which read in part:

> He knew Capitol Hill and how it works and he was a strong advocate for the disadvantaged whose needs were the primary responsibility of the department he headed. . . . When Civil Rights laws were passed, he was there. When legislation to protect farm workers was proposed, his views were sought. He shaped training programs, child welfare standards, and policies to aid the aging and handicapped. He supported Federal aid to education, health insurance, and medical research. And when he left government formally, he did not withdraw from public life but continued to teach and to serve on countless Congressional advisory panels, presidential task forces, and social welfare commissions. Like his friend, Hubert H. Humphrey, Wilbur Cohen cared not only about "the people" but also about individual people. Throughout a lifetime of working to improve the lot of others, he never lost his enthusiasm or his largeness of spirit.

Few people have left such an indelible impact on the American political landscape as this dynamo from Wisconsin, and few have left a greater legacy. In its eulogy, *The New York Times* said: "Wilbur Cohen leaves his own best memorial, the fruits of half a century of energetic effort on frontiers new and old, to help people in need and in pain."

Clearly, Wilbur Cohen was a caring person. He devoted his entire life to helping others. His contributions in the field of health care and aging are matched by few Americans. One measure of his contributions is the fact that one of three major buildings housing the Department of Health and Human Services is named for him. More recently, he was inducted into the Health Care Hall of Fame.

Although Cohen died in 1987, his spirit lives on in the memory of those who loved him and in the form of blessings bestowed on the millions of people he helped through his relentless efforts on their behalf.

Early Years

Wilbur Cohen was born on June 10, 1913, in Milwaukee, Wisconsin, one of two sons of Aaron and Bessie (née Rubenstein) Cohen. His father was a native of Scotland who operated a variety store in Milwaukee. Some of Wilbur's most pleasant memories involved helping his father tend the store. In time, young Cohen attended local schools and graduated from Lincoln High School, where he was editor of the school newspaper, *The Quill*. He attended the University of Wisconsin in Madison, where he studied economics, graduating in 1934 with a Ph.D.

Having completed his studies, Cohen was invited to come to Washington, D.C., by Edwin E. Witte, one of his college professors, who had been named Executive Director of President Franklin D. Roosevelt's Cabinet Committee on Economic Security. Cohen and Professor Witte worked closely with Secretary of Labor Frances Perkins and Arthur Altmeyer in drafting the original Social Security Act. On October 14, 1935, President Roosevelt signed the bill into law, and Cohen became the first employee of the Social Security Administration. His title was Technical Advisor to Arthur Altmeyer, who was named the first Social Security Commissioner.

It is important to understand that the original Social Security bill signed into law by President Roosevelt contained many elements. One part of the bill created unemployment protection, another was a federal welfare assistance program. Only one aspect of this bill, aid to the elderly, concerned seniors. The remainder focused on the working-age population and children. The omnibus bill brought together nearly all existing federal social welfare programs and also contained such features as grants to the states for public health, crippled children's services, vocational rehabilitation, and infant and maternal health. Only in the 1950s did old age insurance emerge as the most important economic security program, important enough to monopolize the term "social security."

Cohen remained Technical Advisor to the Commissioner until 1952. He was in charge of program development and he served as liaison between the Social Security Commission and congressional committees, most especially House Ways and Means and Senate Finance. It was there that he met and worked closely with Claude Pepper; Robert Ball, who later became commissioner; and Arthur Flemming, Secretary of Health, Education and Welfare during the

Eisenhower Administration. "I first met Wilbur in 1942," said Robert Ball, "although we did not become close co-workers until 1946. Cohen came in at the top and always operated at the top level. I came in at the bottom and worked my way up."

From 1953 to 1956, Cohen served as Director of the Division of Research in the Social Security Administration.

Among the victories he achieved were the following: In 1939, he helped enact legislation to include dependents and survivors of workers under the Social Security Act. He helped pass legislation providing federal aid for the construction of new hospitals in 1946. In 1950, he helped enact legislation to cover domestics, farm workers, and the self- employed under Social Security. This same year, he was behind the enactment of legislation to provide federal grants to the states to aid the aged, blind, the disabled, and dependent children. He was a principal architect of 1956 legislation making totally disabled persons age 50 or older eligible for benefits, and in 1958 for the extension of Social Security benefits to children of the totally disabled. During the Korean War, he cooperated with the War Stabilization Board in introducing a plan that allowed businesses to give employees health insurance benefits in lieu of wage increases. That plan resulted in the expansion of Blue Cross and other voluntary health insurance programs.

He left government from 1956 through 1961 to become Dean of the School of Welfare Administration at the University of Michigan. Even so, he continued to serve as a consultant to U.S. Senate Committee on Labor and Public Welfare. In 1959, Secretary Flemming invited Cohen to serve on the Department's Public Assistance Advisory Council. In this same year, he served as a consultant to help establish the White House Conference on Aging held in 1961 and as a consultant to the United Nations.

From the New Deal to the New Frontier: Creating the Great Society

In 1960, Senator John F. Kennedy asked Wilbur Cohen to join his presidential campaign. Cohen was one of 14 key advisors; he advised

Kennedy to make health care for the aged a key issue in his bid for the presidency. Cohen chaired a task force on health and social security. He advised Kennedy to remind voters that Democrats had brought them the most popular government program ever in Social Security and that the unfinished agenda was to extend such social insurance programs to cover health care.

The Senate Aging Committee

In the years 1959–61, Cohen played a pivotal role in the establishment of the U.S. Senate Special Committee on Aging. He persuaded Senators Kennedy, Moss, and others that the special congressional committee was needed, arguing that it would serve to focus attention on the health needs of the aged. The committee would make it possible to develop research data to guide the Congress as a counterpoint to the inaction of the Senate Finance Committee. The Finance Committee in those days was chaired by conservative Senator Henry F. Byrd, Sr., who made it clear that no national health insurance plan would pass that committee whether directed toward the elderly or any other group. Cohen argued, in essence, that a committee made up of younger and more liberal senators was needed to make an end-run around the Finance Committee. Thanks to Wilbur's guidance, Kennedy made Medicare, the need to provide health care to the aged, a central issue in his presidential campaign. Many people think this issue alone insured his election.

In 1961 with the support of the president, the Special Committee on Aging was created in the Senate. President Kennedy made it clear to all concerned that he intended to keep his campaign pledge concerning Medicare. To no one's surprise, Senator Pat McNamara of Michigan, a close friend of Cohen, was named the first chairman of the panel. Cohen himself was named as Assistant Secretary of the Department of Health, Education and Welfare. In this position, he shaped most of the important domestic legislation enacted during the Kennedy-Johnson years.

In the years 1961 through 1968, Cohen hit full stride. He provided leadership and guidance and left a lasting imprint on every major piece of legislation that collectively was called "The New Frontier" and later "the Great Society." In 1968, he reached the pinnacle—he was appointed by President Lyndon B. Johnson to the post of Secretary of the Department of Health, Education and Welfare. He was the first employee of the department to rise up through the ranks to assume the coveted top position.

As *Modern Biography* notes, he established an enviable record. More than half of all legislative programs sent to the Congress between 1961 and 1968 came from the Department of Health, Education and Welfare. By the time he left, the Department accounted for more than a third of the federal budget and an estimated 20 percent of the gross national product. Only the Department of Defense, mired in the Vietnam War, received a larger share of U.S. tax dollars.

Behind the scenes, Cohen worked with the Senate Special Committee and helped engineer a series of congressional hearings to be held in all parts of the nation on the Medicare proposal. The leader of the barnstorming, fact-finding mission and chairman of the hearings was a young senator from Utah, Frank E. Moss. Others who were involved included Senator Edmund Muskie, Edward M.Kennedy and Robert F. Kennedy. The hearings galvanized public opinion and did more than anything else to build necessary momentum for the enactment of Medicare. While significant progress was made, it was only after President Kennedy's death that Cohen and President Lyndon B. Johnson were able to tie up the votes necessary to enact Medicare and a federal-state grant-in-aid program for the poor known as Medicaid.

Throughout it all, Cohen was in the center of the action. He was the glue that held together a coalition of national organizations representing churches, students, the aged, women, labor, and blacks. But Medicare and Medicaid, important as they were, represented only two of some sixty-five major pieces of legislation put into effect during the four and a-half years that he served as Assistant Secretary. In this respect, he worked closely with Senator Hubert H. Humphrey, who was elected Majority Whip, the number two leadership post in the Senate.

Other victories he helped achieve include civil rights legislation, child welfare reforms, mental health programs, veterans' benefits, vocational training and education, and federal aid for education and medical benefits for American Indians. He continued to champion health research with the Heart Disease, Cancer, and Stroke amendments of 1965and to advocate for the health care needs of youngsters through the Child Health Act of 1967. He also helped carry out a reorganization of the department in order to make it more efficient and more responsive to the public.

Robert Ball remembers Cohen as a superb legislative strategist:

> Cohen was nicknamed the "Salami Slicer" because in his legislative dealings he would take one slice at a time. When he introduced a bill, he did not expect great changes overnight, he just kept slicing away, little by little, until, like a sandwich piled high with salami slices, he would get the legislation passed, changes would start to occur, and he would go away satisfied. Cohen combined a sense of where a program should go with flexibility to take less than the ideal. He worked well with people who had great differences of opinion. He was able to pool their ideas and to come away with a consensus. He never ruled people out. He always found a way to include everyone, no matter what their political background. He had a flexible approach to legislation.

On March 23, 1968, Cohen was promoted to secretary of the department. Over the next ten months, he accelerated his legislative efforts. His successes included the enactment of legislation to help fight illiteracy and to support adult education. He won the enactment of anti-poverty programs and helped win federal support for legal assistance programs designed to help the poor. He also spent a great deal of his time preparing the way for what later became the landmark Social Security Amendments of 1972.

On the third anniversary of Medicare, Cohen announced the appointment of a 12-man advisory council to study the possible extension of Medicare to cover disabled persons under age 65. Dr. Henry H. Kessler, Director of the Kessler Institute of Rehabilitation in Newark, was named to serve as chairman. On this occasion, he quoted Lyndon B. Johnson as saying that Medicare was "the most tremendous domestic program ever implemented in the history of government." He added that contrary to the dire predictions, physicians had come to accept

Medicare instead of boycotting it and that it had become "a part of the American way of life." Secretary Cohen argued vehemently that Medicare should be expanded to include the permanently disabled. The task force he appointed came to the same conclusion, and in 1972, Congress made it part of the law.

Educating Future Generations: Saving Social Security

From 1969 through 1979, Cohen helped prepare a new generation of leaders to take up the secular religion of social insurance. He took a job as dean of the School of Education at the University of Michigan. In 1980, he moved to the University of Texas at Austin where he directed the Lyndon B. Johnson School of Public Affairs, a post he filled until his death in 1987.

He remained, throughout his life, the premier expert on Social Security and was its staunchest defender. He was always careful to differentiate "social insurance" from "welfare" programs. Welfare programs are often resented because the tax dollars of all citizens are used to provide for the few who cannot take care of themselves. Social insurance programs, on the other hand, find their acceptance in the fact that all contribute and all benefit, not as a matter of grace but as a matter of earned right.

He compared Social Security to a red traffic light. "You have to weigh the freedom to cross the intersection, even if no cars are coming, against the risks," Wilbur said. "The wisdom of the generations says that in the long run, the red light will save your life. The red light is protection against your own foolhardiness, and so is the seven percent payroll tax."

In 1981, the Reagan Administration proposed deep cuts in Social Security, which Cohen felt would undermine the basic "social contract" between government and the American people. He reacted by pulling together a coalition of over 120 national organizations which he called SOS—Save Our Security. He asked former Secretary Arthur Flemming to join him as co-chair and, together with Congressman Claude Pepper and Robert M. Ball, they created a firestorm of protest that forced the plan's withdrawal. In its place, they argued for a blue-ribbon commission, which ultimately hammered out a combination of tax increases and minor adjustments that will keep Social Security solvent well into the next century.

When asked about his views and why he lead the fight, Cohen said:

> I think of Social Security in a much broader way than Reagan or any of the ideologues who only look at it as a governmental intervention in the private market. I look at Social Security as a social intervention we have created for you to go to work and lessen your anxiety for the future. This has always impressed me as something that is bigger than myself and bigger than life itself because it supports life.

Medicare after 20 Years: Social Security after 50

"If one person can justly be called the father of Medicare and Medicaid, he is Wilbur Cohen, former Secretary of Health, Education and Welfare in the Johnson Administration," wrote *The Washington Post* on Medicare's 20th anniversary in 1985. When asked about his plan, Cohen said that he was pleased with the initial steps, but that more work remained to be done. "My plan was to get health care for the elderly and the poor first, then expand it to cover children, and finally to adults," Cohen told one reporter. When asked to sum up Medicare's impact, Cohen offered the following facts:

- In 1963, more than half of the elderly in the country had no health care care at all. Today 93 percent of the elderly have a regular source of medical care.
- 30 million Medicare beneficiaries would receive $70 billion in benefits in 1985.
- 21 million Medicaid beneficiaries would receive $34 billion in benefits in the same year.
- In 1967, the U.S. spent $51.3 billion annually for medical care and in 1984, health care spending surpassed $370 billion.
- Medicare beneficiaries who turned 65 in 1983 paid an average of $2,690 over their working lives into the program and will ultimately be paid some $34,000 in benefits.
- However, the average out-of-pocket costs facing seniors in 1985 averaged more than $1,600 a year and Medicare still covers only a little more than a third of all their health care costs.

In 1985, Wilbur Cohen also participated in ceremonies marking the 50th anniversary of the enactment of Social Security. Cohen said that Social Security grew out of the Great Depression and that it was an effort to insure that a similar economic holocaust did not again wreak havoc on the American people. He again gave a stout defense for social insurance and so-called "entitlement" programs as opposed to welfare programs. He restated his belief that the notion of an earned and vested right was integral to the success of Social Security. He said that most people look at Social Security and Medicare as an earned right, rather than as a handout. This one factor, he said, explains the acceptance of entitlement programs and the problems facing "means tested" or welfare programs.

He described Social Security as "a labor of love." "I have been involved in practically every aspect of the program, either inside or outside, since 1934. So it's pretty hard to disassociate yourself."

Cohen said that more education was needed. He said that he feared that young people do not understand Social Security and may "junk it because they don't understand it."

"Very few young people know that when a man gets married and his wife has two kids—if he died when he was 33 or 35 his family would have some $200,000 worth of life insurance from Social Security," said Cohen by way of illustrating his point.

Later that year, *The New York Times* reported that Cohen and his wife took a vacation to Hawaii. As was his habit, Cohen took time off to visit the local Social Security office. "I ask employees how they are doing and what are their problems. They are very surprised that a Cabinet Secretary 20 years ago would continue to express that degree of interest in them," said Cohen when asked about the incident.

This one episode does much to describe the qualities of Wilbur Cohen who remained, throughout his life, an inspiration to all those who work for the betterment of society.

Books and Honors

Wilbur Cohen received numerous awards in recognition of his contributions. In 1956, he received the Distinguished Service Award from the Department of Health, Education and Welfare. In 1961, he received the Florina Lasker Award from the National Conference on Social Welfare and the Terry Award from the American Public Welfare Association. In 1962, he received the Blanche Ittelson Award from the New York Social Work Recruiting Commission. In 1965, he received awards from the National Association of Social Workers, the National Association for Mentally Retarded Children, and the Association of Physical Medicine. In 1967, he also received the Bronfman Public Health Prize and the Rockefeller Public Service Award. He received the Murray Green Award from the Volunteers of America in 1968. In 1975, he received the Merrill-Palmer Award and the Hull House Award. In 1979, he received an award from the International Association for Social Security. In 1987, one of three major buildings housing the Department of Health and Human Services was renamed in his honor, and in 1988 he was inducted into the Health Care Hall of Fame. He was given honorary degrees from the University of Wisconsin, the Yeshiva University, and Brandeis University.

Wilbur Cohen has written or contributed to more than 30 books. He has written numerous essays and monographs on Social Security and related fields, including articles for the Encyclopaedia Brittanica. Among his best known works are, *Social Security: Universal or Selective?*, written with Milton Friedman and published in 1972; *Towards Freedom from Want,* co-authored with Sar A. Levitan and published in 1968; *Retirement Policies under Social Security*, published in 1957; *Social Security Programs, Problems, and Policies*, written with William Haber, published in 1960; and *Income and Welfare in the United States,* a project of the Survey Research Center of the University of Michigan, published in 1962.

Views on the Issues

Two months before his death, *U.S. News and World Report* carried a letter by Wilbur Cohen entitled, "Needed: A New Political Agenda for the 1990s." This prophetic communication reads in part as follows:

> The Reagan revolution, with its theme that government is the problem, is over. We have to prepare a forward looking agenda for

> the 1990s . . . look[ing] ahead to the national priorities for the year 2000 rather than back to the less government and laissez-faire economy of the 1920s.
>
> Our new Chief Executive inevitably will have to recommend or accept an increase in taxes to stop the increase in deficits. But even more of a challenge will be the need to meet pent-up domestic needs from the budget cutbacks of 1981–88. Population will have increased and will continue to increase. There will be more aged persons every year. No president or Congress can stop the impact of these unrelenting demographic facts on the need for public services.
>
> A new Chief Executive will find that the extent of poverty will not have been reduced, and welfare reform will remain a national issue. Medical costs still will be rising. Medical technology will continue to develop. There will be millions of persons without any health insurance coverage and millions of others with incomplete coverage. Uncompensated medical services probably will exceed $15 billion by 1990 and medical indigency will be increasing—particularly among those persons needing nursing home care which can cost $25,000 a year per person.
>
> Nationwide adoptions of equal rights and affirmative action for women and minorities will still be a national issue. Comparable worth will still be around. Financing a college education will be a big problem for middle class families and governments. And teenage pregnancy will not have abated by election-campaign rhetoric. AIDS will be an expanding international problem.
>
> We need a new political agenda that erases the terminology of liberalism vs. conservatism and capitalism vs. socialism. We need a pragmatic agenda that meets the nation's urgent problems with courage and innovation. A new generation of political leaders must and will rise to meet the challenges of a nation that will be both more competitive and more compassionate.
>
> As a nation, we must expand both the private and public sector to meet the needs of a high-tech international economy. As a nation, we must be both liberal and conservative simultaneously—but be able to distinguish clearly and effectively which of these qualities apply to basic human needs and which apply to our limited but expanding human and environmental resources.

As is apparent from a review of this insightful letter, Cohen continued that battle for what he believed to be the great problems of society until the very end. Not even two heart attacks would slow him down. He made similar points in other interviews as quoted below.

On Income Security for the Aged

Throughout his life, Cohen argued for private pension protection and increases in retirement income paid through public and private programs. "I don't see for the life of me why people over 65 must live in poverty," he often said.

On Social Security

> There is, of course, no one all-perfect social security system, equally well suited to the needs of capitalist countries, communist governments, unitary governments or federal-state systems . . . . I do not believe that our present social security system is the last word, nor do I believe it should be immune from change. On the contrary, I believe that it can, it should, and it will change and that each generation should be free to remake and remold it to its needs and liking. One key element in social security is being able to count on what you are going to get. Of course, there is no absolute sure thing except for death and taxes, but insofar as possible, a main goal of social security has been to give individual citizens assurance that come what might, he or she will get what was promised them. The second major goal has been to divorce the payment from any need or means test and from any test of relatives' responsibility or other moral criterion.

On Welfare Reform

> The present system is not only inadequate, but has been build over the years in such a way that it fails to benefit all the poor equitably. There are better ways of helping the poor, but all of them involve more costs and more problems, economic, political, administrative, and otherwise. Part of the reason we don't have a better welfare system is because it is difficult in a country as large as ours to agree on what is an adequate standard for both New York and Mississippi and because of the various other complex decisions which are necessary to administer its system in a country as big and diverse as the United States. If one were to attempt a better system to meet the needs of the poor, one wouldn't start with the current system. It's very easy to criticize the system, but it's very hard to find a solution that everybody will accept. The fact is that most of the working poor in the United States are not in the present welfare system, except for food stamps. The solution to the problem is to

find a plan that includes an equitable level for the whole United States and incentives that will encourage work.

On Education

Education is the central solution to the welfare problem. The vast majority of these people on welfare have no education—they're grade school and high school dropouts. They can't make change, they can't take a telephone message. We've got to educate these people, train them for jobs, vastly expand the education of the children.

On Health Care

Cohen continued to advocate some kind of national health insurance plan throughout his life. In his testimony before Claude Pepper and the House Aging Committee on the 15th anniversary of Medicare, Cohen described himself as a legislative incrementalist. "My philosophy is that all social legislation is a matter of process and a matter of development. It is necessary in a democracy to obtain the support of those who will pay the taxes and of those who will receive the benefits," he said.

On Medicare

When asked what he considered the biggest mistakes made in the enactment of Medicare, he responded, saying it was to limit payments largely to hospitals and institutional providers. "I would like to see us spend more on preventive care. I would like to see coverage for prescription drugs, hearing aids, and eyeglasses . . . and I would like to have unlimited home care."

On Long-Term Care

Wilbur Cohen believed long-term care, which is to say chronic disease and increasing disability, were the largest gaps in the American health care system. He spent much of his final years working with Arthur Flemming and Congressman Pepper to bring about the enactment of a long-term care program based on home care. "Home care is the best answer to the question of long-term care. It may cost us a little more to provide it but in the long run, it will reduce costs," said Cohen.

On Quality of Life

> Quality of life, and enrichment of life—that's what I want. I don't mean just to make it so that you can make a couple of extra bucks. I mean, to enjoy the things we have. Clean air so you can walk in a park and breathe, clean water so you can take the kids swimming.

Believed

When asked about his values and beliefs, Cohen told one reporter, "I have a strong belief that deeds are more important than words and I believe all the Biblical injunctions that teach one to love his neighbor." Wilbur Cohen was a man of deeds. His values are apparent from his actions.

He was an advocate of activism rather than withdrawal from life. He chose not to retire but to continue to work 60 hours weeks, even after having two heart attacks. He believed it is better to burn out than to rust out.

He had a benevolent view of life, believing that human beings were basically good and that there was no problem created by humans that could not also be solved by human beings.

He was a man of great enthusiasm; a man of great passion who believed that life was to be attacked every day because time was short. He hated very few things but waste of time and waste of natural and human resources were near the top of his list.

Bill Hutton, former Executive Director of the National Council of Senior Citizens, remembers Cohen for his positivism and his perseverance:

> Wilbur Cohen believed that every single major social reform that is now on the law books was once vigorously opposed as being unwise, unnecessary, too expensive, impractical, socialistic, or un-American. But someone, some group, persisted in the advocacy of the idea until the right historical moment occurred when a political leader welded together a working majority consisting of liberals and conservatives, in a state legislature or in the Congress, to enact it.

Along with historian Charles Beard, Cohen believed that "the wheels of justice grind slow but they grind exceedingly well."

He believed in providing human beings with as many options as possible because choices were fundamental to human dignity.

He believed the solution to most human problems lies in cooperation and collective action.

He believed in fighting hard but fighting fair. He never let emotion cloud his judgment.

He believed in helping everyone he could along the road in life and emphasized the importance of personal action. Personal responsibility was the price we all pay for freedom, he often said.

He believed in leading by example. "The day I have to give an order is the day I am not an effective leader. When you can't persuade someone of something, you may still be the boss but you are no longer the leader."

He also believed in the importance of family and friends. Often on Sunday mornings he took the time to make breakfast for his wife Eloise and their three sons, Bruce, Stewart, and Christopher.

He believed in civility and the importance of small kindnesses. He remembered birthdays and anniversaries and the names of his staff's children.

He believed with Edwin Markham that what you send into the life of others comes back into your own.

Remembered

When asked how Wilbur Cohen should be remembered, his friend, Congressman Claude Pepper said:

> Wilbur Cohen was a legendary figure in the field of social and health care legislation. He was one of those responsible for Social Security and for Medicare, two of the greatest pieces of legislation ever enacted in this country. We should build a Washington Monument or something similar to celebrate what he has done especially for the elderly people of this country.

Robert Ball said:

> As long as I have known him, Cohen was fundamentally a social reformer always striving to make government an instrument

for improving the life of the people. He believed in institutions that helped people at a time in their lives when they needed help the most.

Spencer Rich, the respected *Washington Post* writer, said:

> He was a wonderful loving person with an outgoing personality. I wish he had been my father. I love my father, but Wilbur Cohen was an exceptional, extraordinary person.

There is no doubt but that Wilbur Cohen will be remembered. He was a true visionary with extraordinary leadership and management skills. He had a passion for excellence and a great love of people; he elevated public service to a high art and through his efforts, he made life better for millions of people.

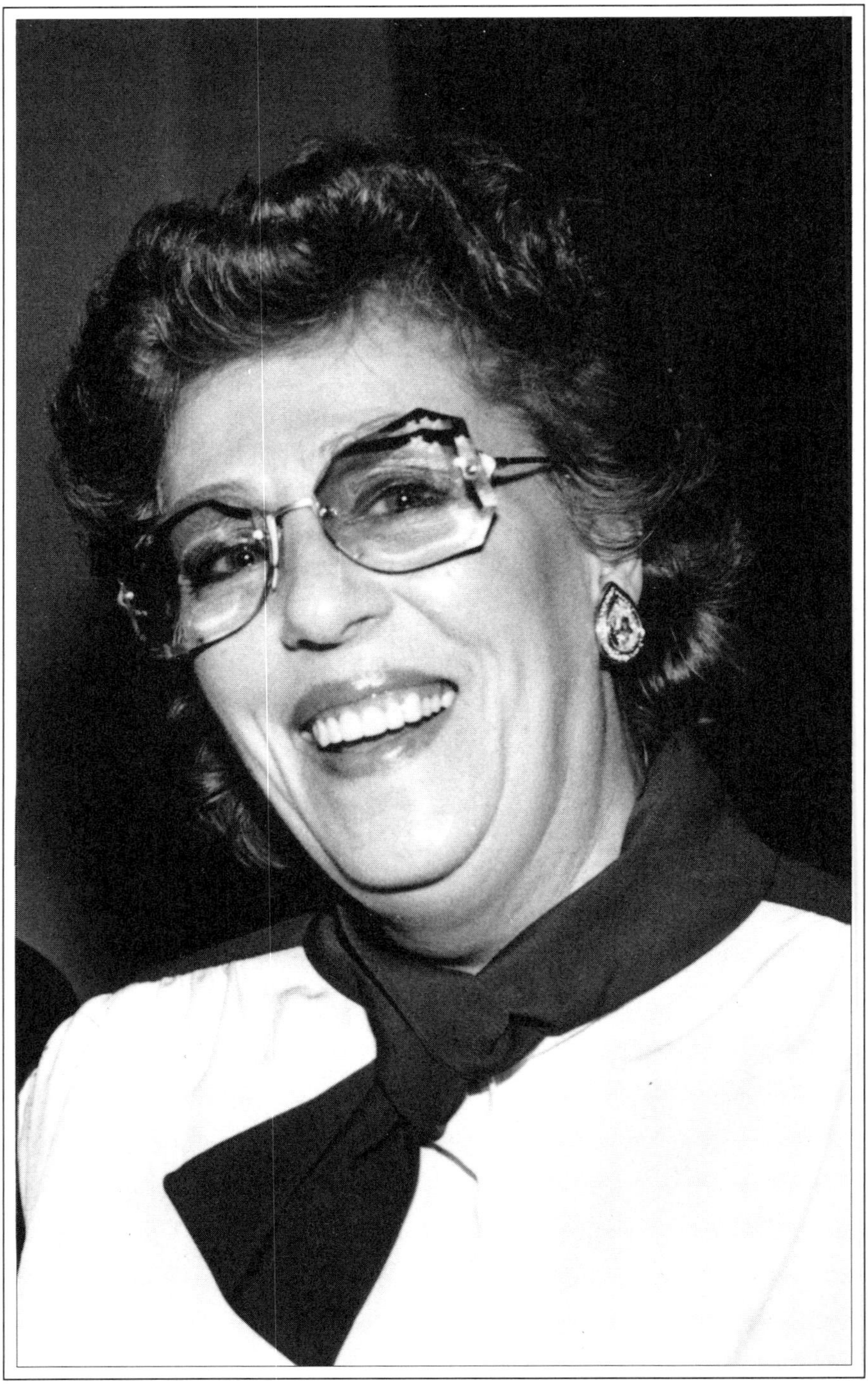

MARILU HALAMANDARIS

TWELVE

Elsie I. Griffith

Elsie I. Griffith is a well-known figure in the field of health care, a giant in the field of nursing, but most people know her as the "First Lady of Home Care."

More than 35 years ago, she anticipated the "graying of America." She realized that the numbers of senior citizens relative to the total population would increase and that seniors, on average, would live to increasingly longer ages. She knew also that those who were blessed with a longer life span were also more likely to suffer from greater disability and therefore have need of assistance to remain in their own homes and perform the essential activities of daily living.

Griffith took a good hard look at the modes of health care delivery in the 1950s and found a great deal was missing, particularly as contrasted with services provided by the British and Scandanavians. She decided that there had to be a better way of dealing with those of advanced age and disability than placing them in institutions. Her search for something better lead her to home health care; in time she became a practitioner providing hands-on care, an administrator supervising the care provided by others, and an advocate with the goal of changing public policy to reverse the existing American bias in favor of institutionalization.

Griffith's long and distinguished career is checkered with an impressive list of "firsts." For example, she was the first to build a viable organization of volunteers in Washington, D.C., a city marked by high turnover and, at times, little community spirit. She was the first to support the extension of Medicare to provide payment for home health services. She conceived and created the first diversified, comprehensive home care agency, which is the model widely used today. She was the first to develop a graduate school curriculum in community nursing and home care administration. She was the first graduate of such a program. She was the first to envision the creation of a home care industry as a full partner in the American health care system. She was the first person who was successful in unifying disparate home care interests into a powerful national organization, and she became its first elected chairman.

First, last, and always, Elsie Griffith is a nurse. Her instinct is always to help. Always she has sought ways to provide more and better services, to be delivered in a more efficient manner to those in need at the least cost, while still maintaining the highest quality.

Griffith's pioneering work revolutionized health care in America. Home care is today the fastest growing part of the health care field. Both insurers and government are beginning to recognize the public's preference for in-home care rather than institutional care. Griffith is the personification of the slogan, "We are bringing health care back home where it belongs." The primary beneficiaries of her work have been the nation's senior citizens, who account for 75 percent of all home care visits. By bringing health care and supportive services to seniors in their own homes, Griffith has helped millions of people to live with a maximum degree of independence and human dignity.

Background

Elsie Griffith was born in Dallas, Texas, and was educated in Texas public schools, including the Ursuline Academy. She was a straight-A student throughout and was the valedictorian of her class.

Her concern for people in need was something she learned early in life from loving parents. Her father, Hershel Ingram, was a civic leader in Dallas with a heart as big as Texas. He was in the life insurance business and was very successful. Each year, he sold more than a million dollars worth of protection, becoming a perennial member of the Million Dollar Roundtable. Griffith's mother, Vivian, came from

French and German ancestry; her family was part of the established aristocracy in Natches, Mississippi. In addition to caring for the family, Vivian also volunteered her time to local organizations.

There were seven children in the Ingram household. Elsie was the oldest, followed by five brothers and a sister. Like all children, they were fun loving. They played together, worked together, and went to school together.

In addition to her keen mind, Elsie was also gifted with athletic abilities. She and her father spent many hours together on the tennis court, where she showed great talent.

After graduation from the Ursuline Academy, Elsie continued her studies, receiving her R.N. degree from St. Paul Hospital in Dallas. She was married shortly thereafter and moved to Washington, D.C.

Washington, D.C.

Griffith lived for five years in Washington, D.C. She remembers going to President Dwight Eisenhower's inauguration in 1956. It was an exciting time. Following her father's example, she became deeply involved in community service activities. She gave generously of her time to one cause after another. She performed so effectively that she was soon in great demand. At one point, she was asked to become the Director of the Volunteer Bureau in Washington, D.C. The Bureau had the task of recruiting volunteers and dispatching them to community organizations.

As is typical of Griffith, she performed beyond all expectations. Numerous programs in the Capital City were able to expand their service at no extra cost, using the volunteers Griffith recruited.

It was at the Bureau that Griffith first learned about home health care. She was greatly impressed by what she saw at the Visiting Nurse Service of the District of Columbia. She appreciated the care, compassion, and support that the organization's nurses and therapists provided to citizens in the community. She saw the satisfaction nurses received from caring for clients in their own homes. The experience left her with a strong desire to use her training as a nurse and provide some "hands-on" home care herself.

Griffith moved to St. Louis, Missouri, where she took a job with the Visiting Nurse Service of that city. She worked as a field nurse, ministering to the needs of the minority groups in a depressed area of Kenlock County. She found youngsters and seniors alike in need of care, but unable to pay. She volunteered countless hours, providing care to indigents.

Kenlock County officials saw something special in Griffith and asked her to be the supervisor of the County Health Department. After a year as the administrator of this agency, she decided to obtain more education and moved to Seattle, Washington.

The University of Washington

In Seattle, Griffith enrolled as a graduate student at the University of Washington. She selected the university because it gave students flexibility in fashioning their study programs. It was here that she designed the first graduate program in community nursing.

In addition to her studies, Griffith completed a nine-month internship at a community home health agency operated by the Tacoma-Pierce County Health Department. Once again, she cared for the poor, the sick, and the forgotten. A great deal of her time was spent working on Indian reservations with the Crow and Blackfoot tribes.

In due course, Griffith received her master's in business administration in addition to her bachelor's degree in nursing. She was the first person in the nation to receive a graduate degree in community nursing administration.

The National League for Nursing

Leaving Seattle, Griffith headed for New York City and employment with the National League for Nursing (NLN). She greatly admired the League's charismatic director, a woman named Hedwig Cohen. Cohen was then one of the best writers and most original thinkers on the nursing scene. Cohen, for example, pioneered the NLN Accreditation Program, which certified to the quality of home health agencies.

Griffith worked for the NLN for about five years. As part of their Community Nursing Branch, she traveled the length and breadth of America. She provided help and consultation in many areas, depending on the needs of those she visited. For example, she persuaded five small agencies in Westchester County, New York, as to the value of unity and merger. The result was the Westchester County Visiting Nurse Service. She also conducted the first NLN accreditation site visit at the Boston Visiting Nurse Association.

During the time that Griffith worked for NLN, the federal government began to implement the Medicare program. In those years, Griffith worked hard to convince providers they should participate in Medicare. Some home care providers at the time had expressed skepticism. They were afraid of excess government control and/or interference in their practice. The states of Indiana and Wisconsin, for example, took the position that they were not going to participate in Medicare. Another problem related to the fact that the existing community agencies were nurse dominated and sometimes resisted the requirement that they hire homemaker-home health aides and therapists as a condition of participating in Medicare.

Griffith helped educate state health departments about how to administer the new Medicare program. States were called on to license and certify home health agencies, hospitals, and nursing homes for participation in the new federal program, but had no idea where to begin. Griffith helped many states set up their programs to train state surveyors on how to go about inspecting and certifying a home health agency. She trained a good number of surveyors personally.

In 1967, shortly after Medicare became effective, Senator Frank E. Moss added an amendment that required states to offer home health services as a condition of their receiving monies under the federal-state grant-in-aid program for the poor called Medicaid. Griffith helped dozens of states implement this program. Moreover, it is no secret that New York moved furthest and fastest in this direction. Under Griffith's prodding, the New York program grew and today account for fully half of all Medicaid home health care payments.

The Dallas VNA

Griffith's return to Dallas, Texas, was an outgrowth of a 1970 NLN meeting in Las Vegas, Nevada. Bea Haggerty, whose husband Pat was the chief executive officer of the Texas Instruments Corporation, was then chairman of the board of the Dallas Visiting Nurse Association (VNA). Haggerty hired Griffith to be the Executive Director of the Dallas VNA. Haggerty worked out a package that was both intellectually and financially interesting to Griffith. She was hired to work two days a week as an administrative consultant to advise the VNA; the other three days a week she was the Director of the Health Planning Council of Greater Dallas.

When Griffith went to the Dallas VNA in 1970, it had a staff of only 35 people, 14 of whom were homemaker-home health aides, and a budget of $350,000. The agency provided only nursing and aide visits, and 30 percent of their service was maternal care. It served only those within the city limits of Dallas. At the time there existed several homemaker-home health aide organizations that would have nothing to do with the VNA, and seemingly this was all right with the RN-dominated VNA staff.

Griffith worked for over a year on a detailed analysis of the VNA. When she presented her report to the VNA board, it sent shock waves through the community. She suggested the need for the agency to merge with the homemaker-home health aide organizations. She suggested adding physical therapy, speech therapy, and other services. She suggested expanding and providing service outside the Dallas city limits. She suggested serving private paying clients. She suggested serving other age groups, including those in their middle years, at their place of employment. In short, she was suggesting the formula for the modern day comprehensive diversified agency.

The board agreed to Griffith's plan and hired her as the full-time executive director to implement it. Griffith began adding services. In addition to traditional nursing, therapy, and homemaker-home health aide services, she added extended services (24-hour available care); patient education; medical social services; nutritional consultation; durable medical equipment; physical, occupational, and speech therapy; and the largest hospice and rehabilitation programs of any home health agency in the nation. In addition, she added vocational rehabilitation and provided nurses aides and others under contract the opportunity to work with nursing homes and other health care institutions.

In her 12 years in Dallas, the VNA increased from 35 staff people to about 1,300 full-time employees. The agency expanded beyond the city limits not only to serve Dallas County, but 10 other counties in North Texas as well. The service area increased from about 600,000, the size of Dallas at the time, to about 10 million people, the population of the 11 counties served. At the end of 1982 when she left, the Dallas VNA had an average daily census of 10,000 clients. In that year, the agency provided over 11,000 nurse and therapy visits and over 118,000 hours of homemaker-home health aide services, with over 1.3 million hours of volunteer, chore, and family care services. During her 12 years, the budget increased from $350,000 to $16 million. This is an enviable record.

The primary reason for this success was the vision and leadership of Elsie Griffith. As many people have said, she is one of those people with the unique ability to see clearly into the future and to set a course to meet and solve not only the problems of the present, but of the years to come. She also has the unique ability to inspire confidence in others and to share with them the enthusiasm for hard work that is so much a part of her life. Griffith is not one to stand still in the face of injustice. If there is a thing that is worth doing, she will find a way to do it.

Another of Griffith's famous firsts illustrates a great deal of her character and courage. When she went to the Dallas VNA in 1970, Texas, the third most populous state in the nation, had never paid for a single home health care visit under the federal-state Medicaid program. It is worth re-emphasizing that states were required by law to offer such services as a condition of their participating in the Medicaid program. Things were so bad that Texas was cited by Washington and threatened with the loss of their Medicaid funds if they did not begin to do so; still they continued to drag their feet. No one knows why. It may have something to do with the tremendous clout of the nursing home lobby in Texas or it may have been reluctance on the part of the state officials to pay out more money in the growing Medicaid program. Whatever the reason, Griffith knew the state of Texas was in the wrong. They were in violation of federal law and they were denying Medicaid beneficiaries what they were entitled to by law. She decided she would challenge the state

Griffith sent her attorneys to meet with state officials and threatened lawsuits. The state Medicaid officials said they would listen to reason. After repeated followup calls and visits, they gave Griffith the criteria for certification. She recalls it was the most elaborate and byzantine procedure possible, ending with the requirement that a physician on the staff of the state Department of Health in the capital city of Austin had to personally sign and give his approval before the Medicaid program would pay for a home visit.

The lawyers wanted to bring suit because of what they felt was an attempt to sabotage the Medicaid benefit, but Griffith held them back. She said that they had been given a criteria and that they would use it. She started with three cases and took them through the state Medicaid maze, and they finally wound up on the desk of the Health Department physician. Griffith personally made the visit with the papers and secured the necessary signatures. This was the first time Texas paid for a home care client under the Medicaid program. This broke the log jam. Today, Texas has a sizable and growing program.

Formation of NAHC

Having worked for the National League for Nursing and its Council on Community Health Associations, Griffith remembers the day in 1968 when Margaret Lewis announced that she was going to form a separate organization to serve the interests of home care providers on the West Coast. She charged that the NLN was East Coast-dominated and that it had paid scant attention to California and other western states. The new group was called the National Association for Home Health Agencies (NAHHA) and it was at that time based in Denver. Griffith thought that Lewis had a point, but felt the future would have been better served if the League had been pushed to become more responsive instead of opening up a rival organization.

For many years, Griffith watched as the two organizations spent precious time, money, and energy competing with each other, instead of getting down to business and making life better for all providers and for the Medicare beneficiaries whom they serve. She also discerned that neither organization was responsive to the needs of large agencies.

In response, Griffith convened meetings of the 10 largest home health agencies in the nation. They were all VNAs and they enjoyed the opportunity for sharing and learning from each other. In time, the list grew to 36 agencies with a combined income of over $2 million. Griffith was the driving force behind the move towards merger and the unification of the home care industry. State associations also pushed merger, having grown tired of competing organizations begging for their support instead of concentrating on the business at hand.

A task force was set up to discuss a possible merger between the NLN Council and NAHHA. Not surprisingly, there was resistance from each side. Griffith found a way to break the deadlock by asking the 36 largest agencies in the nation to join both organizations. Now they were in a position to exert some leverage—and they did.

The groups continued to meet once a month at the airport hotel in Dallas, paying their own way to the meetings. Little by little, differences were resolved. A mission statement for the new organization was finally hammered out and an interim board was appointed, consisting of the full boards of both organizations. Don W. Wortley was elected interim chairman. He and Griffith continued to work out last-minute problems and were in charge of hiring a new executive. Formal merger took place on March 10, 1982. In September the first elections were held and Elsie Griffith was elected chair.

It is testimony to Griffith's ability that the two groups merged in the first place. Even thereafter, the betting line was that the new organization, the National Association for Home Care (NAHC), would not survive. It is a tribute to Griffith that membership increased at a dizzy pace, from an initial membership of 400 established through the merger to more than 4,000 at the completion of her term in 1986.

During her term, two other competitors merged with NAHC. Top-flight educational programs were offered. A public interest law firm and a subsidiary, the Hospice Association of America, were established. A highly regarded monthly magazine called *CARING* and weekly newsletter, *NAHC Report,* were created. The association, through increased clout, enjoyed unparalleled success in the legislative and regulatory arenas.

The secret of NAHC's success was the fact that Elsie Griffith never lost sight of the clients and their needs. She and the organization placed the needs of chronically ill children, the disabled, and dying as their top priority, the rationale being that if these disadvantaged groups benefit, those organizations who care for them will also do just fine. In other words, the concept of service by definition means putting the needs of others first. This is as true for an organization as it is for individuals.

The Visiting Nurse Service of New York

In late 1982, the Visiting Nurse Service of New York, the nation's largest home care agency, had a vacancy with the retirement of the respected executive director, Ann Marie Thom. A national search firm was employed to find the best and most qualified person in the nation to head the program. It was no surprise that Elsie Griffithwas selected for the job, or that she experienced great success in the position.

Griffith joined the New York Visiting Nurse Service in January of 1983. At that time, the full-time staff of 1,200 and numerous part-time employees were spread throughout half a dozen buildings. The agency was making a million visits a year and had an annual budget of some $40 million. Griffith consolidated the offices and brought in top-notch fundraisers, who increased revenues by several million dollars. She diversified the agency's income sources, expanding service to private paying clients and opening for-profit subsidiaries.

Another of her major achievements, which has already paid dividends, is the networking and links to the community. Griffith, like her father before her, has become involved in numerous social causes outside of home care. She has fostered good relations with senior citizen organizations and consumer groups. She worked with hospitals in the New York area, showing them that the VNS was a friend and ally and that it was in the hospital's economic and political best interest that they work together.

Having turned over the reigns in New York to well-qualified people, Griffith returned to Texas in 1990 and enrolled in the University of Texas to study medical ethics. Griffith believes that this will be the next major field with profound effect on the nation's seniors, given the suggestions concerning the rationing of health care, which have grown out of deep concerns about the budget deficit. Griffith has also offered her impressive executive management skills and unparalleled know-how as a consultant to the nation's home care industry. She continues to apply her vision—and the nation's sick elderly, chronically ill children, and the disabled stand to benefit. Elsie Griffith remains today one of the nation's most caring innovators—and most effective managers. It is an extremely impressive combination.

Views

In a wide-ranging 1990 interview, Elsie Griffith was asked for her views on the issues. As can be seen from what follows, she remains as candid and insightful as ever.

When asked who were the most influential people in her life, she cites her father, Hershel Ingram, saying, "He was a real humanitarian. If he only had $5 he would give it to someone who was in need. He challenged me and expected me to be superior in many ways." She also mentioned Hedwig Cohen of the NLN and Bea Haggerty, president of the Visiting Nurse Association of Dallas, as well as Dale Henning, a professor of organizational business planning at the University of Washington in Seattle. Finally, she mentioned Lillian Wald:

> Generally, I have always admired the American pioneers, that is, anyone who opened up new territories. I have always admired Lillian Wald, founder of the Henry Street Settlement in New York, which later became the Visiting Nurse Service of New York. She was the first person who started public health nursing in the United States. She was really the founder of home care and the first one

who took health services into personal care in the home. She was also a woman who was able to attract philanthropy and dollars into home care as well as being a political activist. She was able to inspire a lot of young women to come into the home care movement. In going around the country, I'm surprised to see how many young people still regard her as a role model.

Major Problems

When asked what are the biggest problems facing the nation, Griffith's thoughts go to health care, manpower, and education:

> I think we have fewer young people going into the service fields today. There will be a problem because of this in the future. I think that where the young people will be going is into the technological fields, that these fields will be more attractive. I don't think the service fields have offered the challenges that other fields have offered. We haven't made it challenging and exciting. It could be that there are a lot of tired people in the service area. I also think that, from where I sit and from what I hear, one of the biggest problems is that our educational system is not challenging students enough and not keeping up-to-date with the world. I'm very concerned about AIDS and homelessness and also how we can begin to make strides by using the brainpower of our elderly citizens.

Asked to further comment on her views about the "graying of America," Griffith responded:

> In one sentence, I feel that elderly Americans are the ones who need to have a role in solving their own problems. They need to be involved in coming up with solutions. For too long, other groups—young people, social workers, and so forth—have looked at these problems and come up with solutions. I think the answers lie within elders themselves. I have spoken to different groups and I remember talking to one group of elderly women over 65 who just "wanted to be listened to." I don't think the various national organizations are really doing a big enough job in representing the elderly. They represent the insurance industry and other groups, but not the aged. And I particularly think the frail aged are not represented in any of these groups.

Griffith says she believes that seniors suffer a great deal because they do not know what their role is in society:

> There is no question that depression is one of the biggest illnesses in older citizens and that the suicide rate among elders is higher than among teenagers now. I once met a man who was losing his voice simply because he wasn't using it. But, in a lot of ways, the older population is a whole subculture. They have many supports among themselves. I think that if communication networks were used as much as they could be, we could alleviate a lot of loneliness.

Griffith believes that a great deal more must be done to prevent the degradation of the environment:

> This is a huge concern of mine. One of my biggest concerns is water pollution. This is the biggest crime against the environment that we have. We can't do enough on this problem. I recall a few years ago eating a fish that had come out of one of the Great Lakes. After eating this fish, I had to be rushed to the emergency room because the pollution in the Great Lake had gotten into the fish. On the other hand, we haven't fully explored the good things that all of our bodies of water could do for us. We haven't plumbed the good opportunities that we might.

Opportunities

When asked to talk about the greatest opportunities presently available in America, she responded:

> The greatest opportunities are in communication networks and the types of communications that we have. I don't think that we have begun to scratch the surface of how we can tie people at home into a support network. I think the availability of radio communications presents a lot of opportunities that have not been tapped. There could be an explosion in home care if we were to make use of this technology.

Griffith believes with Buckminster Fuller that we must find ways to convert weaponry into livingry. This means there is a need to cut the defense budget and to increase allotments for social programs, particularly education:

> Certainly, I think a lot more needs to be spent on taking care of societal ills, particularly within the educational system. Our educational system needs an overhaul and an upgrade. It seems to be

> operating just as it was years ago and that the world and the kids are passing it by. In fact, I like Ross Perot's idea that children should go to school like adults go to work—that is, they should go to school year-round. They should have two to three weeks vacation a year just like their parents do and not get three months off each year. Since 75 percent of women will be working (65percent of childbearing women currently are in the work force), there is no one for the kids to go home to. Perot looks toward using more of a child's brain than is currently being used. He believes there should be longer school days, that we should be teaching languages in our schools so our children can become world citizens.

Griffith believes the remainder of the 20th century provides great opportunities for human maturity:

> I think human maturity involves really taking responsibility for the quality of life of other human beings. That taking responsibility is what makes a person mature. This is more what Victor Frankl was saying—that people who give up under the weight of problems are really those who don't take responsibility for moving forward. They expect someone else, some other group, to do this for them.

Griffith believes that the solidarity of the American family should be America's most important value. She believes that bold new initiatives are needed to encourage the development of and support for the family structure:

> I think that there is a cohesion of family no matter where they are. The average family now moves about 10 times in a lifetime, so the chance of having extended family relationships in one area must decrease, but that must be the challenge: how to keep the family unit strong. I do think that it is something the government must be concerned about, it should be at the top of the agenda for the 1990s. We should be sure that the American family has a unit of familial relationships going on, although all the family members are out working and only see each other an hour a day. It is important to forming their backgrounds—what they'll be in the future.

Griffith is an optimist. She believes that America will rise to the challenge. She believes further that the salvation, whether for the individual or for the nation, lies in the love, understanding, and caring of one human being for another:

We can certainly hope that America will rise to the challenge. It is a matter of one plus one plus one plus one. It has to start somewhere. The most important elements are the love and the care, that it's not so important to have the understanding. We can't always wait for ethnic understanding or for the rich to understand the poor. We can try to understand, but even without having that, we can go ahead and take responsibility for other people. It definitely is a matter of neighbor to neighbor; it starts in small cells and moves out from there.

When asked if she has a favorite book, quotation, or poem, she responded:

I especially like *The Metamorphosis* by Kafka because of how the characters handled the disabled, the crippled, and so forth. I still have not read enough of this book, and I've read it many times.

I don't really have a favorite quotation or poem, but I do use something that Dale Henning said. He said that when you can see a giraffe go by your 24th-floor office window and you're able to say, "Gee, I should have expected that," then you've really arrived as a health care administrator. Expect the unexpected; try not to be thrown by things. Using this philosophy helps me get through, especially when dealing with people. It prevents me from putting them in boxes.

Learned and Remembered

Elsie Griffith says the most important lesson she has learned in her life is to look within oneself:

The most important lesson I've learned is that when times are tough or when problems occur, the first place you look is inside yourself. When times are really tough, you have to help yourself first, to look to yourself, before going outside and asking for help.

When asked how she would like to be remembered, she said:

I'd like to be remembered as somebody who pushed out the boundaries of home care—pushed it out further than when I found it. I'd also like to think that I've given some support and encouragement to young staff people in home care and been able to support other home care administrators and boards through difficult times and also helped in getting the service out to the people.

Elsie Griffith will be remembered by future generations for preparing the way for the increasing numbers of Americans who will survive into their eighth decade and beyond. She helped create the highly professional modern day home care industry and managed to do so while keeping all the elements of quality and personal service that have marked home care from its earliest days in America some 100 years ago. She helped educate the media and elected representatives as to the importance of home care, which is today the fastest growing portion of the American health care system. Thanks to her efforts, America, like Europe, is on its way to bringing health care and supportive services back home where they belong.

——— ❧ ———

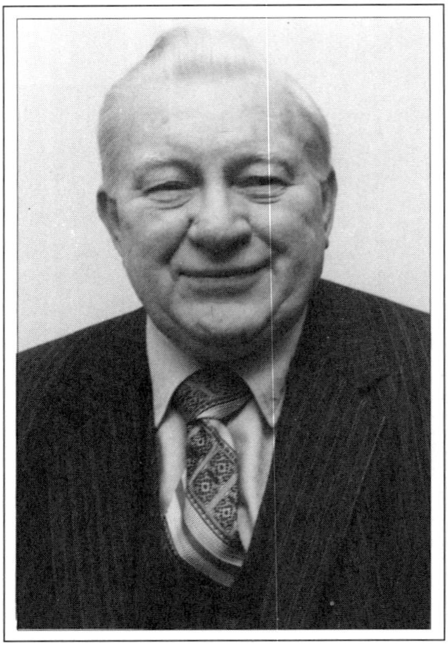

COURTESY OF WILLIAM HUTTON

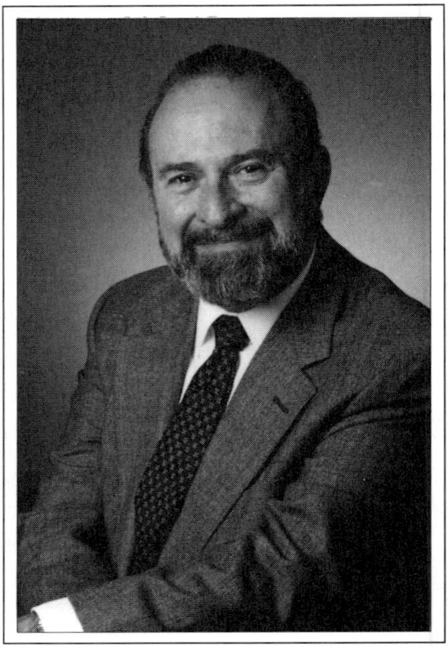

COURTESY OF JACK OSSOFSKY

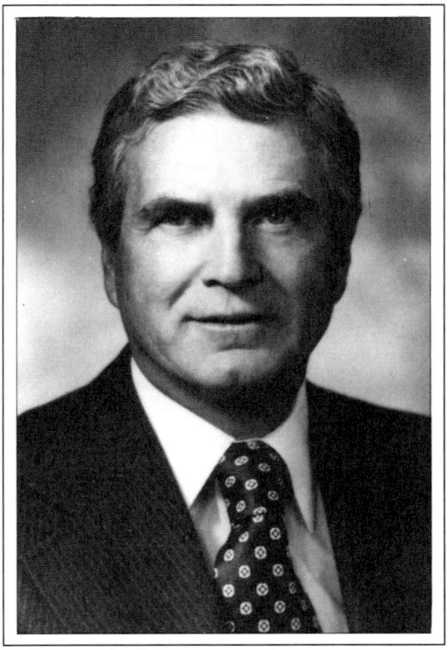

COURTESY OF CYRIL BRICKFIELD, AARP

THIRTEEN

William R. Hutton, Jack Ossofsky and Cyril F. Brickfield

Among insiders in the field of aging, they were known simply by their last names: Hutton, Ossofsky, and Brickfield. More often than not, the names were strung together and uttered simultaneously, giving the impression that they might be a law firm or a stock brokerage. They were, in fact, leaders of the three major organizations representing the interests of older Americans in Washington, D.C., and across the nation.

Each of them played a pivotal role in the growth of their organization. Each of them served in the top position, providing guidance and direction. Each of them served for more than 20 years, providing a measure of continuity. Each of them, although strong individuals with markedly different styles and personalities, was amazingly successful. More to the point, they worked together; they were a team.

They had their differences, of course, and in a way they were competitors; but to their credit, they never allowed minor differences to cloud or interfere with their common goal: advancing the interests of the nation's senior citizens.

William R. Hutton was the colorful and charismatic leader of the National Council of Senior Citizens (NCSC). A newspaperman by training, he produced *Senior Citizen News* and built a powerful grass roots network, which was one of the major reasons why seniors have been so successful in achieving their legislative goals during the last quarter of a century. Under Hutton's leadership, the membership of

NCSC increased from a handful to more than four million.

Jack Ossofsky is the man who forged the National Council of Aging (NCOA), increasing its yearly revenues from $1 million to more than $40 million, and he led the fight against age discrimination in employment. He was the "champion of choices," fighting to help seniors retain as many options as possible and thereby the ability to control their own lives.

Cyril F. Brickfield is the genius who transformed the American Association of Retired Persons (AARP) from a sleepy organization of one million members to a roster of some 30 million people. His publication *Modern Maturity* has the widest circulation of any magazine in America. By some people's accounts, AARP is now the most powerful organization in Washington, D.C.

These three men understood the lesson of Aesop's parable of the sticks: in unity there is strength. Together, they made "senior power" a reality. The organizations they constructed and nourished will continue to serve seniors and the nation for many years to come. Their organizations will continue to conduct research, to disseminate information, to help people, and to educate. Most important of all, they will continue their advocacy role, fighting for legislative solutions to ongoing problems before the Congress and the state legislatures.

Although Hutton, Ossofsky, and Brickfield have retired from their positions, all three are keeping busy, continuing their fight to improve the quality of life for seniors. Because of their contributions past and present, the team of Hutton, Ossofsky, and Brickfield has earned a place in the senior citizens' hall of honor.

William R. Hutton

William R. Hutton was born on November 2, 1916, in the town of Sunderland in the north of England. He takes pride in the fact that his family lived only a mile or two from Washington, Durham County, the ancestral home of the early family of America's first president, George Washington.

Hutton's father, William Renzard Hutton, Sr., was a shipyard worker. His mother, Miriam Griffiths, was a homemaker and a chef.

Both parents were involved in community service. His mother was a volunteer who visited shut-ins and saw to their needs. Mr. and Mrs. Hutton were both very much involved in their church.

> Caring for others was very much a tradition in my family. I remember vividly a man, who was born without the use of his legs, who liked my parents and asked to move in with us. I called him "Uncle Jack" although he was no blood relation. Not only did he move in with us but Father used to carry the man on his back to church every Sunday, which was a distance of two miles to a street car and another two miles down by the river after the street car stop. It was not unusual for the man to attend both the morning and evening service which meant my Father made two round trips carrying "Uncle Jack" on his back. He did that without complaining all of my childhood until the time that I left to go to college.

Hutton's mother was known as a good soul and problem solver. Whatever the problem posed by a member of the community, she would try to solve it. Her fondness for the church rubbed off on, young Bill, who became a boy preacher. He even had the honor of warming up the crowd just prior to public appearances by Amy Semple McPherson, the American evangelist, during her first tour of England.

When Bill was ten years old, his mother told him to bring a lined tablet, some envelopes, and dark pen or pencil and to accompany her on visits to old folks homes. Young Bill volunteered to write letters for the elderly. He also read letters that the seniors received in return from their loved ones. He did this for several years.

> In this way, I became acquainted very early with the problems of the elderly. I identified with them and grew to like them a great deal. I had a great feeling of satisfaction in doing something for people who were crippled with arthritis or otherwise could not write for themselves. This knowledge of the elderly served me very well in my later years and I suppose that I always knew that I would spend some of my life working with the elderly.

Young Hutton was a gifted student. He completed his college education at the age of 19 and set out to follow his dream—to become a foreign correspondent for a major newspaper. Thanks to a strong reference from his mentor, journalism professor John Smithwhite, he received a post on the *Sunderland Echo*, the local newspaper with a daily circulation of about 300,000 people. He worked three years for the *Echo* and then two years for the *London Daily Mail* and simultaneously for *Reuters*, the international news service.

This promising journalism career was interrupted by World War II. Germany declared war on England in September of 1939. Bill Hutton joined the infantry and, following basic training, was immediately assigned to the Middle East. He was involved for the next six years in hand-to-hand combat. He fought behind enemy lines as part of something called the Long Range Desert Group with the British Eighth Army. The idea was counterintelligence and counter-insurgency—the purpose was to destroy as much of the enemy's war machine as possible from behind his own lines. From the Middle East, Hutton joined the 46th Infantry Division, which was sent to Italy and Anzio Beachhead—one of the bloodiest battles of the war. Young Hutton acquitted himself very well and was company commander of the Fifth Battalion, the Hampshire Regiment, which was sent to Greece, where their job was to diffuse the hundreds of thousands of mines that the Germans had placed on the Aegean Sea coastal areas. From Greece it was on to Yugoslavia and finally to Vienna. Major Hutton and many of his troops were demobilized and returned to England in the fall of 1945 after six years of war.

When Bill Hutton returned to England, he was reemployed as required by British law, except that British newspapers at the time were limited to only four pages because of the world shortage of newsprint. This meant there was little in the way of real work to do. Hutton volunteered for the Foreign Service. He was sent back to Vienna where he served as the public information officer for the British Army, the British Embassy, and the British Element of the Allied Commission for Austria.

Hutton stayed in Vienna from 1946 through 1949. It was there that he met his wife-to-be, Miriam Stearns, of Washington, D.C, who was employed in the U.S. Embassy. The couple became engaged in the summer of 1949 and decided to make their home in America following a December 17, 1949, marriage.

Bill Hutton took a temporary job as public information officer with the British Embassy in Washington, D.C., and joined the National Press Club. After two years in the nation's capital, he was assigned to a similar job representing the British government in the Midwest. On August 19, 1952, at the U.S. District Court in Chicago, Bill Hutton took the oath and became a naturalized citizen of the United States of America. It was one of the proudest moments of his life.

Two sons, Griffith and Glen, were born to the young couple; soon thereafter the Hutton family moved to New York City where Bill Hutton established his own public relations firm. For the next years, the firm prospered. Among other things, Hutton developed a series of instructional comic books. One subject was "How to Make Your Home Safe from Fire." These non-funny comic books were paid for by the city government, which distributed them to children through their school system. Additional clients included the U.S. Treasury and General Foods. But Hutton's greatest success was with the Master Newspaper Syndicate.

Hutton pioneered a way to prepare important news stories for distribution to weekly newspapers in ready-to-print form. The receiving paper incurred very little expense in the process of casting a matrix of a prepared story into type-metal. This took only a few minutes to cast and insert into the pages for printing. It was this distribution network and the fact that he wrote often of the elderly that brought Hutton to the attention of the Kennedy Administration.

In 1960, Hutton was asked to meet with the White House staff to discuss problems of the aged and to offer advice about how to bring about the enactment of President John F. Kennedy's proposed Medicare legislation. Hutton was engaged to write a series of articles to be distributed under the bylines of Secretary of Health, Education and Welfare, Abraham Ribicoff, Senator Pat McNamara, and Congressman Aimé J. Forand. He was given the green light to distribute these columns through his newspaper syndicate.

Hutton's stories appeared in some 5,000 newspapers and began a ground swell of interest in the health care problems of the aged.

Hutton also became involved in the building of a grass roots network designed to create pressure for Medicare from the bottom up, rather than assuming the measure could be won from the top down. He became a consultant to the National Council of Senior Citizens (NCSC), which was established in 1960 for the purpose of giving political clout to the nation's growing numbers of elderly. Retiring Congressman Forand of Rhode Island was elected its first president.

In February of 1962, Bill Hutton was hired by NCSC as press director and general manager. He was 46 years old and used his years of experience to set about the task of "giving senior citizens the tools they needed to fight for Medicare." His first move was to create a newspaper, *Senior Citizens News*, which served to unify, inform, and inspire seniors all across the nation. "We got seniors to realize that if Medicare was going to be enacted it had to be by them," Hutton said. NCSC encouraged seniors to establish clubs at the local church or the community center with the goal of both political advocacy and community service. "We told them that you've got to make America what you want it to be," remembers Hutton.

All the hard work paid off. At the Medicare signing ceremony, President Lyndon B. Johnson gave credit to Hutton and his army of seniors. He said there would have been no Medicare law but for the National Council of Senior Citizens.

It was a proud moment for Hutton, who held the reigns at NCSC for 26 years. Throughout his tenure, he put his heart and soul into the job. Membership increased from a dozen people to more than four million. Additional legislative successes followed, such as the Older Americans Act and the Medicare Amendments of 1972, which included the disabled under Medicare and created the Supplementary Security Income program as well as a 20 percent increase in Social Security benefits. Legislation in 1978 and 1988 served to abolish mandatory retirement.

Hutton retired as executive director of NCSC on February 1, 1988. On March 22, 1988, he was honored at a testimonial dinner in Washington, D.C. Jacob Clayman, president of NCSC, said at the time:

> It is impossible to assess his enormous contribution except to state that because of the work that he has done over the years—in

fighting for Medicare, Medicaid, Social Security, and other programs—life is far better for older Americans today than it was 25 years ago.

Perspective

When asked what gave him the greatest satisfaction, Bill Hutton said the enactment of Medicare. Asked if he had any regrets, he answered in the negative, saying that he felt he had been able to help people. He did add that he wished he had been able to spend more time with his family.

His most important role models, he said, were Professor Smithwhite, his father William Hutton, Sr., Senator Edward M. Kennedy, and Congressman Claude Pepper.

When asked what was the greatest need of the elderly, he mentioned long-term care and the need to provide seniors with in-home services. However, he sees this expansion of health care services as something that is equally important for young people as for seniors. The issue in long-term care is disability, not age, he said, while arguing that what is needed most of all is a comprehensive national health care system. He said it was tragic that the only two nations in the industrialized world that do not have such a plan are the U.S. and South Africa. Such failure has devastating consequences, not only to the people involved, but also in economic terms. Escalating health costs serve to increase the costs of many products, putting them at a competitive disadvantage in world markets, says Hutton.

But Bill Hutton is an optimist. He believes that the time for national health insurance is at hand.

> I think we are going to get it. I believe with the late Wilbur Cohen—a 52-year civil servant—that these things go in cycles. We have passed the point where we believed that government was the enemy of the people. People are increasingly coming to understand that government is nothing more than people cooperating to do together for each other what they cannot do for themselves.

When asked what advice he had for young people, he said: "Learn to be honest with yourself and with others. Find some outlet for the goodness within you. Do something that is bigger than yourself, something which benefits all of us. Take an interest in helping people."

In response to a similar question about what advice he has for senior citizens, Hutton, a poet himself, offered the work of William Allen Drumgoole. Drumgoole was a woman who was given a masculine name by her parents, who despaired that their sixth child, like all the others, was a girl. She was born in 1860 and died in 1932, having spent all of her life in Tennessee, where she worked for the *Nashville Banner,* and wrote over 7,500 poems and nine books. The poem, recalled by Hutton is entitled "The Bridge," and reads as follows:

> An old man, going a lone highway,
> Came at the evening, cold and grey
> To a chasm, vast and deep and wide,
> Through which there flowed a sullen tide,
> And the old man crossed in the twilight dim,
> For that sullen stream held no fear for him,
> But he turned, when he reached the other side,
> And built a bridge to span that tide.
>
> "Old man," cried a fellow pilgrim near,
> "You're wasting strength in building here.
> Your journey will end with the dying day,
> And you never again must pass this way,
> You have crossed the chasm, deep and wide,
> Why build you the bridge at the even tide?"
>
> And the builder lifted his old grey head,
> "Good friend, on the path I have come," he said,
> "There followeth after me today,
> A youth whose feet must pass this way,
> This chasm that has been naught to me,
> To that fair-haired youth may a pitfall be,
> He, too, must cross in the twilight dim,
> Good friend, I am building the bridge for him."

The implication of the poem is obvious—that old people must help the young, who in turn will help young people to understand the elderly. "Old people can do wonders with children and children do wonderful things for old people," says Hutton.

When asked how he would like to be remembered, he said, "As

someone who played a necessary role, who made a useful contribution. I wanted to leave the world a better place than when I found it, and I am very satisfied that I have done that."

Jack Ossofsky

Jack Ossofsky was born on September 24, 1925, in the Bronx, city and state of New York. His father, Harry, immigrated from Poland and worked in the garment trade as a dressmaker. Jack's mother, Mary Bugamolney, was born in the Ukraine in what is now the Soviet Union. She, too, worked in the factories of New York City as a blousemaker.

Young Jack attended New York public schools and enrolled in the College of the City of New York (CCNY) in 1943. After one semester, he dropped out to join the army. He was assigned to field artillery and received his honorable discharge in 1946.

Ossofsky returned to New York in that same year and took a job in the construction industry. He was married in 1947, and returned to college at night and later full time. He graduated from CCNY with a B.A. degree in economics in 1950.

Ossofsky volunteered as a union organizer for District 65 of the Retail, Wholesale and Department Workers Union. His efforts as a volunteer proved to be highly effective because of his natural empathy with people. This led to an offer to join the union as a paid staff member. This was an extraordinary tribute to his abilities. The union had a policy of requiring people to prove their mettle before they were hired. Equally unprecedented was the responsibilities they gave him: he was put in charge of the implementation of the union's new pension plan.

"My job was to learn about pensions, and to make ours the best that it could be, to be the union's voice on Social Security and to find a means of organizing retirees into a cohesive structure so that they continued to feel some connection to the workers," remembers Ossofsky.

The union was the first to think broadly about retirement and the first to implement a retirement preparation program. Under Ossofsky's guidance, a trial program was established. In effect, this was a leave of absence granted for the purpose of letting workers see if they would enjoy retirement. The union, with the support of management, also pioneered the first prototype of the modern senior citizen center. The shape of all of these programs was suggested by the retirees themselves. The intent of the programs was to provide a continuity of experience at a time when workers faced wrenching changes in their lives.

The retirees elected their own leaders at the same time and in the same election as the union members chose their shop stewards. Their dues were minimal, but they were still required to pay. The title of the retirees' officers corresponded to that of the union officers who were still employed. Retirees were allowed to participate in meetings with both labor leaders and with management. In short, the retirees were given definite, tangible roles. They were empowered with rights and authority. "My perception was that I was there to serve them as a staff member might serve a congressman. This is when I learned that it was important to do things with the elderly rather than for them," says Ossofsky.

In the course of learning how to do his job better, Ossofsky came into contact with Ollie A. Randall and Geneva Mathiasen, two of the founders of the National Council on the Aging (NCOA), which had been established in 1950. The New York-based organization was created as an information clearinghouse to focus voluntary programs on the needs of older Americans.

Ossofsky became involved as a member of NCOA while he continued his work with the union. The success of his work was such that it soon inspired the work of others. Charles Odell of the United Auto workers and James O'Brien of the United Steelworkers of America soon began to implement some of his ideas at the national level at their unions.

"There were not very many of us working in the field of aging in the halcyon days of the early 1950s, but there were some great leaders such as Ms. Randall, Ms. Mathiasen, as well as Clark Tibbitts and Wilma Donahue of the University of Michigan. It was a period of new knowledge, great solidarity, and the keen sense that we were on to something new and exciting," says Ossofsky.

Ossofsky continued to work for District 65 through 1965 and to volunteer a great deal of his time working with NCOA. He instituted new programs, encouraging retirees to become involved not only in political action, but also in community service. At his urging, retirees created a toy workshop where they repaired children's toys free-of-charge. Volunteers raised money for the American Cancer Society. Arts programs were organized for the community by the retirees, who taught children and adults in the community such things as how to paint and play the guitar. Needless to say, this program created goodwill for the union, which invested still more of its resources in expanding the operation.

In the early 1960s, Ossofsky became more involved in politics. He helped organize a grass roots effort to focus attention on the need for the enactment of Medicare. He was one of the convenors of the New York State Conference on Aging and helped fashion the agenda for the 1961 White House Conference on Aging.

He left the union in 1965 on a one year leave of absence to direct an antipoverty program for NCOA. These were the days of President Lyndon Johnson's war on poverty, and America had focused much of its attention and money on breaking the cycle of impoverishment among its young people. Ossofsky and NCOA pointed out that 30 percent of seniors had incomes placing them below the poverty line and that they should not be ignored in the process. As Ossofsky puts it, the one year leave of absence lasted twenty-three years.

At NCOA he used his inventive mind to create new prototypes which went on to become successful national programs. Ossofsky's Operation TLC became the Foster Grandparents Program in which senior citizens work with young people. Operation Loaves and Fishes was the predecessor of today's congregate meals program authorized under the Older Americans Act. He created Project Find, which was designed to locate and identify those seniors living in poverty and hidden from view. Another program called Medicare Alert helped to locate and sign up seniors who were eligible for Medicare when this new program was created.

Ossofsky's successful programs simultaneously contained several elements. They provided employment and income for seniors. They helped to document the needs of this group and to provide them with necessary services. In addition, these programs created publicity and increased public recognition for the problems of seniors, created a cadre of older advocates, and helped create new professions in gerontology. It is testimony to the success of these programs that they survive today, most of them being administered by the Administration on Aging or ACTION, and yet most people have long since forgotten their origins. "Success has many fathers but failure is an orphan," comments Ossofsky wryly.

As time passed, Jack Ossofsky was elevated to leadership positions at NCOA. First as associate director, then deputy director, and in 1971, he was named to the top post. As executive director, he continued his work to develop new models of service and to convince corporations of the vital contribution that could be made by the elderly if they were given a chance to remain (or reenter) the workplace. He described his mission in terms of developing choices and options for seniors. Individual liberty is meaningless without choices, he once said.

> The greatest loss in aging is not the loss of physical stamina or abilities or economic loss, rather it is the loss of freedom which means a restriction in choices. Personal dignity is intrinsically tied up with the notion of choices and exercising the power of decision. The most debilitating thing you can do to a senior is to take his or her choices away and step in and manage their affairs for them. Work with them, help them develop new options but don't manage them or their affairs.

Ossofsky played an important role in the 1971 White House Conference on Aging, which he said was disappointing by comparison with its 1961 predecessor and yet it was "pretty wonderful" when compared with the 1981 conference. He credits Dr. Arthur Flemming for salvaging the 1971 conference. The 1981 conference, he explained, was marked by political maneuvering by those trying to limit free debate and restrict the recommendations. For example, he cited one committee packed with hand-picked delegates who were programmed to vote for a repeal to the automatic cost of living increases which had been authorized by the Congress in 1972 to help seniors keep up with the pace of inflation. As the leader of the coalition of organizations representing seniors, Ossofsky, together with Congressman Claude Pepper, led a demonstration and protest that garnered national media attention. The onerous proposal was quietly pulled back in the face of a violent reaction from both delegates and seniors across America, who had heard of the scheme through the abundant television coverage.

Ossofsky and NCOA paid the price for standing up for principle. Even though many of the board were Republicans, NCOA lost government contracts, leading many to conclude that the organization was being blackballed. These were tough times, and Ossofsky was forced to do more fundraising among private corporations to makeup for lost government funds. He also had to cut staff, close field offices, and reduce services.

When asked what was his proudest achievement, Ossofsky said it was holding together his organization during these difficult times and the fact that he resisted the political pressure exerted against him, continuing to stand up for his principles. He also mentioned the advertising campaign he developed that received national acclaim and established the fact that a rocking chair was an inappropriate symbol to describe the senior citizens of America.

When asked who were his heroes and role models, he mentioned Ollie Randall, Geneva Mathiasen, Arthur Flemming, and Congressman Claude Pepper. He said that Congressman Pepper taught him one of the most important lessons—how to win and how to lose while maintaining one's dignity. "Most of all don't grind it in when you've won. Leave the other person as much dignity as you can," he remembered Pepper saying.

When asked to name the foremost problems of the elderly, he said that long-term care was the most serious need. He said that there is a need to provide seniors with new options in the form of day care, expanded home care, respite care, and institutional care where necessary. He said that this must be done within the context of a national health system.

Another troubling issue, he said, was the continuing temptation to chip away at the Social Security program. He said what is at stake is nothing more or less than the confidence of citizens in their government. Government must keep its promises if it expects citizens to meet the responsibilities it imposes on them, he said.

He also expressed concern for the current tendency to support "case management" and to see it as a panacea and solution to the escalating costs of health care. "I am not a case and I don't want someone to manage me," he said. He stated that there is something fundamentally wrong with the notion of investing someone with authority and a job title to manage the affairs of other people. He said that case management restricts options and reduces freedom in the area of personal and medical care which cries out for the opposite—namely the involvement of the patient and his family and not just paid caregivers in making the decision as to what medical, nursing, or personal care regimens he or she should receive.

Finally, he said he was concerned about the proliferation of the myth that senior citizens have received an unfair portion of national resources. "The notion that we have done enough for the elderly is false, and through circulation it tends to undermine the self-esteem of the elderly. They begin to feel guilty for receiving the retirement benefits that they have worked so hard to secure for themselves," he said.

When asked what advice he can offer young people, he said:

> I would tell them that you can't do it alone. We so value independence and that is appropriate, but at the same time people should know that there is nothing wrong with interdependence. We cherish the caregiver but we should also cherish the care recipient. All of us in our time play many parts. There are times when we help others and there are times when we should look to others for help. Don't try to do everything alone; learn the importance of doing things cooperatively.

He also said he would teach young people to reject the legacy of the Reagan years, which held government as the enemy of the people and at the same time exalted individualism, exemplified in what sociologists refer to as the "me generation." "Government should be seen for what it is, an instrument of progress through cooperation," he said.

He also said that he would encourage young people to seek to field of aging as a profession because of the rewards it offers and the opportunity for service. He said he would advise them to remember the individual. "Think always of the welfare of individual people and not more globally of some amorphous group of people with common needs. If the needs of individuals are met, then by extension so will the needs of others like them who are similarly situated."

When asked how he would like to be remembered, he said, "as someone who tried to help others, to leave the world a bit better than he found it, and who retained his integrity in the process."

Congressman Claude Pepper said that Jack Ossofsky will be remembered for his role in building NCOA into "the nation's foremost group dedicated to improving the quality of life for older Americans." Ossofsky's entire life and career, he said "has been directed toward how we as individuals and collectively as a society can best work together to help those in need. All of us in America who care about the elderly are deeply grateful for the contributions he has made on their behalf," concluded the Congressman in a March 6, 1985, tribute to Jack Ossofsky carried in the *Congressional Record.*

Cyril F. Brickfield

Cy Brickfield was born in Brooklyn, city of New York, in 1920. His father was a clerk in the local courthouse and a strict Catholic. He raised Cy and his four brothers with a firm hand. He taught the boys to love God and to respect their mother, and the importance of serving other people.

Even though the elder Brickfield made a fair wage, it was still rough raising a family of five boys during the Great Depression. The young men, of course, helped with the chores and took small jobs, when they could find them, to help support the family. Over family dinner, they listened to their father tell them of the value of a good education and hint broadly that the practice of law might offer good opportunities for young men in search of a career.

For Cy, the road to law school was not automatic. He graduated from high school in 1937 and from college in 1941, just in time to fight in World War II. He joined the United States Air Force and became a bomber pilot, flying B-17s into Europe and Africa. In all, Brickfield flew 57 missions, mostly in Germany and Italy. He received his honorable discharge in 1945, retiring from the service with the rank of Major.

When he returned to the United States, Brickfield says he was unsure of what to do with himself. Fortunately, he and his family had a good friend in Judge Albert Conway of the New York State Court of Appeals, which in New York is the equivalent of the U.S. Supreme Court. Brickfield says that the judge, like his father, was one of those people who had a strong influence on his life. He persuaded Brickfield to take the plunge, and in 1948 Brickfield graduated with distinction from Fordham Law School. He passed the New York Bar and went to work as a clerk to Judge Conway in Albany, where he worked through 1951. During this time, Brickfield married and had two children. In 1951, he was courted away by Congressman Emanual Celler of New York, then-Chairman of the Committee on the Judiciary of the House of Representatives, and the Brickfield family moved to Washington.

Congressman Celler was a giant in the landscape of Congress, respected far and wide for his keen mind, his leadership, and his hard work. The congressman was a civil rights activist long before it became popular to be one; he fought hard to protect civil liberties of all kinds as guaranteed to Americans in the Bill of Rights.

"He worked hard in his quiet determined way, he truly believed in social justice and he never compromised his principles," says Brickfield of his mentor. "We all used to strive to be like him. He wouldn't leave each night until all the paper was cleared off his desk and neither would we. Sometimes we would be there until 10 p.m. and we enjoyed it because we knew what we were involved in was important and would make a difference," remembers Brickfield.

In 1961, following the election of President John F. Kennedy, Brickfield was appointed general counsel of the Veteran's Administration. He stayed at the VA for six years, during which time he was promoted to the post of chief benefits director and then to deputy administrator, the number two job in the department. His successes there were many. For example, he was the architect of an ambitious program that for the first time covered long-term care in the context of veteran's benefits. Working with Paul Haber, he developed the VA nursing home and home health care programs that are in existence today. Obviously, this work has been of major importance to the nation's veterans and to their families. His work for the aged veteran was a harbinger of things to come.

During the years in which he worked for the VA, Brickfield somehow found the time to sharpen his educational skills. He went to school at night and obtained a master's degree in law, a doctorate in law, and a masters' in public administration. He gained admission to the District of Columbia Bar and he taught at George Washington University. In 1967, he was hired as Executive Director of AARP.

AARP

The American Association of Retired Persons began as a dream of its founder, Dr. Ethel Percy Andrus, a retired teacher and high school principal from Los Angeles, California. On her retirement in 1944, Andrus became a volunteer director of welfare for the California Teacher's Association. It was in this position that she learned of the needs of the aged and developed her philosophy of the importance of helping them to lead useful lives with a maximum degree of human dignity.

In 1947, Andrus founded the National Retired Teachers' Association (NRTA). She had a gift for writing and she used it to communicate with the American public through the medium of a magazine she called *Modern Maturity*. Eleven years later, Andrus founded AARP saying, "Perhaps we retired persons other than teachers, too, feel the need to have a function in society, to have a respected place in the eyes of others, to be doing something that is interesting and significant in our own eyes, to have a national voice. AARP is a voluntary group which pledges to find for its members the maximum of common interests, to invite older folks to take an active role in meeting resourcefully the needs of all phases of the lengthening life span."

Cy Brickfield speaks reverently of Andrus, who died in 1967, the same year that he was named executive director of AARP. He gives her the primary credit for what his association has become. It was her hard work and vision, he insists, and that of the AARP board of directors, that have made the organization the important force that it is today.

From being relatively equal in size to NTRA when he was hired, AARP soon dwarfed its parent. In 1971, the two entities merged, and the AARP name was carried forward.

Under the direction of Brickfield, AARP increased from about 1 million members to more than 25 million at the time of his retirement in 1988. Total assets, gross revenues, the size of the staff, and the legislative accomplishments of the organization all grew exponentially. Today, AARP houses more than 1,000 staff and countless volunteers in new headquarters at 6th and F Street, N.W., in Washington, D.C. A larger number are housed in AARP's Long Beach headquarters for *Modern Maturity*, the bimonthly publication that boasts the largest circulation of any publication in America.

Exact numbers are a closely guarded secret, but best estimates place AARP's total assets at near $10 billion. Their yearly revenues exceed $500 million a year. While AARP's 30 million members pay only $5 a year in dues, AARP raises money through the mail order sale of prescription medicines, sick room supplies, and other health care projects. They have their own money market fund and generate millions in dollars from the insurance products they sell to the members in cooperation with the Prudential Insurance Company of America.

Among its good works, AARP has established the Ethel Percy Andrus Center on Gerontology at the University of Southern California. The Center was the first of its kind dedicated to research in the field of aging.

Honors

Brickfield has received several significant honors. For example, in 1968 he was elected president of the prestigious Federal Bar Association in Washington, D.C. He has served as chairman of the Leadership Council of Aging organizations, a coalition of 39 organizations representing the nation's elderly. He has served as president of the National Senior Citizens Law Center, which is affiliated with the University of Southern California. He was a member of the Advisory Council for the 1981 White House Conference on Aging, and he was selected to represent the United States as a delegate to the World Assembly on Aging held in Vienna in 1982.

When asked if he has any regrets, Brickfield responded in the negative. Asked what were his most satisfying moments, he mentioned his part in the enactment of major legislative initiatives. Specifically, he mentioned the law barring mandatory retirement, the creation of the Older Americans Act, the extension of Medicare benefits to the disabled, the 20 percent increase in Social Security benefits enacted in 1972, together with the provision that guaranteed automatic cost-of-living increases. When asked what was the low point, he said in 1981—when the Reagan Administration sought to cut $90 billion in Social Security benefits.

In December of 1984, Brickfield addressed a conference jointly sponsored by AARP, the National Association for Home Care, and the National Governor's Conference. The purpose of the conference was to promote long-term care insurance. In that speech, he made it clear that long-term care was a major item on his agenda. He said that he and AARP were committed to providing both public and private assistance to meet the burgeoning costs of long-term care. In his remarks, he pointed out that those over age 85, who are most likely to need long-term care, will double by the end of this century and increase more than five fold by the year 2050. He announced that AARP and Prudential will be marketing an insurance policy to help cover the costs of home care. "Among our members, there was an overwhelming preference for home care rather than nursing home care," he said.

Brickfield went on to say that since "only 5 percent of our older people are confined to the nursing home we need services that will help the remaining 95 percent lead active lives and remain in their homes as long as possible." He added, "The main objective of our Association is to create a society in which older citizens can live with a sense of personal dignity and independence. Our older citizens have made a great contribution to this nation, and the majority of them can continue to make a contribution."

When asked about the most important issues facing seniors in the future, he again mentioned long-term care as the greatest need. He said that ways must be found to insure cost containment and to stretch relatively scarce dollars to cover ever-increasing health care needs. He said that home care and hospice should be encouraged because they provide seniors with options and because most seniors prefer to receive care at home rather than an institutional setting. The fact that such services are generally less costly than institutionalization is an important side benefit, he said.

Asked what he had learned, he stressed the importance of service to others and of perseverance. "I remember Congressman Celler used to say, 'One man who is right is a majority.' I don't think I'll ever forget what he said," remembers Brickfield.

On the occasion of Brickfield's retirement from AARP, Congressman Claude Pepper lauded his achievements on behalf of seniors, saying Brickfield was "a true gentleman and as bright a mind as there is to be found in Washington."

Summary

The senior citizens of the United States have been fortunate indeed to have Bill Hutton, Jack Ossofsky, and Cy Brickfield step forward to center stage at the time that they did. These three men were blessed with the vision and the organizational skills to forge powerful national organizations that became the unified and effective voice for seniors. They gave expression and meaning to the term "senior power" and forever changed the American political landscape. As a result of their increasing numbers and their sophisticated organizational structure represented by AARP, NCSC, and NCOA, the elderly of America grew from a virtual invisible force to one of universal recognition and unrivaled power. Hutton, Ossofsky, and Brickfield left a lasting legacy. If their successors continue to work together and continue to focus not on selfish, institutional goals, but on the needs of America's senior citizens, the result will be still brighter tomorrows for the nation's elderly.

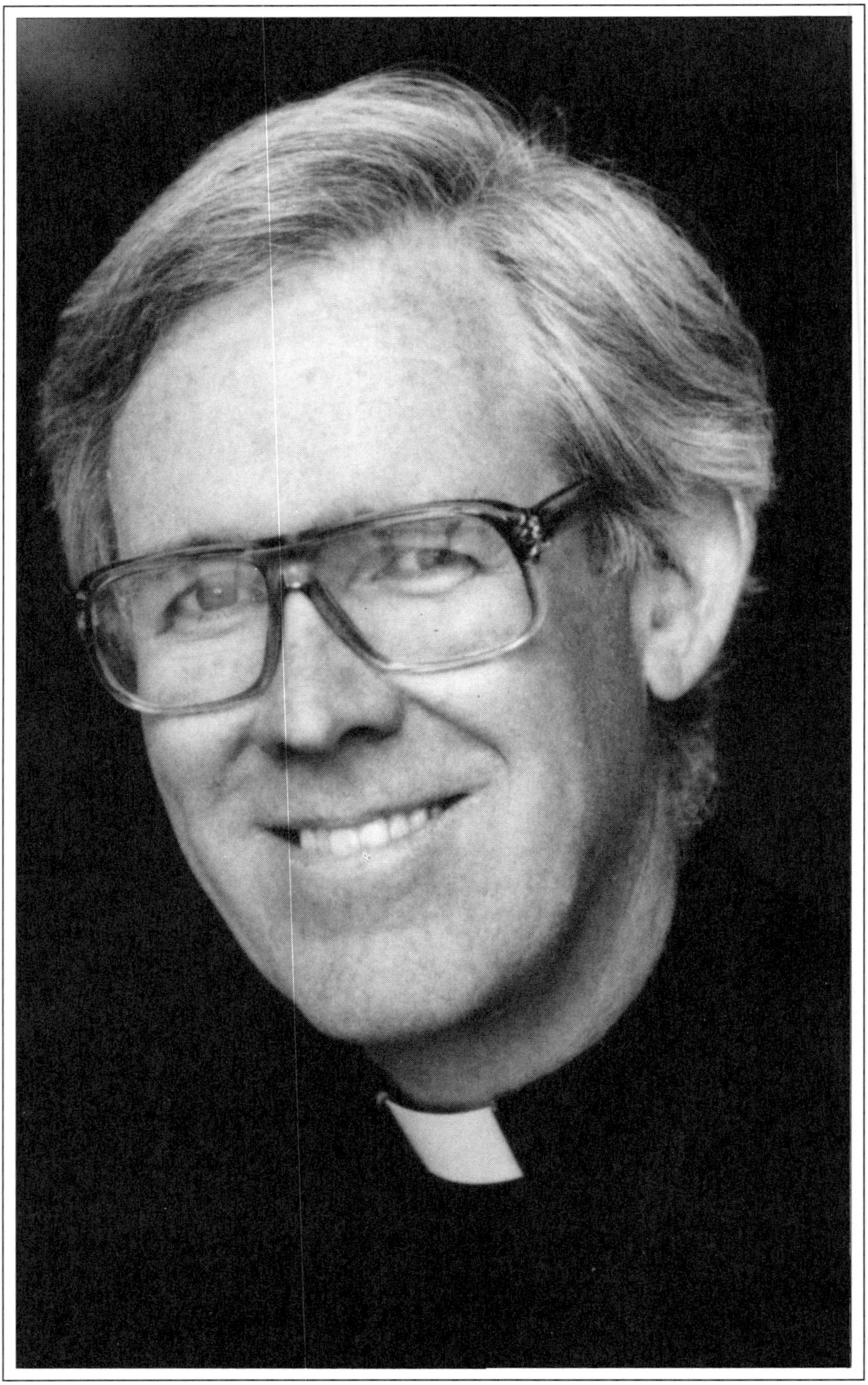

COURTESY OF MONSIGNOR CHARLES FAHEY

FOURTEEN

Charles J. Fahey

Television and the movies have given the world romantic images of Roman Catholic priests. Bing Crosby, Spencer Tracy, Humphrey Bogart, Robert Duvall, and others have all portrayed heroic figures who are the personification of all the great virtues. They are what human beings have aspired to be in the ideal, but so seldom have become in reality. These heroic portrayals based on the lives of real-life clerics have lead some people to believe that perfection in mankind is only found among those who have been ordained as priests.

Whether this is true or not, there is no mistaking the fact that priests, nuns, and religious leaders of other denominations constitute a group of the most caring people on earth. These are the people who on a daily basis come into contact with the miracles of life. They have seen life at its best and life at its worst. They also know the great secret of life: Do unto others as you would have done unto you. They know you get back what you give. They also understand that the true measure of a life is the extent to which it is used to help others.

Monsignor Charles Fahey is in real life the best of what has been portrayed on the movie screen. Not even Spencer Tracy or Humphrey Bogart could summon up the ability to translate to the world the goodness, wisdom, and virtue that emanates from Monsignor Fahey.

Fahey stands tall at six feet four inches. He is thin as a rail, but still a strong and imposing figure. He has the bearing of a scholar and he is, in fact, a great intellectual. He projects a certain warmth and charisma, common to all the world's great religious leaders, and he is one of the most articulate people on the face of the planet.

Fahey has spent his time in service to God and humanity. He has devoted all of his life in service to both. He has been involved in direct, hands-on care; he has supervised the massive Catholic Charities program; and for the last dozen years, he has been a teacher.

Fahey stands tall not only in stature, but in his contributions to the field of aging. He, more than anyone else, has helped focus attention on the question of what seniors should do with their time following retirement. There are only two choices he suggests: contribution or stagnation. He has stood without apology, encouraging the elderly of the United States to choose action over inaction, engagement over disengagement. He believes that there can be no meaning in life unless it is used actively to make life better for others.

Fahey has also helped pave the way for public action on the devastating problem of long-term care. He believes that the time has arrived to come to grips with the problem of disability. He has been an advocate all his life for social and racial justice and for reclaiming those lives that have been relegated to the sidelines of life because of disability.

He has led an exemplary life and he deserves the commendation of the American people everywhere because of his contributions to their common welfare.

Background

Charles J. Fahey was born in Baltimore, Maryland, on April 13, 1933, to Charles and Elizabeth Fahey. Young Charles spent only a brief time in Maryland, moving with his parents to Boston and ultimately to Syracuse, New York, where he spent most of his life.

He attended the Blessed Sacrament School and Christian Brothers Academy, both in Syracuse. From 1951–53, he enrolled in St. Andrew's Seminary, in Rochester, New York, and from 1953–59 he attended St. Bernard's Seminary in that same city. He was ordained a priest in the Roman Catholic Church on February 2, 1959.

His first assignment was assistant pastor at St. Vincent de Paul Church in Syracuse, New York, a post he held from February 1959 through February 1961. "I spent two very happy years in the parish when suddenly the Bishop called me and said, 'You are going into

Catholic Charities,' and that was a fateful time for me," remembers Fahey.

From February 1961 to June of 1967, Fahey was Assistant Director of Catholic Charities, Diocese of Syracuse. A position of this importance necessitated further education; therefore Father Fahey enrolled in the National Catholic School of Social Service at Catholic University in Washington, D.C., receiving his master in social work (MSW) degree in 1963.

> I came to school in Washington, D.C. at the same time as the White House Conference on Aging. My superior, Monsignor Dan Lawler, told me to see what I could pick up in the field of aging. The 1961 conference was the time when we as a country began to recognize the demographics. We learned that the subject of aging was something we needed to follow in a more scientific and systematic way.

From October 1961 to May 1962, Fahey worked in the Social Services Department of St. Elizabeth's Mental Hospital in Washington, D.C. From October 1962 to May of 1963, he worked with the Commission on Aging of the City of Baltimore, Maryland. Afterwards, he returned full-time to his post in Syracuse.

"I went back to Syracuse and Catholic Charities for a number of years, where we were concerned about the full spectrum of human problems. And of course, that was the period of our greatest sensitivity in regard to race relations and community development. I never lost interest in the field of aging, though," said Fahey.

Civil Rights

When asked who were the most influential people in his life, Fahey lists his parents and neighbors, many of whom were from different ethnic and religious backgrounds; Monsignor Lawler, who directed him into the field of aging; and a priest named Monsignor Charles Brady.

> Father Brady was probably the most loving person I have ever met. Just before World War II, he went into the service and became a Catholic chaplain to an all black unit. He went with them all through the South Pacific. Along the way, he learned about the

> problems of black people; he identified with black people and tried to help them. He returned to Syracuse and asked the Bishop if he could do nothing but work in the black community.
>
> Later on, I was privileged to live with him and was deeply influenced by his way of coming at life and by his way of loving people, not only the poor and blacks but everyone.
>
> In those days, it was really painful. Here we were. Our supporters, people who were our natural constituency, were saying, "What are you people doing with all those blacks? They're not Catholics. They're not folks that you really should be identified with. You're trying to destroy our neighborhoods, our parishes, our churches."

Fahey never had a conflict on these issues. Because of his own convictions and the support he received from Father Brady, he became deeply involved in the movement for racial and social justice. "It was natural for me to join the March on Washington, to join protests in Selma and Montgomery, Alabama." Undoubtedly, these efforts made a crucial difference in the battle that ended in 1965 with the enactment of the civil rights legislation by the Congress.

In June of 1967, Fahey was promoted to director of Catholic Charities, a post he held until July 1979, when he was asked to head the Third Age Center at Fordham University in New York City. In 1980, he was named Marie Ward Doty Professor of Aging Studies at the Fordham University School of Social Service.

"I was amazed when I was asked to go to Fordham. I never thought about being an academician. But I was happy to go and direct the activities of the Third Age Center, where I have been ever since," says Fahey.

Involvement in Policymaking at the National Level

Monsignor Fahey has been deeply involved in the fashioning of public policy, particularly in the field of aging, for some 30 years. He has worked to make an impact through cooperative efforts of several major organizations. He began close to home and then reached out to more groups, all of which he helped sensitize as to the importance of these issues.

He began as a member of the Commission on Aging of the National Conference on Catholic Charities. From 1964–67, he served as its secretary and became its chairman in 1967, serving in this position until 1972. During this time, he was elected to the board and later to president of the board of the National Conference on Catholic Charities.

During this same time, he was an active member of the fledgling organization called the American Association of Homes for Aging (AAHA), which represented church-affiliated and other non-profit residences and nursing homes for seniors. He served as president of AAHA and at about the same time was named chairman of the Committee on Aging of the National Association of Social Workers, and chairman of a similar committee established by the National Conference on Social Welfare.

In 1971, Fahey was honored in his selection as chairman of the Special Session on Long-Term Care at the White House Conference on Aging.

In 1974, further honors came through his appointment to the Federal Council on Aging, where he became Chairman of the Task Force on the Frail Elderly and of the Committee on Long-Term Care. In the years 1980–81, he received still greater accolades in his elevation to chairman of the council that helps the White House fashion policy with respect to senior citizens.

In 1981, Fahey became a member of the Advisory Committee on Geriatrics and Gerontology of the Veteran's Administration, serving in this capacity through 1985. In this same year, he became a member of the Subcommittee on Long-Term Care of the American Association of Medical Colleges. Perhaps even more important, he was asked to chair the Technical Committee on Long-Term Care of the 1981 White House Conference on Aging; he also served as vice-chairman of the Technical Committee on Spiritual Well Being.

A year later, he participated in the first World Assembly on Aging, held in Vienna, Austria, as a member of the Vatican Delegation. He has remained active in the field of international aging as chairman of the Washington, D.C.-based American Association for International Aging. Currently, he serves as president-elect of the American Society on Aging.

In the intervening years, Fahey has continued his active involvement as a member of the National Council on Aging, the American Public Health Association, the Gerontological Society, the Paralyzed Veterans of America, the Foundation for Long-Term Care, and the American Hospital Association's Committee on Aging and Long-Term Care.

He was a founding member of the boards of the American Association for International Aging, the National Stroke Association, and the American Federation for Aging Research (AFAR).

He served for six years as a board member of the Catholic Health Association and was a member of two key commissions involving the Catholic Church's involvement in human services: one addressed social services and issued the report "Toward a Renewed Catholic Charities Movement;" the other addressed health, through "Catholic Health Care in the 21st Century."

All of the above, however, still do not adequately reflect the scope of the thought, work, and time that Fahey has put into the field of aging. He has been a consultant to the State Offices on Aging on numerous occasions. Among those states that have called on him for his services are: Arizona, California, Connecticut, Florida, New Jersey, New York, Tennessee, and Utah.

He has lectured at Catholic University in Washington; Yale Divinity School; North Texas State University; Georgia State University; the University of Alabama; St. Elizabeth School of Nursing, Utica, N.Y.; St. Joseph's School of Nursing, Syracuse, N.Y.; Sloan School, Cornell University, Ithaca, N.Y.; Maria Regina College, Syracuse, N.Y.; Onondaga Community College, Syracuse, N.Y.; Mary College, Bismark, N.D.; D'Youville College, Buffalo, N.Y.; LeMoyne College, Syracuse, N.Y.; College of St. Rose, Albany, N.Y.; Georgetown University; University of Pittsburgh; New School of Social Research; Temple University; University of Michigan; University of Southern California; University of Kentucky; University of Buffalo; State University of New York in Albany; Brown University; Columbia University; Einstein Medical Center; and in various divisions of Syracuse University.

In addition to being in demand as a public speaker, Monsignor

Fahey has written numerous articles, which have appeared in various social welfare and health journals. He has been asked to testify before the Congress on many occasions and before the U.S. Commission on Civil Rights.

He has worked extensively with the Robert Wood Johnson Foundation, the Rand Foundation, and the Retirement Research Foundation in the development of original research. For example, in 1985, he worked with Robert Wood Johnson on their "Health Impaired Elderly Project."

In short, Fahey has had a significant impact in the field of aging and long-term care. He has sought to make this impact through cooperation with others. He has used the democratic process and his extraordinary persuasive gifts to fire the imaginations of individuals and organizations. From his great mind have come many ideas that have found their way into legislation. Certainly, few people have done more to bring aging and long-term care out of the closet and into the forefront of public debate.

Progress and Problems

Fahey refuses to take any of the credit for making it happen, but he will agree that things have changed for the better for older Americans over the past 25 years:

> The most dramatic change is in the older persons themselves. It is not just a question of doing away with premature death; we have made great strides. Rather, it is the status of older persons that has improved dramatically. It is greatly encouraging for me to see older persons by and large refusing to live within the stereotypes and cultural expectations and creating new ways of growing old.
>
> It is greatly encouraging to see the greater sensitivity in the field of aging. It is great to see older people organizing themselves. And it is wonderful to see the number of committed people who are advocates for and with the elderly.
>
> We have to be careful that all of this success will not lead us into a trap. We have to live in an age-integrated society, and the very success in highlighting older persons may lead to the perception that older people are a very selfish group of folks.
>
> We must challenge older people and let them know that the

> most important entitlements are not in the law but in the human heart. Somehow, we must let older people recognize that by their behavior in neighborhoods, their behavior in families, and by their behavior in public, they must demonstrate that they are appreciative of what they have received and that they care about the wellbeing of all persons. This will create the entitlement of the heart and bring about caring.

Fahey did not intend by the above to minimize the importance of legislative victories won by seniors, such as the Older Americans Act, Medicare, and Medicaid; "Even though there has been erosion in some of those programs, they are still important building blocks and they give security to virtually every older American. Limited and incomplete as they may be, we have short memories on how difficult it was to grow old before these social investments."

When asked what is the greatest problem facing America going into the 21st century, he spoke of the need to fashion some new metaphors:

> We don't recognize it but one of the most powerful things at our disposal is the use of metaphors. It is really the storytellers who influence our behavior far more than those who come at us with clear, distinct ideas. Jesus continually spoke about rivers, seeds, and fish as opposed to dogmatic definitions or moral prescriptions. One of the sad things is that we have permitted the economic metaphor to drive just about everything. It is almost like what is good for business is good for the country. The use of the commercial metaphor, the economic metaphor, so dominates public life that it really is destroying us as a people. The healing process and supporting care are really a part of a much broader human equation of caring and community. It is a shame we have allowed it to be subsumed by the economic metaphor.

When asked what he would change to make things better, Fahey responded:

> I would change people's hearts and minds. I would hope we could make human beings more caring, more sensitive, and more humble. There is something hypocritical in our reaction to those in public office. We expect good behavior from everyone. But there has to be something that recognizes that there's a lot of weakness in all of us. I say this because only in recognizing weakness can we demand virtue, demand that people be just, loving, and thoughtful,

> as opposed to selfish. We need a broader vision, a more loving approach, love that embraces the people of Central America or South Africa or the Middle East. Big enough to embrace Arab and Jew alike and see the pain in each and try to understand the conflict there. It is so hard today to be intellectually honest; it is so hard to be courageous today.

One of the major problems facing American culture "is the tendency to want to flee death and suffering," said Fahey. "They are both realities. And frankly, the way that we are built psychologically, to say nothing of spiritually, is that we must engage in the suffering of others even as we must engage in and face our own suffering. And it is in facing suffering that we as individuals and as groups are ennobled, and we really grow as a society. To the degree that we become entirely self-centered and selfish, looking for either immediate gratification or try to wipe away all pain, we become a society that is decadent."

The answer to this problem will be found in a lively debate over values and a more organized attempt to transmit these values in society, said Fahey.

> Most of us set ideals for ourselves and constantly fall short; one has to have a great deal of humility. While you strive for virtue, you strive for that which is better and you strive for that which is heroic, but there are going to be moments when you are less than that. You have to be ready to forgive others and to forgive yourself. However, we do expect a basic moral character on the part of people; it is one of honesty, basic generosity, basic thoughtfulness, and basic commitment to social justice.

New Frontiers for the Elderly

Monsignor Fahey believes that there are two basic areas where senior citizens and their advocates must focus in their attempts to secure a better life in the 21st century. "One is in the area of culture. I think the most serious crisis in society is the question: What is growing old all about? The second is the problem of long-term care, which is basically a matter of disability. The good news here is that older people are much better off than they were. The difficult news is the unintended but seemingly necessary concomitant of doing away with premature death is that we have more disability."

Fahey believes, however, that both issues must be seen through the prism of public ethics.

> Moral and ethical questions should begin our discussion, not come later. Ethics is about what we ought to do. There is no way we can escape the development of a public ethic. A public ethic is what society is all about. What we are talking about is the soul of the United States of America. There are lots of things on the record which could be read to characterize us as a very selfish people. I suggest that there is a residual good will and an instinctive generosity in us that we can tap, not just in terms of taxes, but in terms of caring.
>
> We start from the position that there is an ethic which underlies government. The Declaration of Independence begins with an illusion to certain "inalienable rights"—that is certain rights that are secured to us by the very nature of our being. This ancient document is a true wonder. We ask how can we have been able to capture in such a magnificent way this series of statements which corresponds to what we know in our hearts. It is not that the ideas were new, they were not, but they were given a political form so that years later, we can read and say, yes, they were right.

Fahey believes that a public ethic begins with the assumption that men and women by their very nature are interdependent.

> We start from the position that what is necessary and required by our very nature of human beings is that we are responsible for others. Risks must be shared. We must make sure that no one is left alone or left unaided. We must remember that the goods we have are not an absolute right. The things we have are to be shared.
>
> I am the beneficiary of those who have gone before me, of their sweat, blood, tears, structures they developed, culture, and education—because of the investment of generations who have gone before. It continues to be our responsibility that those structures are in place for generations unborn but also for those that built the structures in the first place. It does not start with the question of cost but with the notion of a just society. But sharing burdens in a way that is reasonable, involves public, private, and government efforts. Not merely the preservation of resources but people living out their lives in dignity. We begin with those with resources and ask them to help those who can't care for themselves.

The underlying supposition is that there is more to building a just society that passing new laws. Laws are external, generic, backed up by sanctions, and are minimal in their approach. Ethics by definition go far beyond law. Monsignor Fahey quotes Justice Oliver Wendell Holmes, who said that our whole system of government is predicated on our being a virtuous people.

What Is Aging All About?

Fahey believes that we are battling with a new phenomenon. In years past, few people lived past 60. They had only what he describes as two ages. The first is that of learners, characterized by school, and the second age had to deal with working and earning a living and raising a family. Now, human beings in America and in developed countries the world over routinely live into a third age. The sad part is that this gift of another third of life is often squandered by people who do not know what to do with it. Some people, however, are actively and successfully inventing what it means to be a senior citizen, blessed with the gift of another third of life.

Four- and five-generation families are now common, but the question remains: What happens to the rest of life? Neither retirement nor family provide sufficient status for satisfaction so seniors must look elsewhere, says Fahey. He says one reason why marriages between older people are not particularly happy is because they have not redefined their social roles.

In Fahey's view, the third age should be a time of growth and development. He quotes Chesterton to the effect that youth is so wonderful it is a pity that it is wasted on young people. "I could almost say the same thing about education," he adds. "On the other hand, we ascribe wisdom to old people, and there are a lot of dumb old people, querulous old people, and a lot of non-thinking old people. All things being equal, if one takes life experiences and then works at those in a critical fashion, then indeed one can be wise. Society desperately needs wise people."

People need to grow externally as well as internally. Rather than withdrawal, the third age is a time for greater engagement. The

> human heart has such capacity and need for loving, that it cannot be exhausted within the context of families. In fact, the tendency is, for those instances where a husband and wife zero-in on one another, or linearly through the family, that will create neurotic relationships. Family life is likely to be strengthened, if we see it as sort of a means to an end. So what we need are older people who love other people whether they be the children of the neighborhood, young couples, or whatever it may be. We also need seniors who are involved with societal structures.

To Fahey, the third age should most of all be defined in terms of human maturity and doing everything possible to reach one's potential. He speaks of internal development through study and meditation. External development comes through aggressive engagement within the community. He says that it should be a time of intentionality, consciousness, and decision. He warns that seniors will face decisions that are just as painful going into the third age as the decisions that they made between their first and the second ages. Fahey says that some of the questions which must be asked in order to fashion a successful third age include: What has really made me a decent human being? What things make me less than human? What has brought me joy? What has brought me sorrow? What has demeaned me? What values are significant?

Inherent in all of this is taking control of one's life—making decisions intentionally rather than by default letting choices evaporate. For married people, the most critical question is: What do we do after we have been parents? Most people do not realize it, but they spend more years together not being parents than they do being parents, and yet couples seldom redefine their relationship after children leave home.

Ultimately, the question of what aging is or should be all about is, how to grow old gracefully. Fahey says that the central characteristic of those who grow old gracefully is hospitality.

> Older people who are hospitable, who open their homes and their hearts to those they know and those they do not, to those that they love and those they do not care for, who are ready to be surprised and disappointed to have their flowers trampled upon, who reach out to children, to the disabled, and to those of a different color are never alone. But those who are small and selfish and given to im-

> mediate gratification, who display bumper stickers which bear messages such as "We're spending our grandchildren's inheritance" are often alone and miserable. They unconsciously are creating isolation for themselves and for other older persons as well.

The challenge to older people, says Fahey, is to participate in the fullness of society, to be truly loving people, to continue to grow, recognizing that a lot of them and a lot of kids and a lot of middle-aged people are going to need help from family, friends, neighbors, and from society. "The challenge is to see the whole picture and make an effort diligently to make a difference on behalf of those who share such needs."

Long-Term Care

The problems of disability at any age are enormous, but it is particularly troubling at the end of life, says Fahey.

> Long-term care is basically a problem of disability. It is a multiple problem. It is an economic problem, a psychological problem. It is a familial problem and it is universal. It is a problem that every person in this country faces. We may face it vicariously, through friends, or we face it directly because of parents, or spouses, or aunts and uncles. And we will all face it as individuals. Being frail or being disabled is not inevitable. There will be many people who will live full and complete lives and never require significant assistance from others. But at least one out of two of us will.

Fahey makes numerous points, which he says must be taken into consideration in order to frame a comprehensive long-term care plan for the nation. Among these points are the following:

1. The real issue in long-term care is disability and not age. It is need that is important. How the person became disabled or his or her age is immaterial.

2. The triggering mechanism to qualify individuals for any long-term care program should be functional disability, that is, the ability to perform essential activities of daily living.

3. Care should be offered to people first in their own homes, with adequate institutional alternatives available thereafter when this is desirable or necessary.

4. Any public program that is created must not supplant care presently given by friends and family.

5. Any new program must cover both physical incapacity and mental disability.

6. Any system that is put into place must include both social supportive services and medical interventions. "Much of the hurt of long-term care is social, and we must be willing to address these needs."

7. Any new program must be built on a cooperative model, rather than the present competitive model which treats health care as an economic exchange. "Can we really afford the competitive model and what real price are we paying for invoking its use exclusively?" he asks.

8. The delivery of services must be coordinated at the local level. The decision-making mechanisms must be as close to the people as possible and serve to empower them, that is give them information and explain options and otherwise act as advocates for clients.

9. Long-term care is more of a problem of community organization than a problem of service delivery. "Any new program must look at the client in totality. This means evaluating the whole environment, the house and the neighborhood; the need to development of a community that cares is what is needed, and yet few communities are organized this way."

10. Every possible measure must be taken to insure the quality of services. Providers must go beyond the law, beyond what is required. "They must meet ethical standards to help clients live with a maximum of human dignity—not only to live but to flourish and to keep control over their own lives."

11. The problem of long-term care is so great that a mixture of public financing, private financing, and private health insurance will be needed to address the problem. A residual Medicaid program will be needed as a matter of social justice.

12. Those who claim the burden of caring is too great are wrong. "It is quite one thing to talk about heroic and esoteric kinds of interventions that may prolong life for a day, a month, or a year. It is quite something else to talk about dealing with people in a decent manner with basic food, clothing, and shelter and having a caring person

present. The real issue in society isn't the former. In fact, there are relatively small resources being expended in what many would judge an inappropriate way. The huge cost to society and individuals, both in economic and opportunity costs, and in emotional costs, is the question of supporting persons who are not dying but who are disabled and basically need the presence of another human being, and the stimulation to do what they can do within the physical and psychological limitations that they have."

Fahey summarizes the issue:

> Nobody is born by themselves, and nobody dies by themselves. And surely, throughout life, no one is self-sufficient. In fact, one of the ironies of modern society is, it becomes increasingly complex—the more complex it becomes, the more we have to make life enjoyable, the more interdependent we become. But somehow, we tend to think that, when one is disabled, and particularly at the end of life, that one has to fend for oneself, and one has to be independent. Autonomy and commitment to autonomy can be the last refuge of a non-caring people. So we're struggling with this notion between autonomy, freedom, independence, community, caring, and being involved with others.

Public and private interventions along with a reshaping of community are all necessary, according to Fahey, so that no husband, wife, family, or individual need fear that they are going to be alone, that they are going to be abandoned, or that the work of a lifetime is going to be wiped out because of an illness.

The Future of Seniors in America

Monsignor Fahey believes the future looks bright for seniors in America. He believes that individual seniors will continue taking over control of their own lives, looking for satisfaction, and making creative contributions to society. There will be more seniors and more disability, which means a greater need for long-term care services. Major breakthroughs are possible with continued research. However, he does not believe that massive increases in government funding for long-term care will come soon; this makes it all the more important to marshal community resources. Community development will be exceedingly important in the delivery of services to the aged in the 21st century, he believes.

Honors

Among the honors that Monsignor Fahey has received have been an Honorary Doctor of Laws from St. Thomas University, Fredericton (New Brunswick), Canada, and D'Youville College, Buffalo, New York, and Honorary Doctor of Divinity from St. Bernard's Institute in Rochester, New York. He was appointed by New York Governor Hugh Carey and reappointed by Mario Cuomo as a member of the prestigious New York Public Health Council. He received a special recognition award from the Interfaith Coalition on Aging and was honored to be chosen to deliver the first annual John McDowell Memorial Lecture. He received the Seltzer Award from the Daughters of Jacob Geriatric Center for Excellence in the Field of Gerontology; he was honored by the National Association of State Units on Aging in 1980 when they chose him to deliver the annual Arthur Flemming lecture. He received the Community Service Award of the American College of Nursing Home Administrators. He also received the National Award of Honor from the American Association of Homes for Aging. In 1967, he was chosen "Man of the Year" by the Junior Chamber of Commerce. He has been elected to membership in the Institute of Medicine of the National Academy of Sciences.

Volunteering

Despite the heavy load that he carries at the University and his involvement on important policymaking committees, Fahey still finds time to provide volunteer clerical duties at the following Catholic Churches: St. Catherine's Church, Vernon, New York; St. Patrick's Church, Oneida, New York; St. Joseph's Church, Oxford, New Jersey; St. Paul's Church, Oswego, New York; Immaculate Heart of

Mary Church, Liverpool, New York; Holy Family Church, Syracuse, New York; St. Ann's Church, Syracuse, New York; St. Margaret's Church, Syracuse, New York; St. Rose of Lima Church, North Syracuse, New York; Charlie Borromeo Church, Syracuse, New York.

Heroes

When asked who he most respects for their contribution in the field of aging and long-term care, he mentioned four people. Senator Frank E. Moss, whom he said had done "more than any other person to bring the question of long-term care to the public eye;" adding that Moss was "a tireless champion of the underprivileged, who worked to bring quality nursing home and home health care to all Americans who were in need." He said that "Claude Pepper was everyone's hero" and that Arthur Flemming is one of the most impressive people that he has ever met. He also included Nelson Cruikshank, formerly of the National Council on Senior Citizens, saying these people were "the quintessence of public service."

With respect to the broader question of which citizens of the world he particularly admires, he named three: Barry Goldwater (with whom he disagreed on many issues), Pope John XXIII, and Mother Teresa. He sees in all of these people a fierce independence and a sense of choosing to meet life on its own terms. There is also the notion of openness—remaining respectful of life, continuing to learn and grow, and to share the joys and the sorrows of others as a full participant in life's many miracles. To Fahey, these people share a quality that he calls hospitality. By his definition, they are excellent examples of people who age gracefully.

Remembered

When asked how he would like to be remembered, he responded that it mattered little whether he was or was not. He offered a variation of the quotation: "Your life is your gift from God. What you do with your life is your gift to God." If the quotation is true, there is little doubt but that the Supreme Creator has good reason to be pleased with

Monsignor Charles Fahey. There is also little doubt but that he will be remembered for his contributions to help improve the quality of life among the poor, the aged, and the underprivileged in late 20th century America. He will be remembered as the pioneer who taught Americans and citizens of the world to make use of, rather than squander, the great gift from God, the third age of life, and to use this time in service to others. In a very real sense, he will have helped redefine what it means to be an older American. In his terms, this will be for future generations a time of learning rather than a time of stagnation; it will be a time of growth rather than retraction; it will be a time of engagement rather than disengagement; and most of all, it will be a time of caring. For millions of Americans, this will mean little more than following the example that Monsignor Fahey has established in his own life.

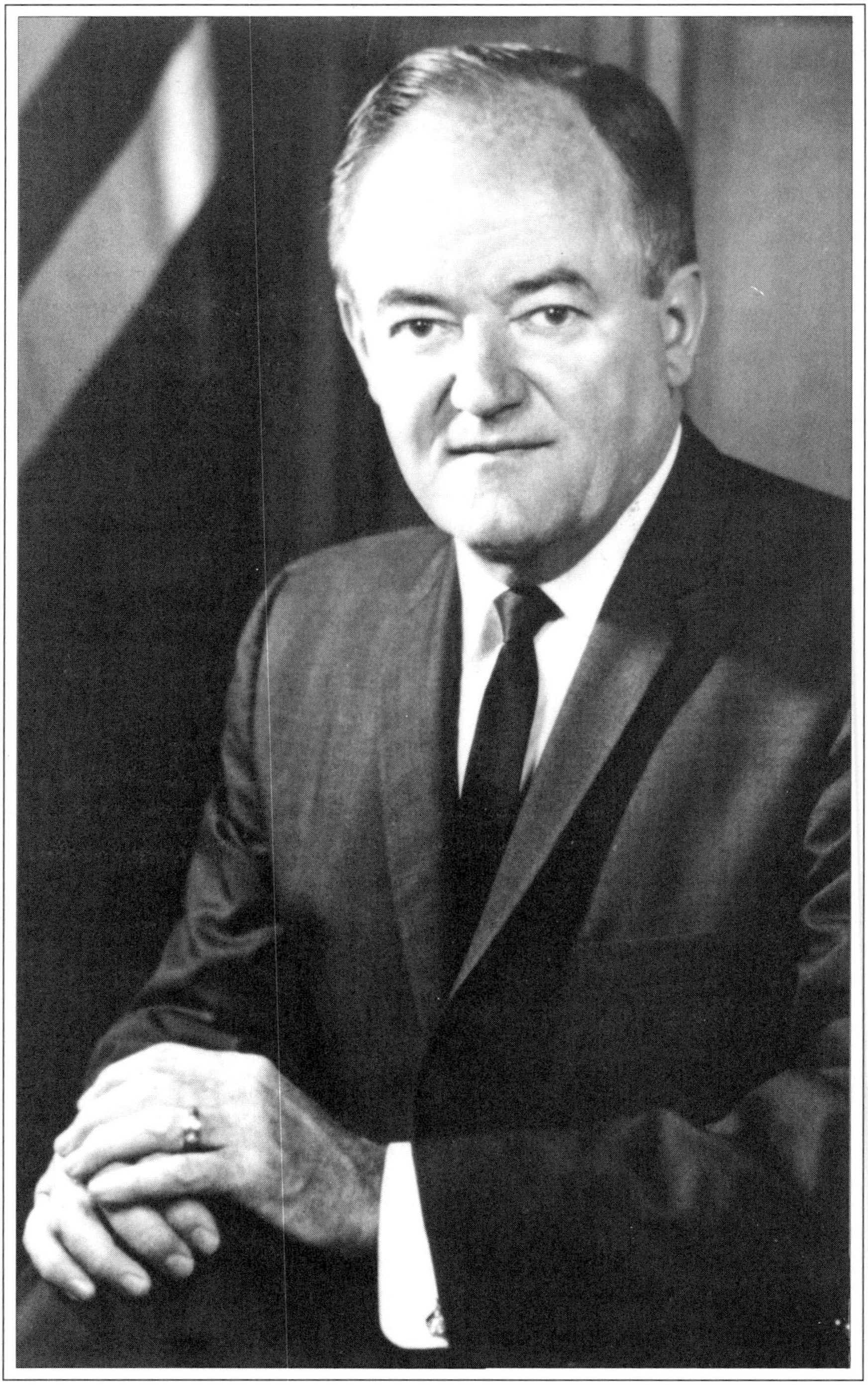
COURTESY OF THE HUBERT HUMPHREY LIBRARY

FIFTEEN

Hubert H. Humphrey

People such as Hubert H. Humphrey enoble the human race. By any standard, he ranks among the best of God's creations. The measure of any human life, said one Greek philosopher, is the extent to which it has been used to help others. In this sense, Hubert H. Humphrey was preeminent. No one cared more deeply than did he and no one tried any harder to help.

Hubert H. Humphrey gave of himself to others; he continued giving irrespective of whether they reciprocated. He gave to those who agreed with him and to those who did not. He gave to those who asked and to those who didn't. He gave and he kept on giving even when he was physically exhausted and seemingly had nothing left to give.

He was the champion of the underprivileged, the restorer of rights, a great and powerful voice for peace and justice in the world.

He was the advocate of civil rights and human rights. He was the enemy of discrimination whether on the basis of age, sex, religion, color, or creed; he fought this great evil with the strength of a thousand armies.

He became the conscience of the nation. If Americans did not always listen to him, they knew in their hearts that he was right.

His courage was forged scrambling to earn a living in the plains of South Dakota and tempered by the cold Minnesota winters. It was severely tested when as mayor of Minneapolis he crushed the power of the mob and threw them out of the city. His courage was tested again when he broke the back of communist-dominated trade unions that were paralyzing his city with strikes. Through it all, he not only survived, he gathered the strength he would need for still greater battles to come. As Lyndon B. Johnson observed, he seemed to gather strength from adversity, not be crushed by it.

Stories illustrating Humphrey's warmth and caring nature abound. In one case, he stopped his car en route to a speech to help an elderly woman carry two bags of groceries what turned out to be a dozen blocks. He helped ex-cons get a job. He went out of his way to help a sick child, sending his personal physician to a Minneapolis home and anonymously paying the bill himself. Similarly, he aided the author who was suffering from severe back pain, without request making appointments for him to see the best orthopedic physicians at the Mayo Clinic.

If a poll were taken of the most caring members of Congress in the last century, there is little doubt that Hubert Humphrey, Claude Pepper, and Frank E. Moss would rank at the top.

Hubert H. Humphrey, in a 1977 poll, was voted the most effective senator of the 20th century. Some people have gone so far as to suggest that he invented the concept of the modern U.S. senator. There is no doubt but that he set the standard for others to reach.

No man ever loved more people than Hubert Humphrey and in return no one was more beloved by the nation.

Hubert Humphrey served in the U.S. Senate for 23 years, more than one-third of his life. Without making a single enemy in the Chamber, he fathered more important pieces of legislation from origin to enactment than any member of Congress. Among his achievements was the Civil Rights Act of 1964. He conceived it, and worked 16 years to see its enactment into law. Some historians believe this is the single most important piece of legislation enacted in America during the 20th century.

But there is another achievement that looms just as large. The first bill he introduced when he joined the Senate in 1949 provided health insurance for the aged through Social Security. He called it Medicare. He worked with Senator Moss to make sure the program included coverage for home health care as an alternative to nursing homes and the preferred way of providing long-term care for the infirm elderly.

His third achievement was the enactment of a Nuclear Test Ban Treaty with the Soviet Union, which in 1963 represented the first real control on the arms race.

For these and other achievements, Hubert Humphrey received the Medal of Freedom, more than 40 honorary degrees, and the everlasting affection of his country. In doing so, he reached his boyhood ambition "to add something significant to the nation's history."

Hubert H. Humphrey: The Man

What kind of man was he, this man of legends? For one thing, he was tall at five feet, eleven inches, but he seemed taller. He was jolly, with a constant smile and an infectious laugh. His face had a certain cherubic quality, round and innocent.

He walked in quick steps with speed and determination, which suggested he not only knew where he was going but also that he was impatient to get there. Impatient he was. Impatient for progress in the area of civil rights; impatient with excuses of those who failed to see problems or failed to lift a finger to help those in need. If he was short on patience, he was long on determination. Once he set a goal, he would never quit until he reached it.

He was a man of extraordinary vision. He was fully grounded in the present and yet he could see into the future. His legislation anticipated the inevitable changes that occurred in problems. He had a finely tuned sense of what the public wanted and an instinct for doing just the right thing at the right time.

He was a highly positive man who loved life and gave full measure of himself to the people. He seemed to draw his strength from those he served.

Humphrey, more than most people, was what he appeared to be: affable, kind, happy, hardworking, and full of enthusiasm. He could be moody, but not for long. At times he talked too much; he was too glib and on television he projected a certain softness which caused many people to tell him he didn't look like a senator, a vice-president, or whatever. He responded by saying that Franklin Pierce and Warren Harding were two of our most handsome presidents but undoubtedly were among the nation's worst.

When asked to explain his prodigious energy, he said, "It is just there." He was a man who carried the Puritan work ethic to the extreme. He had a fire in him which burned brightly, often to the point of being out of control. He was compelled to do the things he did; obsessed might be a better word for his behavior.

When urged to relax, he responded, "Relax? I don't know how." He loved his family, but sacrificed time with them to serve the nation.

There is one story that illustrates Humphrey's obsession with work. Neighbors reported that Humphrey, returning home late, would sometimes be found at two in the morning scrubbing the kitchen floor. His dedication to work, said one author, was his strength. He was willing to pay the price by working longer and harder than anyone.

The downside of this is that he worked so hard himself that he sometimes missed the fact that others needed to be supervised. He did not understand that subordinates did not always share his vision and invariably he would be disappointed in the product they produced.

He was always in a hurry and always late. This was because of his disrespect for the tyranny of schedules. He wanted to live life a little spontaneously. This meant that at times he appeared to be (and probably was) a little disorganized. Already late, he would stop to chat with children, sometimes keeping senators and heads of state waiting.

Commentators agree that Humphrey's best ideas came to him when he was speaking. He seemed most alive when he was giving a speech. He was inclined to talk off the top of his head, throwing out dozens of ideas. He was less inclined to subject these ideas to analysis in the cold light of reason. He was spontaneous, not calculating; open, not closed; outgoing, not reserved.

His speeches had a spiritual quality about them. "He makes you feel good about yourself," was the most common response when people were asked about the phenomenon. When asked about his speeches, he said:

> You have to give to people. I don't make a speech, I give a speech. I try to give people a lot of knowledge and perhaps a useful idea or two.
>
> Truman won the White House because he gave to people. He was a terrible speaker but he took the time to go down and pat the kids on the head and to say a few kind words to Mama.

He was a nice guy, meaning by that that he trusted everyone. He was totally incapable of being vindictive. As President Lyndon Johnson once told him: "The trouble with you, Hubert, is that you are just too good. A person can kick you in the teeth and you would reach over and pat their leg."

He was the ultimate Christian in the sense that he kept turning the other cheek no matter what the insult. His political allies and foes alike abused him, and he responded by loving them back. He was not afraid to make himself vulnerable even if this meant that he was continually going to be disappointed in people. He could be tough and he was certainly determined; he was a good fighter for causes in which he believed, but he lacked the killer instinct.

For many people who met him for the first time, he was simply too good to be true, but the longer they knew him, the more apparent it became that he was the genuine article.

He was intensely ambitious. He took his issues seriously, but not himself. He was unusual in the sense that he did not have one enemy in the Senate. He fought hard against special interests, but he found a way to do it without alienating those who were on the other side of the argument from him. He was also a man of grace, spending much of his time being thoughtful and considerate of the other person.

He was a man of humor as well as intelligence. "In the Senate, what you say is not as important as how you say it. A sense of humor is mighty important. If you don't kid around, you'll go crazy," he said.

He was also an internationalist. He said that the policy of isolationism was the one flaw of the New Deal. "The world is getting smaller and smaller," he said. "What happens in any part of the world ultimately affects all of us."

He believed in a strong defense, but believed the strongest possible defense was the education of children. Moreover, he stressed the importance of values. Most major civilizations were not conquered by armies from without; rather, they lost their values, lapsed into anarchy, and withered from within, he said.

He was a man who was well educated, particularly in political theory. He was able to fuse classical political theory and adapt it to use in the modern American democracy, thus becoming the greatest social architect of our times.

Background

Hubert Humphrey traced his roots back to Jonas Humphrey, a Puritan from England who settled in Dorchester, Massachusetts in the early 1700s.

Hubert's paternal grandfather, John Humphrey, ran a sawmill in Granite Falls, Minnesota. He married Addie Register, the first schoolmistress in the town and soon they had five children. The oldest, Harry, obtained his Ph.D. in agriculture science from Stanford University and worked for many years with the Department of Agriculture in Washington, D.C. The second son was Hubert's father, Hubert H. Humphrey. Both Hubert's father and his Uncle Harry had a profound effect on the future vice-president.

Humphrey's maternal grandfather had been a sea captain in Norway and was lured to the United States to work for friends, with the expectation that he would find ready work on the wide Mississippi. When this turned out to be a false hope, he turned to farming, at the age of 38, in Dakota territory some 80 miles north of Sioux City, Iowa. Andrew Sannes was a hard worker who prospered in the face of adversity; his wife, Minna, was something of a frontier superwoman. Their second daughter, Christine Sannes, married Hubert H. Humphrey, Sr. in 1908.

The family took up residence in Wallace, South Dakota, where Hubert, Sr. worked as a pharmacist. Young Hubert, born on May 27, 1911, was the second of four children.

It is reported that Hubert's mother was shy and introspective. She was very serious about life but even more serious about the life hereafter. She had great hopes that Hubert, Jr. would grow up to be a minister of the gospel. It was a hope that she clung to even after her son had obtained his office of vice-president.

Hubert, Sr. was a gregarious man who worked for a time as a traveling salesman and then worked his way through pharmacy school. He was a man who believed in hard work. Good natured, he opened several pharmacies in various Dakota towns during the Great Depression, somehow managing to make a go of it. Hubert, Jr. said of his father that he was "a rebel in a politically orthodox town but they elected him mayor." The elder Humphrey, like his son, was an excellent speaker. This and other political skills got him elected as a state representative. For a time he was also head of the Democratic party in South Dakota.

The elder Humphrey exorted his children to stay out of bed because "most people died there." He idolized President Woodrow Wilson. His ambitions were strong, but he always seemed to find time for his family. He was a positive man who never once compromised his political principles. He urged his children to dream. "Before the fact there is the dream," he used to say.

Hubert Humphrey, Jr. as a child was straight out of "The Little Rascals." He enjoyed teasing and having fun. He had boundless energy and an entrepreneurial spirit, which surfaced not too long after he learned to walk. As a youngster, he sold eggs, delivered newspapers, helped out in his father's drugstore, shot rabbits or pheasants to put meat on the family table, and somehow found time to excel in his studies. In 1929, he graduated as the valedictorian of his high school and left behind him a trail of achievements in forensics, dramatics, journalism, and athletics. If this was not enough, he taught Sunday school and was a Boy Scout leader. As one commentator put it, "Young Hubert had a zest for life, he plunged in full throttle, grinning all the way." In his autobiography, Humphrey himself says that he had a wonderful childhood and that his only fears were that he might disappoint his father.

College Years to Mayor

Young Hubert entered the University of Minnesota in the fall of 1929. He worked his way through his first year, washing dishes, waiting on tables, and working in the campus drugstore. But the depression intervened, forcing him to drop out of school to help his father in the drugstore. The entire family worked in his father's pharmacy, where the hours were seven in the morning until eleven at night. Humphrey postponed his college education for seven years, working without a salary to help his father keep afloat the little country pharmacy which was the family's sole means of support.

Along the way, Humphrey had acceded to his father's wishes and enrolled in the Capital College of Pharmacy in Denver. In a frantic effort to get back to help his father and family, he sprinted through two years of courses in six months. He passed the exam and, like his father before him, became a licensed pharmacist.

All this noble sacrifice, however, took its toll. The young man was thin as a rail, troubled by ulcers and fainting spells. It wasn't until 1936 that young Hubert could bring himself to tell his father that he didn't want to be a "pill pusher"—that he wanted to be out on his own.

The year 1936 was a special one in Humphrey's life for many reasons. It was the year he came of age, beginning to assert himself and to make his own course in life. It was the year he led a troup of Boy Scouts to Washington, D.C. where he and the children were fascinated by things political. In his memoirs, Senator Humphrey says that this was the point at which he made up his mind that he would come back to Washington and that he would find service in the Congress of the United States. As it happened, President Franklin D. Roosevelt's train stopped in Huron, South Dakota in 1936. The elder Humphrey, the Democratic committeeman, was escorted onboard to meet the president and he brought the wide-eyed Hubert, Jr. with him. Much impressed with the meeting, Hubert, Jr. promptly founded a Young Democrats Club.

But 1936 was even more important for another reason. In September of that year, Humphrey married Muriel Buck whose father bought and sold produce in and around Huron, South Dakota. The young couple both worked and managed to save up $675 in a year. In the fall of 1937, they moved back to the Twin Cities where Humphrey again took up his studies at the University of Minnesota at the age of 27.

In order to pay for his tuition and support his family, Humphrey took every job he could get, from swabbing toilets to tutoring students in French (a language he had learned only the previous semester). On completion of his B.A. degree, magna cum laude, the Humphreys set out for Baton Rouge, Louisiana where Hubert had been awarded a fellowship in political science. He ultimately received his master's degree based on the completion of a thesis that evaluated (favorably) the philosophical underpinnings of Roosevelt's New Deal.

In the summer of 1940, the family returned to the University of Minnesota. Humphrey had the promise of a fellowship, but by now he had a child to feed and needed a little more money in order to survive. He took a job with Duluth State Teachers College teaching adult education courses for the Works Progress Administration (WPA). The idea was to help retrain the unemployable for new jobs. What started out as a summer job soon became permanent. He did so well that they made him the statewide director of the WPA. With the advent of World War II, he worked for a time with the War Manpower Commission, the successor to the WPA.

Beginning with his return to Minnesota in 1940, Humphrey's college professors and those who worked with him in the WPA had been nudging him to run for political office. In 1943, he made his first bid, running for mayor of Minneapolis. He lost, but he laid important groundwork and eventually brought about the unification of the Farmer Labor and Democratic Parties in Minnesota; the DFL, as the new party was to be called, soon became the dominating force in Minnesota politics. In 1945, he ran a second time for mayor and was elected.

By all accounts, Hubert Humphrey was a wonderful mayor. He led a forceful campaign to clean up the city. He appointed a new incorruptible police chief and threw the mob out of the city. The city's criminal element put up a fight both in the courts and in the streets. Mayor Humphrey was offered bribes, threatened, and even shot at by gangsters. He pushed ordinances through the city council that guaranteed the rights of blacks to equal access to schools and housing. He led a campaign against racism, discrimination, and antiSemitism. He also intervened aggressively to end the seemingly endless series of labor strikes that had paralyzed the city. In short, he restored order and justice, and he restored public confidence in government. Not surprisingly, he was reelected overwhelmingly in 1947.

Bursting on the National Scene

Hubert H. Humphrey first came to national prominence with a speech delivered on the final day of the 1948 Democratic National Convention. The convention had decided to renominate President

Harry S. Truman, who had succeeded to the office in 1945 following the death of President Franklin D. Roosevelt.

The Democratic party was badly divided. Liberal Democrats were holding onto the hope that Henry Wallace, Roosevelt's vice-president in the 1940–44 term, would be selected. But Truman had won renomination by a narrow margin with no one giving him much of a chance of reelection against the well-financed campaign of Governor Thomas Dewey.

A group of southern conservatives controlled the Platform Committee and not surprisingly, they reported out a status quo framework from which Truman was to launch his candidacy. Mayor Humphrey and others had tried in vain to get the group to accept a plank in the platform that would commit the party to action on civil rights. Losing his fight before the committee, Mayor Humphrey decided to take his case to the convention floor. He introduced a minority plank committing the Democratic party to aggressively fight to end discrimination on the basis of race, creed, or color.

It is reported that this eight-minute speech so moved the crowd that they rose in a spontaneous demonstration that lasted several minutes. Among the lines he delivered that night are the following:

> To those who say that we are rushing this issue of civil rights — I say to them that we are 172 years too late.
>
> To those who say this bill is an infringement on states' rights, I say this — the time has arrived in America. The time has arrived for the Democratic party to get out of the shadow of states' rights and walk forthrightly in the bright sunshine of human rights.
>
> People — people — human beings — this is the issue of the 20th Century. In these times of world, economic, political, and spiritual —above all spiritual — crisis, we cannot and we must not turn back from the path so plainly before us. That path has already led us through many valleys of the shadow of death. Now is the time to recall those who are left on the path of American freedom.
>
> Our land is now, more than ever before, the last best hope on earth. I know that we can — know that we shall — begin here the fuller and richer realization of that hope — that promise — of a land where all men are truly free and equal, and each man uses his freedom and equality wisely and well.

The consensus among historians is that this speech and the Democratic party's advocacy of civil rights was pivotal in giving the election to President Truman. Hubert Humphrey's singular act of courage also made him an instant national figure and facilitated his own election to the U.S. Senate later that year.

U.S. Senate

The election of 1948 had brought the Senate such giants as Estes Kefauver, Paul Douglas, and Lyndon Baines Johnson; yet *Time* magazine elected to bypass them in favor of Senator Humphrey. In putting him on their cover, they marked him as a man of extraordinary gifts, the member of the new class of 1948 most likely to succeed. The result of the *Time* cover, together with Humphrey's judgmental and moralistic style, soon resulted in his being shunned by the established power elite in the Senate.

He had to learn that the Senate was an old men's club where new senator's were seen and not heard. What newcomers did not do is to threaten the establishment by challenging the "evils" of the seniority system or questioning the "unwise and inappropriate waste of taxpayers dollars" by senior senators. Most especially, junior members should know enough not to throw the nettlesome issue of civil rights in the face of the southern conservatives who ran the Senate. But Senator Humphrey was undeterred. He kept coming at them, challenging their ideas, shattering their taboos.

For example, he took the Senate floor to explain to the American public the existence of "tax loopholes," which were created to allow certain wealthy groups to escape taxation. He made enough of a clamour that a tax reform bill was quickly drafted. But whatever was done was done in such a way as to exclude Senator Humphrey. So great was his ostracism that none of the 57 bills and the dozens of amendments that he introduced in his first session of Congress were accepted.

However, Senator Humphrey had a way of growing on people. The longer they knew him the more his fellow senators liked him. Historians such as Carl Solberg, who has written the best biography on the senator are in agreement that it was Senator Lyndon Johnson who took Humphrey under his wing and taught him the unwritten rules of the Senate. LBJ, cunning and relentless, had a good feel for Humphrey's abilities and sought to use him toward the attainment of his own goals: becoming Senate Majority Leader and then president of the United States. It was LBJ who helped remove the crown of ostracism from Humphrey's brow, but he also wanted and received help from the Minnesota senator. Sometimes it was in the form of information, sometimes it was his vote. LBJ made himself the broker between the conservatives and the small band of liberals that gathered around Humphrey. LBJ would call on both sides to compromise in the name of party unity and/or the good of the country. He made the deal and got everyone to support it in the name of unity and compromise.

LBJ went out of his way to raise funds for Senator Humphrey. He was careful to say that their political views were 180 degrees apart but insisted that Humphrey was a vitally important cog in the Senate machine. It was Senator Johnson who was instrumental in helping Humphrey get a post on the coveted Foreign Relations Committee; for the first several years, Senator Humphrey had been relegated to the political Siberia of the Post Office and Civil Service and Government Operations Committees.

As it was, the legislative action in the Congress during this period proceeded at a snail's pace. The only major activity consisted of blocking President Eisenhower and the Republicans from dismantling portions of the New Deal. Attention instead was focused on what to do with Senator Joseph McCarthy and his assertion that a Communist was lurking under every rock in government. The result, after much travail, was his ouster by the Senate.

The Race for Higher Office

Having failed to take the presidency in 1952, the Democrats were determined to take it back in 1956. Governor Adlai Stevenson of Illinois, the candidate from four years before, was back and looking fit. The real question facing the 1956 Democratic Convention was who was to be selected to be the party's candidate for vice-president.

Senator Hubert Humphrey stepped forward seeking the nomination. He had the support of powerful individuals with views on all sides of the political spectrum, from Lyndon B. Johnson to Eleanor Roosevelt. Among those he counted as his supporters were two U.S. senators with high name recognition: John F. Kennedy and Estes Kefauver. Unfortunately for Senator Humphrey, both Kennedy and Kefauver recanted their support and began running for the position. To make matters worse, the presidential nominee broke his promise to support Humphrey, throwing the nomination to the convention floor. After a tough fight, Kefauver emerged victorious over Kennedy by the slimest margin. Ironically, it was Senator Humphrey and the Minnesota delegation who were called on to the break the tie, and gave Kefauver the nomination.

It was a bitter defeat for Senator Humphrey, who felt that he had been betrayed by several close friends. The backlash of the decision to choose Kefauver over Kennedy set the stage for what happened in 1960. To Humphrey, the unsuccessful run for the number two spot on the ticket brought support for the conclusion that only Lyndon Johnson had stood by him when the going had been tough.

The Democrats lost the White House in 1956 but continued to add to their support within the Congress. Then-Senate Majority Leader LBJ quickly saw that Humphrey's liberal allies were growing in number while the old southern block was beginning to lose its hold. LBJ made his move. He made Senator Humphrey vice-chairman of the Democratic Senatorial Campaign Committee, the committee designed to help elect Democrats to the Senate. He retained actual control of the moneys raised through his conservative soul mate, George Smathers, who he appointed as chairman of the panel. In a second move by way of positioning himself for a run for the White House, LBJ broke with the southern block on civil rights. He gave the nod to the introduction of a bill and quietly allowed it to be neutered. In doing so, he lectured Humphrey on the necessity of incremental change and compromise; to the southerns, he argued that this action was needed, perhaps it would serve to stave off more serious reforms. The bill passed.

The next year, 1958, was a memorable one for Humphrey. He founded and ascended to the chairmanship of the Subcommittee on Disarmament of the Senate Foreign Relations Committee. In this capacity, he traveled to the Soviet Union, where he was received by

Premier Nikita Kruschev. Senator Humphrey made major headlines upon his return with the assertion straight from Moscow that the Soviets would favor some sort of a ban on the testing of nuclear weapons. The fact that Kruschev received Humphrey with the ceremony usually reserved for a head of state served to boost his stock at home in America. He became a household word, respected from Maine to Moscow and back again. Another event, just as important, was the November election. A huge Democratic tide rippled through America, bringing with it the largest class of progressives ever to hit the Senate at one time. Among them were some giants, men such as Edmund S. Muskie, Phillip Hart, Frank E. Moss, Gayle McGee, and Senator Humphrey's protégé, Eugene McCarthy. Humphrey now had an army to lead.

To Hubert Humphrey, the 1958 election, his ascendency within the Democratic campaign committee, and the avalanche of favorable press seemed like the wind of destiny that he thought just might pick him up like Dorothy and Toto and drop him in the Oval Office.

The year 1960 soon was at hand. Senator Humphrey had on his track shoes. As one senator put it, he had been bitten by the presidential bug, a disease that only embalming fluid can cure. In looking around, it soon became clear to him that he was on the outside with further to run and that the inside poll position was being held by Senator John F. Kennedy. JFK had generated mountains of publicity and television coverage through the publication of his book, *Profiles in Courage*, which extolled the values and virtues of some of America's early statesmen. The book was a clarion call to return to good old American values. JFK avoided debates or head-to-head competition with Humphrey, working behind the security of a multi-million dollar campaign organization. JFK was not the least bit bashful to borrow a good idea when he heard one and Humphrey had too many not to be liberated of a few. Senator Humphrey, by contrast, had virtually no money and no organization; he arrived in airports a lonely figure carrying his own baggage.

The promised help from LBJ never came, and it soon became clear why. Senator Johnson was quietly running for the nomination himself. If Kennedy's appeal was to the public, LBJ's was to the pols who frequented smoke-filled rooms where promises were exchanged more often and honored less than in a Las Vegas wedding chapel. The result was that Humphrey was forced out of the race and JFK was nominated over LBJ. In a shrewd move against his brother Robert's advice, JFK selected Senator Johnson as his running mate. This may have been the single most important decision in bringing about his election.

The aftermath of 1960 was bittersweet for Senator Humphrey. He mourned the loss of what might have been but he rejoiced in the election of two good Democrats. He decided to make the most of it. Having failed in his bid for the presidency, he had run and been reelected to the Senate in 1960. With determination he set his sights on becoming the best United States senator in the history of the Republic.

Once again, Vice-President Lyndon B. Johnson came into play. He was instrumental in helping Senator Humphrey reach the number two post in the Democratic leadership. As Majority Whip, he was second in command to the pipe-smoking, silent man from Montana, Mike Mansfield. Hubert Humphrey reveled in his new role. He singlehandedly supplied the ideas and the steam to enact a significant body of legislation, which came to be known as the New Frontier.

He became the grandmaster of Senate manuevering. He used the rules like a fan dancer used feathers. He pushed through Humphrey bills to create the Peace Corps, the Youth Conservation Corps, the Food for Peace Program, the Tax Reform Act of 1963, the Occupational Health and Safety Act, and a Nuclear Test Ban Treaty that bars the testing of nuclear weapons in the atmosphere by either the United States or the Soviet Union. In 1964, he successfully broke the back of a southern filibuster and opened the way to the enactment of major civil rights legislation. The icing on this impressive list of achievements was the enactment of Medicare, a Humphrey bill proposed in 1949 shortly after he joined the Senate.

In November of 1963, President John F. Kennedy was gunned down in Dallas. No one took it harder than Humphrey. However, he pulled himself together in time to meet a shaken former vice-president, now President Lyndon Johnson when Air Force One landed at Andrews Airforce Base. It was Senator Humphrey who wrote the president's first speech to the nation and who authored LBJ's prayer and plea: "Let us continue."

The Vice-Presidency

Lyndon Johnson ran for election as president in 1964. It was something that he had planned and worked towards for most of his life. Based on his relationship with the Congress, the inside support of Hubert Humphrey, and the sympathy created by the death of President Kennedy, the Democrats enjoyed a commanding lead in the polls. The election of the president over Senator Barry Goldwater was a foregone conclusion. Even though this was true, LBJ played cat and mouse with the press with respect to his choice for vice-president. He dropped names with the frequency of a Hollywood gossip columnist.

Ironically, two senators from Minnesota, Humphrey and his colleague Eugene McCarthy, emerged as the frontrunners. LBJ selected Humphrey only after extracting an oath in blood that he would render complete, blindly faithful loyalty to the president. It required him to sacrifice his identity and to merge it with the president's—a price he soon found to be quite heavy to pay.

The Democratic Convention of 1964 will be remembered by historians for three reasons: the 20-minute standing ovation for Robert F. Kennedy following a filmed tribute to his late brother, the nomination of LBJ, and the fiery speech by Hubert H. Humphrey accepting the vice-presidential nomination. Humphrey said in part:

> Most Democrats and Republicans in the U.S. Senate voted for the nuclear test ban treaty, but not the temporary Republican spokesman.
>
> Most Democrats and Republicans in the Senate voted for a $11.5 billion tax cut for American citizens and for American business. But not Senator Goldwater.
>
> Most Democrats and Republicans in the Senate, including four-fifths of his own party, voted for the Civil Rights Act. But not Senator Goldwater.
>
> Most Democrats and Republicans in the Senate voted for an expanded medical education program. But not Senator Goldwater.
>
> Most Democrats and Republicans in the Senate voted for expanded education legislation. But not Senator Goldwater.

The speech was greeted with wild approval, as were the candidates. The team of Johnson-Humphrey won the election in a landslide, the dimensions of which had been exceeded only once in history—by President Franklin Roosevelt.

The historians have recorded, however, that Humphrey was miserable during much of his term as vice-president. President Johnson left him in the dark, deprived him of fundamental information available to other cabinet officers, and yet demanded a stout defense of his politics from his vice-president. To President Johnson, independence of mind in a vice-president was tantamount to treason.

Thus it was that Humphrey spent much of 1965 and 1966 in LBJ's doghouse. The denigration of the vice-president took place in both public and private. For example, LBJ refused to send him to represent the United States at the funeral of Winston Churchill, sending Chief Justice Earl Warren instead. He refused to let the vice-president have staff for the use of aircraft his express permission. Humphrey's speeches were censored and he was sent off to make peace with business leaders. LBJ wanted business to contribute to the Democratic party war chest, and he wanted to show that Humphrey had recanted some of his populist beliefs. Humphrey continued to assert some independence; but the straw that broke the camel's back was when he openly opposed the president, arguing against the bombing and against a wider U.S. involvement in the war in Vietnam. This move resulted in his being barred from Security Council meetings. Humphrey became almost a prisoner in the Executive Office Building.

So fierce was the president's displeasure and so cold was his shoulder that somehow, Hubert Humphrey managed to persuade himself to be a good scout and do things the president's way. He even adopted the president's hawkish view on the war and became its staunchest defender. The more he blazed away in support of the president's policies, the more rope, access, authority, and perquisites that LBJ gave him. However, even Humphrey's eloquence could not turn the tide. By 1968, resistence to the war had grown so great that sit-ins, riots, and violence among students was daily fare for the national television networks, which juxtaposed these images with the death and destruction broadcast live from Vietnam.

The first major sign of trouble for President Johnson came when Senator Eugene McCarthy received 46 percent of the vote in the New

Hampshire primary. The president had won that race but barely. It showed how vulnerable he was within his own party to say nothing of how vulnerable he would have been in the general election. The results in that state encouraged Robert F. Kennedy, then a senator from New York to run for the nomination against LBJ. In one of several violent shock waves that hit the nation in 1968, the president announced on March 31, 1968, that he would not be a candidate for reelection; he needed all of his energies, he said, to pursue peace in Vietnam. The vice-president had been informed that this announcement might come only the day before it was made. The president told him flatly and without enthusiasm that if he were going to run, he had better move quickly.

In Pursuit of the Presidency

The vice-president entered the race. He left it to Senators McCarthy and Kennedy to slug it out in the primaries while he went around collecting votes from the deal-makers. The other two candidates had offered themselves as advocates of change while Vice-President Humphrey staked out the status quo. He became the candidate of the establishment. Firmly tied to President Johnson's apron strings, he did not dare to split with the president on the crucial issue of Vietnam.

The second major shock of that fateful spring came in April when Martin Luther King was assassinated in Memphis. Dr. King's death set off riots in a number of major cities. Angry blacks looted and burned buildings; the authorities countered by calling out the police and the National Guard. It was a serious and a sad time, the wrong time for a politician to proclaim "the politics of joy" as his campaign theme.

The death of Robert Kennedy following his dramatic victory in the June California primary further heightened the national malaise. A nation that was sick to death with war was now sick to death with death and more than a little sick of government.

RFK's death opened the way for Vice-President Humphrey to receive the nomination of his party at the forthcoming Convention being planned for August in Chicago. The Convention was a disaster by anyone's reckoning. Mayor Richard Daly's riot police overreacted and beat a park full of anti-war protestors to a pulp in full view of the national television cameras. Not surprisingly, the American public was presented with an even more negative view of the party of Lyndon Johnson.

Hubert Humphrey and Edmund S. Muskie lost that 1968 election to Richard Nixon and Spiro Agnew by a whisker. Historians looking back agree that victory was within Humphrey's grasp if he had only disassociated himself from the president and the unpopular war. The irony was that this amounts to saying that all he had to do was to be true to his principles and announce that he was against continuation of the war. And yet he was grateful to — or afraid of — President Johnson. Other scholars blame Lyndon Johnson for the loss saying he refused to turn over money and support to the vice-president. One theory holds that President Johnson had a secret plan to line up a Summit Conference with the Soviet Union to settle the Vietnam War. The Soviet's assent to it was to be announced at an elaborate birthday party that had been planned for the president by Mayor Daly. The choice of the convention site and dates was anything but accidental. Some hold that LBJ fully expected to pull this off and march triumphantly into the convention hall where wildly cheering delegates would demand he accept renomination for the presidency. Still another theory is that a settlement was at hand and it was undercut by the China lobby, which persuaded the South Vietnamese leaders that they should hold out because they could get a better deal from the hawkish Nixon rather than from Humphrey.

Whatever the reason, the Humphrey-Muskie ticket lost. Humphrey returned to private life for the first time since 1945, teaching at the University of Minnesota. He ran and was reelected overwhelmingly to the U.S. Senate in 1972.

In 1972, Edward Kennedy was the odds-on favorite for the Democratic nomination to oppose President Richard Nixon, but Chappaquiddick changed all of that. Senator Edmund Muskie sought the nomination as did Humphrey and Senator George McGovern, another Humphrey protege. Muskie pulled out early and Humphrey won some primaries, but McGovern ultimately was selected as the nominee. Senator Humphrey was asked to run for vice-president with McGovern but turned it down. Nixon was reelected only to resign in the face of impeachment over Watergate.

The party regulars came calling to Humphrey again in 1976 and for awhile the old warhorse tried on the political armor. He reserved time in the Senate Caucus room and it was largely expected that he would agree to enter the race against Gerald Ford. Instead, he announced that he had little appetite for running in all of the primaries in order to obtain the nomination. He told party leaders to look elsewhere. They did, to a largely unknown peanut farmer-engineer and former Governor of Georgia, Jimmy Carter. In September of 1976, two months before Jimmy Carter was elected, former vice-president Hubert H. Humphrey was diagnosed as having terminal cancer. During this painful time when he was undergoing chemotherapy, it was a source of pride to him that one of his own, Walter F. Mondale, had been selected to run for vice-president and that the Democratic team of Carter-Mondale won the election.

During 1977, the last year of his life, Hubert Humphrey was showered with honors both from within the United States and from overseas. The Senate honored him by creating a new post of Vice President Pro Tempore. This position carried with it a luxurious office in the capitol, a car with a driver, and other such amenities. A shower of cards, gifts, and letters sent by well-wishers from every corner of the globe flooded his office.

Hubert H. Humphrey died on January 13, 1978.

In fitting tribute, Humphrey was chosen as one of only 13 Americans ever to be accorded the honor of lying in state in the Capitol rotunda.

At his funeral service, which was attended by an impressive array of political leaders and celebrities from around the world, his student and friend of many years, Walter F. Mondale said of him:

> Above all, Hubert was a man with a good heart; and on this sad day it would be good for us to recall Shakespeare's words:
>
> "A good leg will fall; a straight back will stoop; a black beard will turn white; a curled pate will grow bald; a fair face will wither; a full eye will wax hollow; but a good heart, is the Sun and the Moon; or, rather, the Sun, and not the Moon; for it shines bright and never changes, but keeps its course truly." Hubert's heart kept its course truly.

He taught us all how to hope and how to love, how to win and how to lose. He taught us how to live and, finally, he taught us how to die. At critical times in our history, the United States has been blessed by great people who, just by being themselves, give us a vision of what we are at our best and of what we might become. Hubert Humphrey was such a man.

Learned

As one writer put it, for Hubert Humphrey, "The American dream wasn't just a dream. It happened every day. Money alone wouldn't make it. Talent, energy, some luck, and a willingness to try. These were the qualities that shaped such dreams, and this was the country where they came alive."

When asked what was the single most important key to success in politics, Humphrey said: "You have got to show people that you care about them. The main thing is that you have got to like people."

When asked what was wrong with politics, he said the lack of public financing. The present system, he said, corrupts because it forces politicians to go with their hands out to the very interest groups that are seeking legislative favors. As far as individual officeholders, he advised:

> The worst thing that can happen to a man in politics is to be vindictive or to reminisce too much. The main thing that you have got to keep in mind is that everything is not as important to other people as it is to you.

When asked what advice he would give to students and the younger generation, he said:

> What you do, what each of you do has an effect on the community, the state, and the nation and the world. There is so much to be done to build a better life. Whatever your views, don't jeer from bleachers, pitch in for what you think is the best team. Take an interest. Get into politics.

He emphasized the importance of adopting a positive attitude. "The key to winning is believing with all your heart that you can do it." Adding a comment about his battle to run the mob out of Minneapolis he added: "The toughest job was not beating down the hoodlums but overcoming the cynicism of my friends and sideline critics who told me that it couldn't be done."

He advised youngsters to "be themselves" and not to be afraid to express their emotions. It was a theme he returned to in his last speech before he died. He told a Minnesota labor audience as he cried that, "A man without tears is a man without a heart."

Hubert Humphrey loved his family and he especially loved children. He advised his colleagues to spend time with them. "Spending time with children nourishes my soul. Spending five minutes with a kid is like going to the beach. It helps me that much. It really does. You get as much as you give."

He said that good health was the strongest asset that anyone could have. "I've always felt that you can't really appreciate happiness until you've known pain, just as you can't appreciate health until you've suffered illness. There is an old saying, 'He that has health has hope and he that has hope has everything.'"

Finally, he was asked what was the test of good government and he replied:

> The moral test of government is how it treats those who are in the dawn of life, the children; those who are in the twilight of life, the aged; and those who are in the shadows of life, the sick, the needy and the handicapped.

The Humphrey Legacy

As noted previously, no man has ever matched Senator Humphrey's legislative achievements. His range of interests was tremendous. The power of his ideas and his success as a legislator is indicated by a partial recitation of some of his achievements below.

Certainly no man has ever done more for the nation's elderly. Medicare was the first bill that he introduced after joining the Senate in 1949, but he also pushed legislation to broaden the scope and benefits of Social Security, to bar discrimination on the basis of age, to create the Administration on Aging and the National Commission on the Aging.

No one can match his record in civil rights from early laws to outlaw lynching and abolish the poll tax to the landmark Civil Rights

Act of 1964, and the subsequent Voting Rights and Fair Housing Laws.

His achievements in arms control included establishing the first Senate Subcommittee on Disarmament, creation of the Arms Control and Disarmament Agency, and winning Senate approval of the Limited Nuclear Test Ban Treaty.

No one has done more to establish jobs and provide job training. His legislation created the Job Corps, the Youth Conservation Corps, and the Peace Corps. He sponsored the Manpower Development and Training Act, the Youth Employment Act, and the Migrant Families Assistance Act.

In the area of labor-management relations, he scored a number of victories related to wages, hours, and working conditions. He sponsored the Occupational Health and Safety Act in order to bring about improved safety and working conditions.

Many of the nation's housing assistance laws bear his name. It was his legislation that created the Department of Housing and Urban Development.

He sought to help the states with the Area Redevelopment Act, the Economic Opportunity Act, and with his revenue-sharing program.

He fought hunger at home with legislation that created the food stamps program, and he fought it abroad with the Food for Peace program. In an effort to stop abuses in the trading of commodity futures, he authored the bill creating the Commodities Futures Trading Commission.

In order to assist expecting mothers, he pushed through the WIC (Women, Infants and Children) program and the Headstart program, as well as substantial improvements in the federal School Lunch Program.

He assisted veterans with the Cold War G.I. Bill of Rights and provided comparable assistance to the disabled through the Vocational Rehabilitation Programs, the program of Disability Benefits to the blind under Social Security, and by establishing the Community Mental Health Centers Act.

No one can match his record in the area of education. He sponsored and pushed through the first bills to provide federal aid to elementary and secondary education. He created the federal Scholarship for Youth Program, the Library Services Construction Act, the Health Professions Training Act, and the Nurse Training Act.

He worked hard to protect the environment. Among his successes include the Wilderness Preservation Act, the National Forest Management Act, and the Land Use and Conservation Act.

In the area of consumer protection, he authored legislation to require certain auto safety standards including seat belts and to protect consumers from habit-forming drugs.

He made his mark in crime and law enforcement with minimum sentencing legislation as well as legislation such as the Juvenile Delinquency and Youth Offenders Control Act.

He was in the forefront of space exploration as chairman of the National Aeronautics and Space Council.

Some of his most significant reforms were visited on the Senate itself. He introduced legislation to revise Senate rules on cloture and the selection of committee chairmen, and introduced a bill that created the Joint Committee on Organization of Congress. His legislation required members of Congress for the first time to disclose their finances, and he helped create standards of ethics. His legislation also extended some of these concepts to the executive branch.

He was also a patron of the arts. His legislation helped create the Kennedy Center, the Museum of African Art, the National Portrait Gallery, and created the National Council on the Arts as well as the National Foundation on Arts and Humanities. In addition, he served as a member of the Board of Regents of the Smithsonian Institution.

Finally, some of his most important legislation were amendments to the Constitution itself. His legislation established the right of 18 year olds to vote, provided for the direct election of president and vice-president and provided procedure for filling the office of vice-president in case of a vacancy and clarifying presidential succession procedures.

Since the above list is illustrative and not exhaustive, it is little wonder that Hubert Humphrey is the consensus choice for best senator in this century, and it is no wonder that buildings are named after him in several government departments. He obviously was an extraordinary man.

Remembered

When asked how he would like to be remembered, he said: "As an effective man of government." There is no doubt but that his wish will be realized. Former President Harry S. Truman had his own thoughts on the subject:

> His assets were — character — intelligence — energy and an inborn sense of public service. His was the hard road and he deliberately chose it. He threw his political lot and future with the little fellow — the farmer — the worker — and the everyday people who worked for a livelihood.
>
> He never waivered from his original commitment. He had to overcome the natural hostilities of the people of privilege and much of the press. He fought the hard battle and he won — all on merit.
>
> I salute him as a man truly of the people and for the people. A man with a profound sense of public service, a man of probity — integrity and —above all — as a man of peace.

It is the responsibility of all of us who loved him to keep his dreams alive, to learn from the lessons he taught us, to honor his memory and preserve the legacy he left us all.

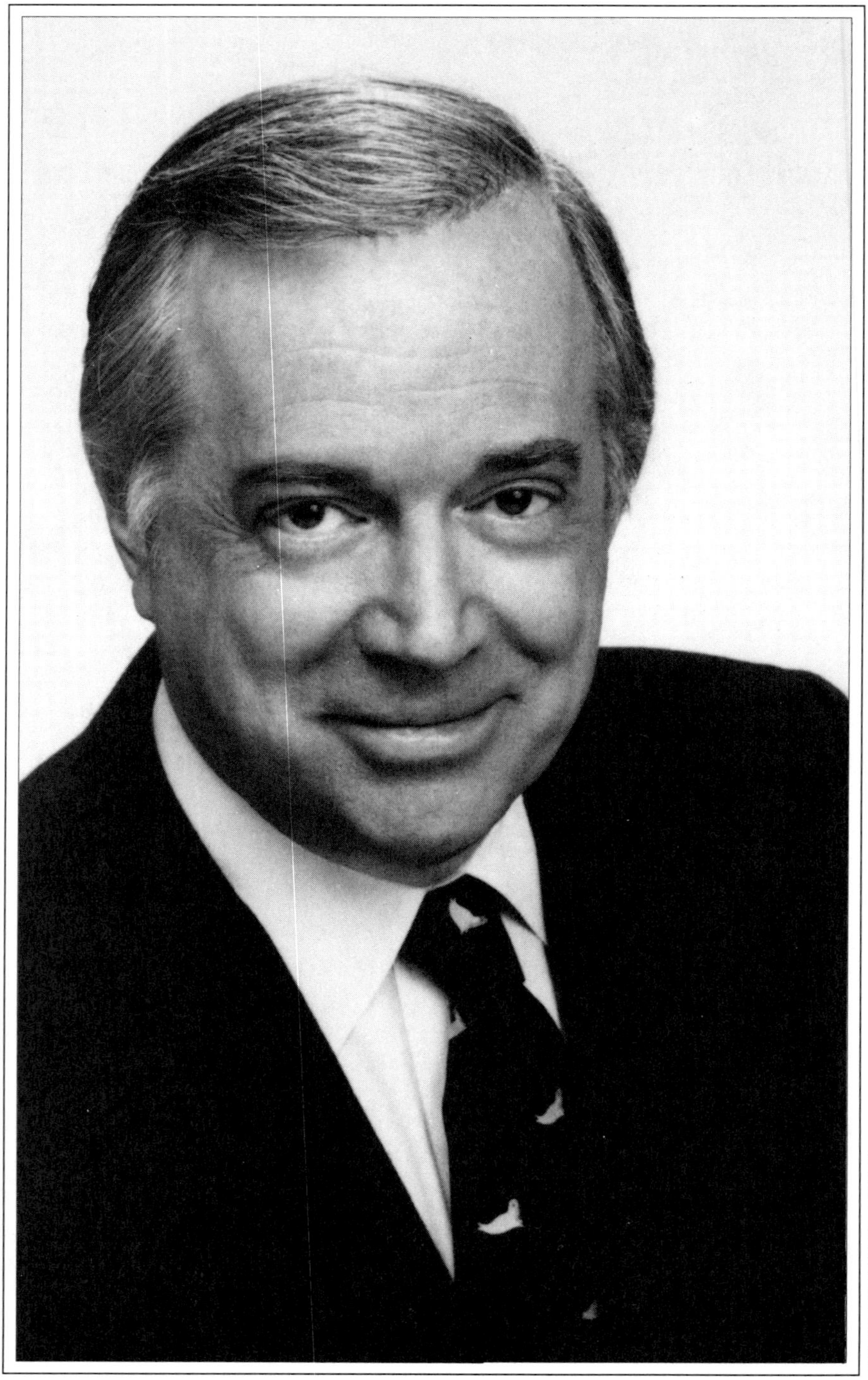

COURTESY OF HUGH DOWNS

SIXTEEN

Hugh Downs

He is the world's most familiar television personality; a legend in his own time for several generations of television viewers. At the comparatively young age of 69, he has already spent 51 years in broadcasting, holding the Guinness Book of World Records certificate for on-air longevity; he has spent more than 10,000 hours in front of the camera. It is a record to which he adds every week and one which probably never will be broken. Not only is he the most recognizable person on television; by most measures, he is the best in the business. He is the consummate professional, arguably the most beloved and most trusted figure on television today.

He helped make the "Tonight Show" the accepted institution that it has become. He took over as host of the "Today Show" when the program was in trouble and restored it to its highest ratings. After nine years as host of "Today," he left commercial television, only to return to the air as the host of the highly acclaimed "Over Easy," a program directed at senior citizens that he helped transform into the second most popular program ever broadcast on public television. Then he accepted an offer from ABC News to rescue their new magazine program entitled "20/20 " after what can only be called its disastrous beginning. He helped make the program what it is today—one of the longest running and most respected of network news programs.

His name is Hugh Downs, and his efforts have been recognized within the television industry, which has bestowed on him Emmy Awards and other accolades. Impressive as these achievements may be, however, they only begin to define this modern-day renaissance man.

Hugh Downs is the author of seven excellent and thought-provoking books. He is an expert in matters of science, astronomy, aeronautics, ecology, and aging. He has written articles and regular columns on these subjects for years. For example, along with such notables as Isaac Asimov, he was a regular columnist in *Science Digest.*

He is a teacher, having taught courses in communication, science, and aging. He is in demand as a public speaker, having lectured all over the world.

He is a father and a grandfather; a man highly devoted to his wife of 46 years.

He is a pilot, having flown everything from a glider to a F-104 fighter, the latter at twice the speed of sound. He even made five simulated landings in the U.S. Space Shuttle.

He is a race car driver, or at least it can be said that he has driven an automobile at more than 175 miles an hour at the race track that yearly hosts the Indianapolis 500.

He is a composer who has created not only simple songs but symphonies for full orchestra.

He is an excellent scuba diver, having explored the Great Barrier Reef in Australia and searched for buried Spanish treasure off Tortola in the British Virgin Islands.

He is an excellent sailor; he challenged and crossed the Pacific Ocean in a five-month journey in a small sailboat.

He is an explorer who, on December 10, 1982, traveled to the South Pole with a National Science Foundation expedition. Once there, he was given the honor of moving the bamboo stick marking the southern tip of the world about 10 meters to its proper location as determined by calculations from satellites. In the course of that adventure, he helped save the life of a fellow scientist who had fallen into a hole in the ice and was headed for certain death.

In addition to all the above, he is a man of issues and a man of action. He believes that something must be done to control the arms race, to end pollution, to increase justice, and to eradicate disease. He is a strong advocate of improved education and of helping individuals and society in general reach a state of maturity, which he says is possible only through selflessness and love. He has a special affinity for the elderly, having taken a post-master's degree in gerontology from Hunter College in New York City, and he has similar concerns about children, having served as chairman of the U.S. Committee for UNICEF.

Little wonder that he is known as the mild- mannered Clark Kent of journalism. His achievements are such that they could very properly be attributed to Superman. The fact is, however, that Hugh Downs is a mortal, a human being, albeit a quietly amazing one.

Downs has done more for older Americans than just about anyone. For example, he was among the first to research and broadcast a special on the subject of aging as far back as 1952, when the topic was considered taboo. Television executives argued that Americans did not want to see or hear about the vicissitudes of old age; they were embarrassed by thinking about their own mortality. Hugh Downs shattered the taboos and proved network executives wrong. Second, three of his seven books are devoted to the subject of aging and maturity. One offers practical help to those planning for retirement, another seeks to shatter the myths about aging, and the third points the way to effective aging—to greater maturity for both individuals and society. Third, Downs, at age 69, provides an excellent role model for seniors, having demonstrated in his own life that growth and emotional maturity continue with age; that age is no barrier to achievement; and that action is the preferred method of retirement. Fourth, Downs lent his considerable prestige to the program "Over Easy," which did more than any program before it to increase understanding of the problems of the elderly. By lending his name, he gave the program acceptance and excellence; he elevated the nation's seniors to a new standard of importance on television. Finally, Downs continues to be a strong advocate of the elderly in his capacity as correspondent and anchor for ABC's "20/20," he has repeatedly used this powerful platform to fight the injustice and discrimination perpetrated against the elderly.

Downs says in his autobiography, "I came to the reluctant conclusion that my generation has caused many of the problems for my parent's generation. We were the ones who tried to deny the problem, shunting our older citizens off into nursing homes and forgetting about them." Even if the premise can be accepted, Hugh Downs has more than made amends. He has been a one-man army who has helped to dissolve problems and thereby insured a better life not only for the nation's 32 million seniors, but for generations of seniors to come. For this alone, quite apart from his other Herculean achievements, Hugh Downs deserves the commendation of the nation.

Background

Hugh Downs was born in Akron, Ohio, on February 14, 1921. When he was two, the family had moved to Lima, Ohio, where he spent his formative years. His father, Raymond, was a machinist with the Lima Locomotive Assembly Company until he was almost killed in an accident; this event caused him to leave the job and take employment as a distributor of automobile batteries.

Young Hugh helped around the house and began his education in a one-room schoolhouse. When he was nine, the family moved to a small farm so that they could supplement their income. Hugh helped raise chickens and sold eggs to bring in a few more dollars.

After graduating from high school, Hugh won a one-year scholarship to Bluffton College in Lima by taking first prize in a public speaking contest. Hugh had to drop out of college after his first year in order to help out at home.

One afternoon in July of 1939, Hugh, then 19, was passing by the local radio station and on impulse walked in and asked for a job. Jobs were impossible to find in Lima during the depression, but to his surprise he was hired as staff announcer at the full-time rate of $12.50 a week.

In short order, he became the program director; he was given the authority to hire three more announcers and his salary shot up to $25 a week.

In 1940, he made his move, accepting a post with WWJ in Detroit, Michigan, as one of six full-time announcers. Pearl Harbor interrupted his career. Downs tried to enlist, but was turned down because he is color blind— only to be drafted by the Army. He was released from the service in May of 1943 and returned to his old job in Detroit. A year later, he landed a job with NBC in Chicago. At the age of 22, he became the youngest network announcer in America.

It was at NBC that he met Ruth Shaheen. They were married on February 20, 1944, and soon had a son, Hugh Raymond (H.R.), and a daughter, Diedre Lynn. Hugh Downs stayed at NBC for 11 years, reading the news, announcing music and drama, conducting interviews, and narrating programs. His next major move was to television.

"Radio was kind to me," says Downs. "It gave me a life's work and my life's love."

Television: Today and Tonight

In 1954, Hugh Downs left the security of the network to become a free lance announcer on a television show called "The Home Show" with Arlene Francis. The program was a kind of televised economics class and it stayed on the air until 1957.

Never one to let grass grow under his feet, Downs also took on an assignment as the announcer for the "Sid Caesar Hour" from 1956–57. In 1957, he was chosen to be the announcer of the "Tonight Show" on NBC. Steve Allen had brought that program to some prominence until he was cancelled in 1956. An obscure comedian named Jack Paar was hired as host, and together with Downs, they helped make the "Tonight Show" into a national institution.

Downs calls Paar a genius. He credits Paar for inventing the talk show as we have come to know it. Under Paar, the program became a kind of verbal free-for-all. The television audience was allowed to eavesdrop on the living room conversations of some of the nation's most interesting celebrities. In three short years, the program was broadcast on 76 stations, it reached 30 million viewers, and at any one time enjoyed an average of nine major sponsors.

The "Tonight Show" became the talk of the nation. Its success was measured by the fact that each of the other networks soon copied the format. It became the place to be seen for movie stars, celebrities, and political figures. And thanks to Jack Paar's eye for talent, it helped more than a few people break into show business. Among the "Tonight Show" discoveries are: Carol Burnett, the Smothers Brothers, Shelly Berman, Phyllis Diller, Flip Wilson, Don Rickles, Joey Bishop, Nipsey Russell, Mort Sahl, Mike Nichols and Elaine May, Woody Allen, Bill Cosby, and Jonathan Winters.

Downs speaks fondly of his days with the "Tonight Show," but adds that the program was a little bit like riding a bronco. One never knew what the mercurial Paar was going to do next. On February 11, 1960, Paar took offense at some network censorship and reacted by telling the network executives on the air what he thought of their actions, promptly walking off of the show. A month later, differences had been reconciled and Paar returned at his feisty best. He left the show for good in March of 1962.

In the clamor to decide who should replace Paar as host, Downs was mentioned by several commentators as a natural. He had presided as guest host more than any other person and those sessions in Paar's absence had received rave reviews. In the end, the network executives decided to go with another comedian, Johnny Carson, and Carson in turn brought with him his sidekick and announcer, Ed McMahon.

The "Tonight Show" had served the valuable purpose of bringing Hugh Downs to the attention of the American public. He was perceived as Paar's resident Plato. He was as solid as Paar was fragile. Eminently likable, well-read, and well-spoken, Hugh Downs demonstrated the kind of personality that wears well. The longer people know him and the better they know him, the more they like him.

If Hugh Downs had any disappointment in not being selected to host the "Tonight Show," it was short-lived. NBC tapped him to host their prestigious early morning fare, "The Today Show."

Beginning at 7 a.m. on September 22, 1962, and every weekday morning thereafter for the next nine years, Hugh Downs hosted "The Today Show." For Downs, this meant a radical adjustment to his biological clock; it meant getting up every morning at 4 a.m. and going to bed in the early evening. It also meant a switch from tape delay to live broadcasting. Finally, it meant a move away from the programming to the news side of broadcast journalism.

Throughout the turbulent 1960s, Downs was there every morning, as certain as the rising sun, reassuring the nation with his ready smile and positive demeanor.

It was the era of the Vietnam War or protests, civil rights demonstrations, and political assassinations. Downs comments:

"From my vantage point it looked like the country might really fall apart. The mood of the 1960s was so tinged with outrage, fear, anger, and violence that it was a real demonstration of our national resilience that the country was not more badly damaged."

For comic relief, Downs brought on board former baseball player, Joe Garagiola, whose good humor was welcomed by audiences shaking the sleep from their eyes. He also championed the cause of women by bringing Barbara Walters onto "The Today Show" as a regular contributor. Until that time, women had been relegated to minor roles on television, such as reading the weather forecast. It was Hugh Downs who helped Barbara, and women in general, make the transition to full-fledged, equal status.

In 1965, Downs broke another taboo. He had a hair transplant to banish male-pattern baldness and he talked about it on the air. Within weeks, Joey Bishop, Frank Sinatra, and Senator William Proxmire made news by having the same surgical procedure.

In his nine years as host of "Today," Hugh Downs made television history. He had rescued an NBC flagship program when it was in deep trouble and he raised it to the pinnacle of journalistic excellence. While he was doing so, he found time to host other television programs such as "Concentration," a popular daytime game show, and to continue his formal education. Having scaled the television pinnacle and at the very height of his popularity, Hugh Downs chose to leave it all behind.

Sabbatical: "Over Easy"

On October 11, 1972, Hugh Downs severed a three decade-long relationship with NBC, turning "The Today Show" over to Frank McGee. Hugh and Ruth Downs relocated to Carefree, Arizona, a quiet spot in the mountains some twenty miles north of Phoenix.

Hugh Downs took this time to study, reflect, write, teach, and to devote himself to one of the dozens of humanitarian causes which are so important to him. For example, he taught communication at Arizona State University. He wrote books such as *Rings Around Tomorrow*, and *Potential: A Guide To Human Maturity*. He participated in the work of the Center for Democratic Studies and succeeded Dr.

Wernher Von Braun as president of the non-profit National Space Institute. He took a course in astrophysics, served on the board of Planned Parenthood and UNICEF, and agreed to host the first network talk show specifically directed at the elderly called "Over Easy."

Hugh Downs's interest in gerontology dates back to 1952 when, at the age of 31, he and Jules Powers, a young producer, prepared a program for NBC entitled "How Long Can You Live?" In 1975, this same man approached Downs about hosting "Over Easy." The Department of Health, Education and Welfare (HEW), through its Administration on Aging, was putting up $4 million for 39 weeks of half-hour programs, five days a week. KQED, the public television station in San Francisco, had applied for the grant, which meant that the programs must be produced in that city.

"It struck me immediately as something I ought to do. The subject intrigued me. It was for PBS; pay was a fraction of commercial television but I was glad to oblige if the project was right. I believe in non-commercial broadcasting but never got the chance to try it. I felt a series on aging could be successful on a non-commercial basis," said Downs.

Unfortunately, problems soon developed. Powers was insisting on network production values, which was a standard that the PBS station found hard to reach. The original hope, that the five half-hour programs could be done in one day or two, soon evaporated. Hugh Downs spent more and more of his time in San Francisco or in the air between Arizona and California. Finally, he and Ruth moved to San Francisco, with the Arizona home again becoming a vacation respite.

Other problems developed. HEW, which had put up the money, was asserting more and more control. It seemed to some people that HEW merely wanted its services promoted on television. Downs says HEW wanted "Over Easy" to focus on problems of the elderly, not broadcast inspirational material depicting successful aging.

The wrestle for editorial control continued and when the money ran out, it had to be raised privately in order to have the program continue. In the end, Downs and Powers won out. "Over Easy" became a landmark. In addition to seniors, the program attracted a significant number of 18- to 30-year-olds. "Over Easy" helped to shape a new ethic concerning aging. It soon became the second most popular program on public television, right behind the "MacNeil/Lehrer Hour," it was broadcast on over 200 stations. In May of 1981, Hugh Downs was honored with an Emmy Award for his involvement with "Over Easy."

Hugh Downs served as the host of "Over Easy" from 1978 through 1981. In June of 1978, he responded to an SOS from Roone Arledge, CEO of ABC News, who asked him to take over ABC's new magazine show called "20/20." Downs agreed to do this, but he would not break his contract with "Over Easy." What this meant was that for three years he flew coast to coast, spending two and a half days doing each of the programs. He did both and he did them well. It was a prodigious feat by anyone's standard.

ABC's "20/20"

It is no secret that the other networks long envied CBS the success of their highly acclaimed program, "Sixty Minutes." The other networks tried numerous times to replicate the formula but not until "20/20" came along did they succeed. It almost didn't happen that way. The fact that it did is in large part due to Hugh Downs.

The premier program of ABC's "20/20" was a disaster by anyone's measurement. The core of the problem was an offbeat team of hosts who anchored the program. Many people take for granted what a television anchor is supposed to do. Some assume that the person is simply an announcer or, at most, an interlocutor. The term is really closer in its television application to its sports use as the strongest runner in a relay race.

A television anchor is the person who sets the tone for the broadcast, offers the audience reassurance, introduces the program and the correspondents, and generally provides the glue that holds the entire program together. The premier "20/20" program had become unglued because the wrong people had been chosen to anchor the broadcast.

It was no wonder that Roone Arledge would try to hire the most polished anchorman of all time to save his show and the network from yet another embarrassing failure.

With his many years of television exposure, including his nine-year stint as host of "Today," Hugh was, along with Walter Cronkite, the most trusted person in broadcasting. His presence at the opening of the second "20/20" program was an immediate signal that what was to come was serious and high quality broadcasting. The public knew that this was so or Hugh Downs would not be associated with the program. He gave the program instant credibility and acceptance, as well as some greatly needed professionalism.

Those who had not seen him since he left "Today " welcomed him back like an old friend. Those who were watching him on "Over Easy" were delighted to see more of him in a sparkling new format. New, younger viewers who were drawn to the program with its sporadic emphasis on teen rock stars found that Downs was easy to like.

While Downs credits Arledge, former Executive Producer Av Westin, Barbara Walters, and others, a fair share of the credit for the success of "20/20" belongs to Hugh Downs.

ABC's "20/20" had its 10th anniversary in June of 1988. The occasion was marked with a three-hour retrospective. As the highlights indicate, the program has provided entertainment and education in equal measure. Some of its strongest contributions relate to its exposure of fraud, abuse, and the waste of taxpayers' dollars. The program, like Hugh Downs himself, has been the advocate of the underprivileged and it has done good work in bringing serious problems to the attention of the American public and to the Congress.

ABC's "20/20" has had a significant effect on the legislative process at both the state and the national level. Numerous pieces of public interest legislation, having languished for years before the Congress or state legislatures, magically found their way into law after being highlighted on "20/20." Thanks to Downs, Walters, Westin, and others, the program has developed a high degree of credibility and it has become a force for good as well as an entertainment or educational vehicle.

Having filled his anchor role so well, it might seem to some that Hugh Downs would sit back and let his producers and correspondents bring stories to him. Not so. Every year he insists on going into the field and directly helps prepare about a dozen stories. The stories in which he has chosen to act as both correspondent and anchor are extremely powerful because of the attention he gives them and his choice of themes. Not surprisingly, many of his stories relate to the elderly. In 1988, one memorable offering was a story about thousands of seniors forced to accept retirement in clear violation of the statute that bars age discrimination in employment.

Commenting on his career in broadcasting in his book, *On Camera*, he says:

> In looking back over four decades in television, I have tried to put myself into perspective. . . . When I first joined "The Home Show," I realized that if I were ever going to survive on this new medium I would have to play myself on camera, nothing less and nothing more. In a medium full of flashy entertainers, brilliant comedians, superb actors and honey-throated announcers, I was none of the above. I was a well spoken kid from Ohio with an absolutely ordinary personality.
>
> It took me a few years to realize that if the 20th century is the era of the common man—as H.L. Mencken so acerbically put it—then television is the medium of the 20th century.
>
> I think the important part of what I do is to try to represent the viewer. In a free society the media will rise and fall according to the power granted to them by the people.

Impressions

What kind of man is Hugh Downs? The answer is that he is very much what he appears to be on television. He is intelligent, sensitive, and a little shy. He is so positive one writer described him as a "puddle of sunshine."

He has a childlike, unquenchable curiosity. He loves to read, to learn, and given the opportunity, he loves to teach. He is extremely calm, so much so that one writer said he makes Perry Como look like a nervous wreck. He is cool and collected, although he admits sometimes to having butterflies underneath.

> The calmer approach has always worked for me, first in preservation of my health, in audience acceptance and in allowing me most of the time to do more than one broadcast series simulta-

neously. I am proud of my record of more than 10,000 hours on air. I've taken precautions to make sure that I didn't burn out like some of my colleagues.

He is blessed with great energy; he has the stamina of a man half his age, a fact that led one writer to say that he moves in more directions than a centipede on ice.

He enjoys his work, there is no doubt about that. He has found ways to make it fun. He has used his job as a means of opening up new experiences and furthering his education on a host of subjects. He learned to dive, for example, in connection with one of his programs and he learned to fly as part of another.

He is a man who pushes himself to the maximum, often to the point of putting his life on the line. He says he became a daredevil, if that is the right word, as a means of overcoming his many fears. "I have always been intrigued by people who push themselves beyond the supposed limit of human endurance." He also notes that he adopted this aggressive approach to life as a reaction to his relative timidity as a child.

He notes that he is not much of a sports fan because he is not very competitive. "I hate to lose and I am embarrassed when I win." However, when it comes to competing with himself, it is a whole other matter. There is no doubt but that he pushes himself to scale the lofty heights of excellence.

He likes classical music and has read (and understands) the great books. He has the ability to speak to men of science in their own terminology, whether that might be aeronautics or nuclear physics. Some of his knowledge was obtained in college through one of the dozens of college courses he has taken; much of it is also self-taught.

He is genial, modest, and by his own definition, mature. The latter implies that he is selfless rather than self-centered; he puts the needs and interests of others first.

He is a man of integrity; his word is his bond. He is also a man of principle. He works actively for the causes he espouses instead of merely paying them lip service. No matter what the pressure, he remains true to his beliefs. They are, after all, usually well thought-out. Most people simply do not take the time to fashion their personal philosophy, to sort out their values and beliefs. Hugh Downs took the time to do this and it has served him well. At a time in life that others find turbulent, he remains very well grounded.

He is fun to be around, down-to-earth, and pleasant; he is a charming conversationalist, in part because of his vast storehouse of knowledge and in part because of his genuine interest in other people.

Hugh Downs is also blessed with an excellent sense of humor. For example, when someone described him as a walking encyclopedia, he amended the statement to "a walking pamphlet." Another example comes from his autobiography:

"I really wanted to be an artist," he says of his youth. "Then it was a fireman, railroad engineer and an astronomer. Mother hoped that I would become an Episcopal bishop. I became what I was supposed to be all along, an adult human being expert at nothing but curious about everything."

Hugh Downs sees himself primarily as a communicator who has the ability and the opportunity to get ideas of worth across to his audience. He believes that a communicator can reduce stress because merely knowing the truth has the effect of diminishing fear. "For we have learned that unknown dangers are far more disquieting than the known."

His friends and colleagues see him as a wonderful person; and as is so often the case, it is the judgment of one's peers that is most accurate. For example, Barbara Walters, his co-anchor, acknowledges the debt she owes to Downs:

> I have had the pleasure—and believe me, it is that—of working alongside Hugh Downs for a great part of my own career. Indeed, were it not for Hugh's encouragement and support, I would never have been on television.

Marion Golden, formerly senior producer with both CBS's "Sixty Minutes" and ABC's "20/20," says that Downs is "one of the rarest forms of life in network television these days ... a gentleman."

Karen Burnes, now of ABC News, and previously a star of CBS's "West 57th" and producer of "20/20," termed him a "gentleman of the first order."

> To say that he is gracious is an understatement. In my years at "20/20," and in hundreds of days under enormous pressure, I have never seen him raise his voice or lose his emotional calm. That he is

> a true professional is obvious to all. That he is funny, very funny, may be less obvious to the viewing public. But he is wry, witty, filled with wondrous anecdotes and all kinds of obscure facts. This is one man who has not lost his sense of himself or his compassion for others despite the brutal business he's in.

Peter Kuhnhardt, another former "20/20" producer who recently collaborated with Downs to make "Eldercare," a half-hour home video tape designed to help seniors and their families with the difficult decisions of long-term care, comments about Downs.

> Hugh has a genuine commitment to the elderly. . . . He is committed to the elderly in his head and in his heart. By communicating the problems to the rest of the country, not only has he become an unofficial spokesman for the cause, but a leader in the field.

ABC News anchor Tom Jarriel added:

> Never have I known a person whose life so genuinely spans such a broad spectrum. Hugh Downs is ageless. He is as much at home with kids as he is with younger colleagues or the elderly. . . . Sometimes he talks about subjects which are so complicated I don't have the faintest idea what he's talking about. But on the "20/20" set he has the ability to be the clearest communicator in the broadcast business. In one area of Hugh's character I have found no ambiguity; he is genuinely one of the nicest human beings I have ever known.

Major Problems of Our Times

Hugh Downs has thought long and hard about the major problems of our times. Among those problems he lists the arms race, ageism, degradation of the environment, overpopulation, failures in education, the breakdown of the family unit, and the failure to find a national sense of purpose. Downs believes that this is a time of crisis. "We are on the spearpoint of the world's drive to live," he says.

With respect to the arms race, he says:

> The task is one which will make all previous endeavor seem small. Our animal instincts, our competitive drive, coupled with our newfound intellect, have given us dominance and propelled us onto the field. Man now finds himself in the position of the dog who

chased the locomotive and caught it. What does he do with it? In a sense, man has seized evolution and is stuck with the responsibility for managing it. Man is now on the throne and must trade his aggressive habits for cooperative ones or perish.

He adds:

> Humanity is somewhat like the toddler who has found the meat cleaver and is waving it above his head. He may drop it on the floor or he may drop it on his skull. The point is that he is not equipped with enough sense to handle it. It has often been observed that though man is a social animal he has not developed sufficiently sophisticated social machinery to handle safely the tools and weapons he has recently produced.
>
> The Gods were mad at Prometheus not because he stole fire but because he and his kind were not ready to make the sort of use of it that showed progress in God-like direction. Now that we have stolen fire from the heart of the atom, we will have to show such cause. We already have an inkling of the punishment we'll suffer if we fail.

Downs also sees overpopulation as a threat. "Nothing in evolutionary history has ever made reproduction a threat to survival. It was always the other way around. The more children who were born and survived, the more safety the community enjoyed. This has been true until quite recently."

He has strong concern about the degradation of the environment.

> A sudden and dramatic disaster is an unfortunate and unsettling circumstance but still worse that there is the situation where a real and ghastly danger to all humanity comes only slowly and undramatically and realization and remedy are stifled by human apathy and inertia. Humanity is threatened in just such a way right now. The industrial smokestack, symbol of America's muscle and technical plenty, is endangering your life whether you live in or out of Los Angeles. Often we breathe more poison in very light smog than we get from smoking cigarettes, cigars, and pipes. Living in an environment that is polluted means that every breath you take has harm in it.

He is critical of the established educational system which in America is not geared to provide knowledge and help people learn how to think. Rather, he says, it is directed to the production of minds conditioned to preserve the established order, to serve the state or the economic order, and to force conformity.

He says the most pernicious pattern in our culture is the belief that "You can't teach an old dog new tricks. We still cling to the idea that a child has a 'learning period' laid in roughly from the age of six through adolescence and then it is over. The formative years should last until the end of life."

Downs believes strongly in self-teaching. "Most things that people think you have to have a teacher for, you can teach yourself."

He believes that it is particularly important for individuals to teach themselves emotional maturity, "which will bring them great reward and at the same time contribute to setting the whole human species on a parallel cosmic path." He says that unless this happens on an individual level, it will not happen. "No legislation, no law enforcement, no courts, no dispensations to the poor and indigent and no school system will accomplish the task that faces humanity."

He adds that physical and mental maturity apparently slack off with time, but emotional maturity apparently does not. He says the aim of the mental health movement is not only to care for those who have collapsed under emotional strain, but to provide preventive measures and guidance to maturity.

He criticizes the "me generation," with its emphasis on acquisition of things material, as a sad waste of human resources and potential. "The sickness of the 20th century could be that we have not found a sense of purpose commensurate with the liberating effects of political freedom and leisure that our age has ushered in."

Increased leisure, according to Downs, does not mean having more time to spend in the tavern; it means more time for inviting the soul, for planning one's destiny, for civic and government involvement, and for heightening individuality.

Science has brought us great progress, but it also has its downsides, he asserts. "Our progress lulls us to sleep and makes us flabby. The conquest of the moon and Mars is an endeavor cut from the fabric of immortality but the pop-up toaster and the electric nutcracker are proffered to us by the bony hand of the Ferryman."

Another item of concern for Downs is the breakdown of the home and the extended family unit. "The home still contributes the principle shaping of human mental and emotional character. . . . Parents set examples. Children imitate. If parents are seen to be learning, children will be motivated to learn. No utopian scheme, no social experiment, no commune has yet proved superior to the domiciled family unit."

He feels strongly that health care in America must be improved; that health care is a basic civil right and that the failure to emphasize wellness is a serious shortcoming.

Hugh Downs is also sharply critical of ageism—that is, the discrimination against the elderly that is present in American society. He says:

> Today, the older people who have accumulated something like wisdom find themselves neither revered nor consulted by anyone of lesser age. And in the confusion, civilization itself drifts ponderously toward the rocks.
>
> There is no aging problem except that created by social injustice. We refuse to employ the aged and infer from their joblessness that they are unemployable. We deny them the dignity of being taken seriously as students and say they are uneducable.
>
> We force them into poverty and then, in studying their expenditures, conclude that they don't need much money. We shame them into impotence and declare they are not interested in sex. When they are righteously indignant at our neglect or unfairness or confused through overmedication, or simply reluctant to conform, we write them off as "senile." When they hurt from injury or illness, we say it is because they are old, as though old is a disease.
>
> What we do to our elderly is really quite reprehensible.
>
> Let's face it, there is more than a hint of ice-floe ethics in our attitude towards the old. When elderly Eskimos could no longer hunt, or even sew skins or build shelters, obliging to society their relatives placed them on ice floes or otherwise exposed them to extinction so as not to diminish the food supply needlessly. Cruel as this may seem, it had communal survival value. But when a society becomes industrialized, and one farmer can feed many people, the practice becomes anachronistic. Still we insist on placing older people as a group in the ice floes of retirement or rest homes or loneliness or otherwise expose them. This all reflects prejudice, not survival value.

To Hugh Downs the answers to these problems are self-evident. The answer to age discrimination is to end it. The answer to the arms race is arms control. If pollution is the problem, the answer is to clean up the environment. Population control is the answer to overpopulation. If the educational system does not help people learn how to think and does not give them the knowledge base they need, the answer is to change it to do so. Likewise, the erosion of familial responsibility can be changed by the establishment of new norms in behavior. Finally, if there is no sense of national purpose, one must be established around the concept of preserving the benefits of freedom and individual liberty to generations of as yet unborn. "Humanity is surely on the brink of finding some way to supercede the nation-state and the old balance of power relationships," he says.

Learned

Ask Hugh Downs what he has learned and he will begin by telling you the importance of having a positive attitude about life. "We see a social problem and we get overwhelmed by it. We say to ourselves, 'Gee, there is nothing we can do about it.' And that is not true. To say something is bad may be factual but to say it is hopeless is an opinion. By taking the positive approach we can often make significant inroads and help bring about a solution."

He will tell you how he learned to conquer fear. "I was always full of fear. First, I was a terribly timid child. When I started out in radio, I had a murderous case of stage fright, and then, on television, of camera fright. I discovered that there is only one way to handle fear: Go out and scare yourself!" He adds that fear can only be faced head-on because, "Being alive is being vulnerable."

He advises young people to dare to dream and to act on their dreams. "Try the impossible. Think the impossible. Entertain any idea that comes to you. You must believe it will work at the outset. If you believe it can't work it becomes a self-fulfilling prophecy when applied to any motivational problem."

He advises young people to be active and not passive. "The world imprisons us with conventional ideas. A self-motivated person helps create his own environmental change. Meddle with fate. Go for a walk in the rain."

He advises others to forsake anger, guilt, and hatred. "We are never angry unless something is threatened. Reaction is because we think deep down that the critic may be right. Guilt is almost thoroughly useless; it is worse than useless, it is self-destructive." Don't carry past hurts on your back; forget the past, he says. One of the sources of anger, he says, is the fear that we might lose our prejudices. "Hatred is an emotion more dear than grief. We clutch our prejudices to our bosom like loved children. They justify our cruelties and provide a rationale for our dislikes. We don't have to stop hating, it is a matter of redirecting it. In general, if we hate certain things, conditions, actions, and ideas, we are still free to feel kindly towards all people."

In a reversal from traditional advice, he advises young people to mix business with pleasure. He has certainly done so in his career and it has apparently worked very well for him. "Always mix business with pleasure. If you don't find pleasure in your work, you won't find pleasure. I never made a name or any money in television until I started having fun with it. A 'You can't fire me, I quit' attitude somehow diminishes the punishments that fate hands out."

Asked about happiness, he will quote Victor Hugo: "The supreme happiness of life is the conviction that we are loved." He will add that "A happy person is not a person with a certain set of circumstances but rather a person with a certain set of attitudes." He is fond of telling the Zen parable about the fool who went searching for fire with a lighted lantern, with the obvious point that the potential for happiness is within us all the time; it is simply a matter of how we look at things.

"The attitude of the advised is more important than the advice," he says. "The real cause of any emotional unhappiness is within your power to be dealt with and since it is clearly not in your power to change the world, try the other."

He advises young people to adopt a "zestful attitude not only to make the world more fresh but to make ourselves less stale." In most cases, he says, this involves abandonment of the preoccupation with self. He tells a story attributed to Helen Hayes, who managed to keep her performance fresh even after hundreds of performances of the same play. When asked how she did it, the actress said: "I focus on the audience for whom this play is opening night. If I thought about myself, the play would have been stale after the tenth performance." Downs adds, "Great inner security is needed to keep other people in mind in everything we do, but ironically, self is best served by looking away from self." He cements the point by offering the lines of Dr. Zhivago, which related to a locomotive with its headlight on backwards in an attempt to see itself. "This is futile since it cannot see itself and it can't illuminate the track ahead, which is what it needs to do."

Maturity

Hugh Downs believes that the mark of a mature person is dissolving the ego shell so that excursions outside of it are possible. Human maturity involves being selfless rather than selfish; it involves having empathy for all other living beings.

Like his hero Albert Einstein, he believes that "the most mature human insights come from one's introspection rather than from exterior research." Einstein said he had learned more from the world of imagination than from all the great books of the world.

"Human maturity," says Downs, "is nothing more than moving along the line from competitive habits to cooperative ones. We must move along this line as a species. We must move along this line as individuals."

"In the shift from autocentrism to allocentrism—that is from self-centeredness to other-centeredness—all tears may be idle but maturity is measured by what makes them flow." He adds that a highly mature person often has a magnetic quality about him or her that attracts disciples. Mature people, he says, are generally happy despite a penetrating awareness of reality. "The mature person comes to regard himself more and more not as a thing but as a process."

To cement his point about maturity, Downs tells the story of the man who was bereft following the death of his wife and three children in an automobile accident. He says that salvation was found in one word. At first, the man asked selfishly, "To whom can I turn for comfort?" Then he found the answer and asked, "To whom can I turn with comfort?" Downs says that grief was converted into efforts on behalf of other people whose problems were susceptible to understanding and love. The man became a volunteer in a mental hospital and as he grew to care about helping others, he reestablished his interest in life.

"Our job," says Downs, "is to get more individuals in society to maturity, at which time we will see an explosive social progress analogous to the explosive character of technical progress touched off by the advent of the machine."

Love

Hugh Downs believes that love and maturity are strongly linked. He presented a paper on this topic a few years ago at the Center for Democratic Studies in Santa Barbara, California.

> It seems to me that the next big step in civilization will be the emotional maturing of man. Imagine what would happen if you had a society mature enough to choose its leadership from the wise instead of among the powerful.
>
> You and I could easily name ten people we know who would never break into our car or home and take something, not for fear of retribution but because they wouldn't want to take something. Imagine now if a whole society achieved that level of maturity.

The key to the attainment of maturity is love. "Somebody once said there is only one heroism, to know the world as it is and to love it. Perhaps the great of history, certainly the spiritually great, gave evidence of this ability, which I think is strongly linked to maturity."

Downs quotes Thomas Merton, "Power always protects the good of some at the expense of all the others. Only love can attain and preserve the good of all."

A man in love can perform miracles and rise to incredible heights of ingenuity and endurance, or in sublimating his sex drive can bring prodigies out of his obsession, says Downs. "Love must start with love of self," he adds. "Anyone who does not love himself cannot love anyone else. Loving oneself has to do with self-respect and this has to do with accepting oneself."

The mature person loves beyond need, says Downs. "It is futile to love in order that we be loved in return. As soon as it is recruited in some other service, it ceases to be love. Love is an outward act, an end in itself. Love is limitless and ennobles anything it touches. It has to do with cooperation not competition. It is the main characteristic of normalcy, health, and maturity."

He continues, adding: "If religion has anything to offer man, it is the idea of cooperation through caring which runs through all the doctrine, quietly, stubbornly insisting that man will save himself individually and collectively only in this way."

He concludes that it is significant that most major religions have a common tenant: It is necessary to love. "The Spanish Inquisition was short lived. The concept of love persists." He adds that true Christian love "involves loving the unlovable, which requires a real sense of charity that is caring, a genuine caring even for genuinely unlikable people."

Downs believes that the biblical story of Jesus advising the rich man to sell all his possessions and give them to the poor has been misinterpreted. "What he urged us to do was to care so intensely about the poor and all mankind that his wealth would have meant nothing to him. In this circumstance, he would have given it willingly. No sacrifice is involved. Nothing is forced. Who can hinder you from loving, from caring?"

"At the deepest seat of our being," he says, "is the knowledge that 'to be loved' is not in our power, but to love always is . . . love is like a fire, it reproduces and expands itself" and one cannot stress too strongly the tangible results that come even from very small moves at getting outside oneself.

Aging

Hugh Downs has written extensively on the subject of aging. In one book, *Thirty Dirty Lies about Old*, he shatters many of the popular myths about growing older. In another, *Best Years Book—How to Plan for Fulfillment, Security, and Happiness in the Retirement Years*, he offers practical advice to seniors on how best to prepare for their life after age 65. Some of his excellent advice is carried here.

> I have come to the conclusion that when we speak of old age, we really don't know what we are talking about. There is no neat,

airtight definition. The final stage of life is not without its limitations but most of them are socially concocted and not at all intrinsic.

There is nothing wrong with getting old or being old. There is always something wrong about being ill or injured. There is nothing wrong with retirement or retiring. There is something wrong and destructive about being forced into uselessness because of calendar age: Everyone ages but few have learned that:

(a) there is no fixed timetable for a decline of powers or impairment of faculties; (b) impairment and limitations gradual or sudden can be dealt with less painfully than we generally think and up to a point can be accommodated with no net loss of happiness; (c) the risks of encountering these losses can be modified and something can be done about them. There is no longer such a thing as a hopeless disease. There are irreversible impairments but there are also a growing number of ways to offset them and go on functioning; (d) we need not shackle ourselves with the expectations of society that mistreats and misunderstands age. We can raise hell. We are at the dawn of an era in which elders are beginning to move toward center stage again: and society will gain by reinstating what went dormant when citizens became consumers.

When all the myths, injustices, and prejudices are retired, age will be seen in its true light: as a triumph over the forces of decay and dissolution, a time for a well -earned reward and respect, and a time for choice as to one's satisfaction including the right to savor the memories, the friends, the kin, the accomplishments, the honors, skills, techniques, and landmarks that have accumulated in the course of a lifetime. When age is viewed in this light by the whole community, it will be seen that there is no aging problem.

When asked about retirement, Downs responds, "A sensible person does not retire. He or she changes activities or actions. One who retires to do something else, to live life in a positive, new way is still in command. One who has been 'retired' is a victim."

He tells seniors that what their life is like after age 65 is largely up to them and it depends on how well they plan for it. "Unlike other societies, the United States has yet to institutionalize a proper role for its older citizens. So each retiree in America has the challenge of creating his or her own lifestyle. This can be a problem or an opportunity, because there are many subtle issues involved in retirement. It should be a period of renewal and purpose. Most successful are those who have let go of their old roles, opened themselves to broader personal perspectives and who have reached out to grasp the new opportunities."

Downs says the three major pitfalls related to aging are financial insecurity, uncertainty about where to live, and post-retirement letdown. With respect to income, he is sharply critical of Social Security and Medicare gaps. He makes the point that the U.S. ranks near the bottom of the top 30 industrialized countries in terms of the percentage of its gross national product that it pays out to retirees. The average of the 30 nations was about 14 percent of GNP spent on old age pensions, while the U.S. came in below five percent, "barely above Portugal." "None of the systems is ideal; ours lags behind adequacy." Downs says our failure to come to grips with this problem is like walking blindfolded off a cliff. We are cheating not only today's elderly, he contends, but all of the rest of us as well. Given the fact that greater numbers of people will have more years in retirement, the system needs reform at once, he asserts.

He points out that good health is the rule and not the exception at age 65-plus. "Anything that reinforces the idea that sickness of any kind is synonymous with oldness is a lie. Nobody ever died of old age. Disease, accident, body abuse, what have you but not old age. Old age is hardly a cause of death. On the contrary, it stands as a symbol of victory over all the forces of destruction, decay, and dissolution that threaten us throughout life." Downs notes that something is amiss with our health care system in that there are tremendous gaps, services that are not provided, and yet the U.S. spends a higher percentage of its GNP on health care than any other nation.

Downs notes that recent scandals involving nursing homes have singled out some really horrible examples of abuse and neglect, motivated by greed. "These places are dreadful and they should be spotlighted and changed or closed," he says.

Hugh Downs is a strong advocate of home care, which serves to keep the elderly in independence in their own homes as long as this is possible. He believes in home care not only because it is more cost effective, but because it serves to help keep families together. In October of 1983, Downs received the Lois Lillick Award, the highest award from the National Association for Home Care, in recognition of his lifetime devotion to improving the quality of life for the nation's elderly. He said at that time:

> There is never anything wrong with getting older or being old but there is always something wrong with being sick or alone or broke and discriminated against or being shunted off in warehouses for the dying when an enlightened culture would tend more toward taking care of its own.
>
> There are societies in the world where home care is so much a part of the culture that they don't think about needing someone to do something about it. Home care is the norm in many parts of the world. Admittedly the techniques and some of the clinical aspects could be enhanced but this is the concept that we need to reestablish in our culture. . . and we are moving in the right direction.

When asked about sex and the elderly, he says he sees little reason why it should be limited. He offers reference to Faust who, he says, apparently was not a wise man for all of his learning. He wanted to be younger so badly that he sold his soul to the Devil in exchange for a fling with Marguerita. "I've always thought the real tragedy of Faust was that he could have made it with Marguerita at his real age had he come on properly."

When asked what the elderly can expect in the future, he says, "An older person's loss of strength and flexibility will be offset by personal environments that will amplify power and mobility and aid the failing senses. Above all, the wishes of the individual will govern efforts to 'care' for him or her. . . . Finally we can begin to expect in our later years justice and comfort. If we get these at any age, there is little else that we need ask for." When this happens, then in the words of Longfellow, "age is opportunity no less than youth itself."

Remembered

In an interview that dates back to the mid-1970s, Hugh Downs spoke in general terms about the concept of a renaissance man.

> I have often thought that if some kind of renaissance man were to appear in our midst just now, he might not be recognized because

> American society would tend to require that he pin a label on himself, and then everything else that he did would be considered merely interesting hobbies—in other words, the person wouldn't be taken seriously. More and more young people today are tending toward the desire to do things rather than to be things.

Hugh Downs may be correct about these judgments. American society has not always valued its greatest citizens—at least not in their lifetimes. However, history has already made the judgment where he is concerned. Hugh Downs will be remembered for what he is, one of America's true national treasures, a 20th-century renaissance man.

Conclusion

The purpose of this chapter is to identify the common elements among the people profiled in this book. Each of them in their own way is a hero or heroine. Their individual achievements have been great and their collective impact has been vast. They helped shatter the myth that incompetence and decrepitude are a natural state among the aged. In doing so, they liberated America's seniors and gave them freedom from fear. In guaranteeing freedom, hope, and opportunity for seniors, they also removed the shackles from younger generations who will all too soon be old themselves.

The key questions are: What do they have in common? What has made them so successful? What have they learned? and What do they regard as the great secrets of life?

The answers are important to both young and old. Both will look to this book for role models. Seniors can take heart in learning that Maggie Kuhn's achievements came after she had retired and that Claude Pepper was 63 when he began his service in the House of Representatives. Similarly, youngsters can see in Pepper, Robert Butler, and Elisabeth Kübler-Ross people who were very focused—who knew what they wanted to do at a very young age.

Young people will also find in these elements of commonality many of the great secrets of the universe. Like all truths, they are simple. Readers will quickly see that the truths disclosed below are common not only to the people who helped move aging from the back pages to the front pages of the American consciousness, but also to the greatest people who ever lived on the planet.

One of these great truths, for example, is that self-realization is only possible through caring for others. Whether for the individual or for the nation, self is best served in transcending self. Albert Einstein, perhaps the brightest man of the 20th century, expressed this truth by saying, "Only a life lived for others is worthwhile." Mother Teresa of Calcutta said her life has been built on this one principle: "Love one another, there is joy in transcending self in order to serve others."

What is implied from the last paragraph is that people have intrinsic value, and beyond that they should be measured by what they have done for others. In other words, success should find its meaning in caring and public service and not in the selfish acquisition of wealth and material possessions. Judged by this standard, the people in this book have been inordinately successful. Each of them is the personification of the word "caring." All have used their time on earth and devoted their full energies to making life better for others.

Following is an analysis of many of the points these wonderful people have in common:

1. They are senior citizens.

At the time that this book went to press, all of the individuals profiled except Claude Pepper, Hubert H. Humphrey, and Wilbur Cohen were living. They continue to live exciting, vibrant lives as valued members of society. With the exception of Monsignor Fahey, Elsie Griffith, and Daphne Krause, they all qualify as senior citizens. Virginia Henderson is the oldest member of the group, having been born in 1897. Their average age in 1990 was 74, which means they have a natural affinity for problems of older Americans. They are living proof that old age is not synonymous with powerlessness and decrepitude. They are, in fact, excellent examples of graceful aging.

2. They all have strong family backgrounds.

All of the people in this book have strong convictions about the importance of family, which they see as the fundamental building block of society. Most of them were fortunate enough to be raised by caring parents who provided them with excellent role models. Dr. Albert Schweitzer made the point, saying that when it came to education, example was not a factor it was the only factor that mattered.

In the case of Frank E. Moss, it was his father, Jimmy, who was the role model. Jimmy Moss was a teacher and the father of high school athletics in Utah. He was a man who was revered by generations of Utah citizens. Bob Ball's father was a Methodist minister. Arthur Flemming's father was a lawyer with a strong social conscience. Bill Hutton's father gave him a quiet example of courage and caring by carrying a disabled man two miles on his back to church twice every Sunday. Similarly, Hutton's mother visited shut-ins and did her best to comfort those in nursing homes.

Hugh Downs explains the importance of the home environment, saying: "The home still contributes the principle shaping of human mental and emotional character. Parents set examples. Children imitate. If parents are seen to be learning, children will be motivated to learn. No utopian scheme, no social experiment, no commune has yet proved superior to the domiciled family unit."

Elisabeth Kübler-Ross says it this way: "You have to serve as a healthy example for the best values and ideals. The parents' greatest gift to their child is to work out his or her unfinished business. If you want to raise healthy children, you must first heal the child inside of you."

Given their rich family backgrounds, it is logical that the people included in this book would support the extended family concept. Most of them also oppose age-segregated housing. The comment of Helen Hayes is typical: "I have always been of the opinion that separating the generations is a gross injustice to all concerned."

3. They have strong religious convictions.

The people in this book are both spiritual and religious. They believe in God and credit a higher power for the successes that they have achieved. Most of them, though not all, find expression for their beliefs formally through a particular religion. All of them, however, subscribe to the fundamental tenets that are common to all the world's great religions. Wilbur Cohen, for example, said, "I have a strong belief that deeds are more important than words, and I believe the

Biblical injunctions that teach one to love his neighbor." Both Elisabeth Kübler-Ross and Daphne Krause made the point that the only people they had ever seen who could face death with calm were those with tremendous, unshakeable faith. Hugh Downs adds: "If religion has anything to offer man, it is the idea of cooperation through caring which runs through all the doctrine quietly, stubbornly insisting that man will save himself individually and collectively only in this way. The Spanish Inquisition was short-lived. The concept of love persists."

4. They are highly positive people.

All of the people in this book are disciples of Dr. Norman Vincent Peale. They believe in the power of positive thinking, particularly when it is coupled with positive action. It is hard to imagine that anyone could be more positive than Claude Pepper or Hubert H. Humphrey or Wilbur Cohen. Like all the others in this book, they were always optimistic. They went through life with positive expectations and surrounded themselves with positive people. They worked very hard and more often than not, they achieved positive results. Humphrey, Pepper, and Cohen loved life and gave full measure of themselves to others. They seemed to draw strength from those they served.

Hugh Downs is so positive that one writer described him as a "puddle of sunshine." Downs comments, "By taking the positive approach we can often make significant inroads and help bring about a solution to problems."

Frank E. Moss has an equally benevolent view of life. He believed that human beings are basically good and that there is no problem created by humans that could not also be solved by human beings.

Elisabeth Kübler-Ross says, "Negativity feeds on negativity; you must be positive." Much of her work involves eliminating the negatives from the lives of people, what she calls their "unfinished business," in order that they might become completely positive. "Each of us has within us a Mother Teresa or a Hitler and it is through positive action," she says, "that we are able to become like Mother Teresa,

Gandhi, or whoever is our private saint."

Helen Hayes also cites the importance of having a positive attitude. Along with Norman Cousins, she believes that negative mental attitudes manifest themselves in physical problems. "We have learned, for example, that great and continuing stress or shock lowers the immunological activity of the body, making us susceptible to illness."

Hubert H. Humphrey stressed the importance of positive belief with respect to his success in running the mafia out of Minneapolis during his term as mayor. He confessed that the task had not been easy, but he said what was many times more difficult was convincing his friends and supporters that it could be done.

5. They believe in the work ethic.

All of the people presented in this book have worked hard, and they continue to believe that people should do so right to the end of their days. It is better to burn out than to rust out, they reason.

As far as Humphrey, Pepper, Hayes, and all the others are concerned, the American dream is not just a dream. It happens every day for people with talent, energy, and ideas who are willing to work hard. In their view, it is work that transforms dreams into reality.

All of the people in this book believe that doing the work is what matters. It makes no difference whether it is paid or volunteered. They see no job as menial. Each job in its own way benefits society and confers dignity and pride upon the person who performs such activity. Helen Hayes is right on point when she says:

> We neglect to teach our children the pleasure of work and we rear them in an environment that doesn't encourage or admire hard work for its own sake. To get away with a minimum amount of work is the ideal. Leave it to machines, robots, services, gadgets, electronics, automatons. If we continue to fail our children, this negative approach to work will also stifle creativity and progress. The satisfaction of working to the limit of one's capacity has to be reinstilled in our society. Those of us who are older and remember the time when everyone worked, children included, have a lot to contribute.

6. They have a burning desire to make life better for others.

All of the people in this book have chosen to dedicate their lives in service to the public. Several have chosen to do so directly through the medium of government service. Others have done so informally. However, what unites them is idealism, a certain fire within and a passionate desire to make the world a better place.

Arthur Flemming describes this in terms of helping people to reach their highest potential. Elsie Griffith speaks in terms of empowering individuals. Elisabeth Kübler-Ross talks of removing obstacles in their path.

When asked how they would like to be remembered, the answer was similar for all: As someone who made life better for others and left the world just a little better place than when they found it.

When they were asked their philosophy of life, most of the people in this book echoed Pepper, who said simply: "Make it better. Do whatever you can to make life better for others."

7. They believe that it is a privilege and not a burden to serve.

There is a consensus among the people in this book that service is a privilege. The response of Daphne Krause was typical. The following paragraph, she said, incorporates the most important lesson that she has learned in her life:

> In my youth sometimes I was denied this honor. One time I remember I was caught by the nuns as I was swinging on the bars of the cubicle which surrounded my bed when I should have been asleep. The Mother Superior came in and caught me; she gave me demerits and I was not allowed to feed the poor who used to gather outside the convent gates. I learned that you had to be good in order to serve; that it definitely was a privilege.

8. They have great compassion.

The people in this book share an extraordinary degree of compassion. They have great empathy for others. Hubert Humphrey was known for his compassion. This quality finds illustration in his most famous quote:

> The moral test of government is how it treats those who are in the dawn of life, the children; those who are in the twilight of life, the aged; and those who are in the shadows of life, the sick, the needy and the handicapped.

"I'm naturally a very compassionate person. I suffer a lot when I see people in trouble," says Virginia Henderson. "I think I would suffer myself if I had time to think about myself."

"I became acquainted very early with the problems of the elderly. I identified with them and grew to like them a great deal," said Bill Hutton. "I had a feeling of satisfaction in doing something for people who were crippled with arthritis or who could not write for themselves. This knowledge of the elderly served me very well in my later years."

Compassion implies being able to step out of one's ego and imagine what the other person experiences. Claude Pepper continually thought about those less fortunate than himself. He also credited Franklin D. Roosevelt with this trait. Pepper said: "Compassion, genuine concern for one's fellow man, should be at the heart of every man or woman who assumes the responsibilities of public office."

9. They are dreamers and visionaries who do what is impossible.

All of the people in this book could fairly be characterized as dreamers and visionaries. They are able to see the world as it is and imagine it as it could be. They have the ability to hold that image in their minds and work to make it become a reality. In short, they have the gift of creativity.

Moss, Humphrey, Pepper, Hayes, Maggie Kuhn, and all the rest believe that, "If you can dream it, you can do it." All of the people in this book are capable of doing the impossible. In fact, Claude Pepper used to say that doing the impossible was easier than doing the remotely possible.

Hugh Downs put it well when he said: "Try the impossible, think the impossible, entertain any idea that comes to you. You must believe that it will work at the outset. If you believe it can't work, it becomes a self-fulfilling prophecy."

10. They have a childlike innocence and curiosity.

The people profiled in this book believe with Aldous Huxley that, "To carry the spirit of childhood into old age is the secret of genius." All of the people in this book could fairly be described as childlike and open. They have retained a childlike innocence and curiosity, which is another way of saying that they have not allowed themselves to become jaded or cynical.

Claude Pepper believed in keeping alive the child within himself. Walt Disney had the same view, which led his protégé, Mike Vance, one-time Dean of Disney University, to retrofit a term from biology to describe this phenomenon. Vance calls this quality "neoteny" and describes this as the source of all creativity. Vance, who now teaches creative thinking, encourages people to spend time with children, to seriously listen and learn from them. Hubert Humphrey had the same idea: "Spending time with children nourishes my soul. Spending five minutes with a kid is like going to a beach. It helps me that much. It really does. You get as much as you give."

11. They are balanced in their sense of time.

Another common denominator among this group is that they are balanced in their sense of time. In other words, they are able to draw from the past without dwelling on it, to live in the present and savor each moment, and at the same time to plan for the future and imagine it unfolding.

"You cannot simply live for today, that is the height of selfishness," said Senator Moss. "You should enjoy the present, of course, but at the same time one must look to the future and make use of past experience as a way to prepare for what is to come."

12. They are blessed with great energy.

Anyone who has walked through an airport with Claude Pepper,

Hubert Humphrey, or Virginia Henderson (even at age 92) will have an appreciation for this point. It is common to Wilbur Cohen, Elsie Griffith, Arthur Flemming, and all the rest. Hugh Downs, for example, has such great energy and stamina that one writer concluded he "moves in more directions than a centipede on ice." It should also be said that Downs does everything he tries exceedingly well.

When asked about her own prodigious energy, Elisabeth Kübler-Ross gave a response which perhaps is applicable to the group as a whole. She was asked how she could continue to generate such energy, given the fact that she works 15 hours a day, seven days a week with dying children. She says the answer is in eliminating negative emotions and influences, which she calls "unfinished business." It takes energy to worry; it takes energy to be afraid and that energy can be recaptured once people become totally positive, she says, citing such examples as Mother Teresa and Albert Schweitzer: "When people are free of their fears, they inevitably have prodigious energy."

13. They are joyful and have great senses of humor.

Humphrey, Pepper, and Moss were three of the most joyous people to serve in Congress. They were usually smiling and happy. Humphrey, in fact, earned the sobriquet, "The happy warrior."

"If you are not happy yourself, you can't possible lift up other people who are discouraged and down on their luck," says Moss.

Helen Hayes and Hugh Downs have much the same demeanor. Downs says a happy person is not a person with a certain set of circumstances, but rather with a certain set of attitudes. He is fond of telling the Zen parable about the fool who went searching for fire with a lighted lantern.

All of those profiled also have an excellent sense of humor. For example, when someone described him as a walking encyclopedia, Downs amended the statement to "a walking pamphlet." Pepper used humor effectively, often turning it on himself. When someone told Hubert Humphrey that he did not have presidential looks, he responded by saying that Franklin Pierce and Warren Harding were two of our most handsome presidents, but undoubtedly among the nation's worst.

Elisabeth Kübler-Ross and Robert Butler, both of whom are psychiatrists by training, point out that a sense of humor is a sign of mental health. They also believe that it is a very useful tool to help people navigate through the problems that appear in old age.

14. They have a passion for excellence

When people speak of Helen Hayes, they inevitably refer to her as "the first lady of the American theatre." What is behind the title is the fact that she is generally considered to be the best in her profession. Within the Congress of the United States, Hubert H. Humphrey, Frank E. Moss, and Claude Pepper are universally ranked at the top. When it comes to the media and the field of journalism, Hugh Downs has no peer. In the field of nursing, Virginia Henderson and Elsie Griffith rank at the top. If the field is public administration, then Arthur Flemming, Robert Ball, and Wilbur Cohen are the best. The same is true of Robert Butler and Elisabeth Kübler-Ross in the field of medicine.

The people in this book have scaled the heights of their professions because they care about others and this compassion pushes them to strive for excellence. Claude Pepper illustrates the point when he said, "I have always tried to do my very best, to be the best I could be. To do less would be to disappoint my family, my teachers, and those friends who have invested so much of their time to help make me what I am today."

15. They believe in taking action.

There is a broad consensus among the people in this book that action is better than inaction. "Healthy people don't react, they control their lives," says Elisabeth Kübler-Ross. "If you spend your entire life reacting to others, you never live your own life and you become a cripple." Maggie Kuhn is also an activist: "Do not go gentle into that good night, / Old age should burn and rave at close of day; / Rage, rage against the dying of the light," might well be her theme song. Wilbur Cohen was a man of great passion who believed that life should be attacked every day because time was short. Senator Moss decided many years ago that if he were to make errors in his life, they would be errors of commission and not of omission. If he were to fail, it would be because he tried too hard, he said, not because he didn't try hard enough. Claude Pepper was a firebrand who said in a 1941 speech:

> Give me the young men at Arcola, and at Lodi, who went forward in the face of the enemy's hail of bullets, and not the shrinking men at Waterloo. So long as life lasts, men hope to go forward and upward in their course, to dream dreams, and eventually to soar beyond the summit of the highest clouds.

16. They are advocates of individual responsibility.

There is a broad consensus among the group that individuals must take responsibility for making the world a better place. "Because the world is so nasty, you can be a little island of love, of peace and light," says Kübler-Ross. "The only way to heal others is to heal yourself."

"The most important lesson I've learned," said Elsie Griffith, "is that when times are tough or when problems occur, the first place you look is inside yourself. You look to yourself before going outside and asking for help."

Hugh Downs believes that it is important for individuals to teach themselves emotional maturity, which he says will bring them great reward and at the same time confer benefits on the entire human species. He says that unless this happens at the individual level, it will not happen. "No legislation, no law enforcement, no courts, no dispensations to the poor and indigent, and no school system will accomplish the task that faces humanity."

Daphne Krause believes that one cannot walk away from problems. She believes they must be confronted head-on and that only through the action of individuals can society prosper. "You must be outraged and you must challenge evil and injustice wherever you find it."

Claude Pepper also believed that one could not sit idly in the face of injustice. "Indignation, outrage, and individual action are all appropriate responses," he said.

17. They all have great determination and perseverance.

All of the people in this book believe that one man or one woman can make a difference as long as he or she stays focused and perseveres. Claude Pepper required great perseverance to win the enactment of his "lend-lease" bill and legislation to abolish mandatory retirement. "One man who's right is a majority," he said.

Wilbur Cohen believed perseverance was essential because every single social reform now enacted into law was at one time "vigorously opposed as being unwise, unnecessary, too expensive, impractical, socialistic or un-American, but someone, some group, persisted in the advocacy of the idea until the right historical moment occurred when a politician welded together a working majority in a state legislature or in the Congress to enact it." Senator Moss was fond of quoting historian Charles Beard, who said, "The wheels of justice grind slow but they grind exceedingly fine."

18. They have great courage, having overcome tragedy and pain.

The people in this book have great courage. Sometimes this courage was expressed in standing up for a principle and doing what they thought was right. Often, it was expressed in their survival of personal tragedy and pain and becoming better people through suffering. What Pepper said of Franklin Roosevelt is equally applicable to him. "Roosevelt," he said, "had a soul sweetened by suffering." He said that polio made Franklin Roosevelt sensitive to the problems of others. Pepper suffered a crushing blow when he was defeated to the re-election to the Senate in 1950. But years later, Pepper was able to say that he had learned more and grown more as a result of his defeats than through his victories.

"The secret to surviving tragedy," says Helen Hayes, "is not to keep to oneself. When you love other people, they leave you and they perish, but one must love again; one must adventure endlessly in loving, never fearing loss or pain."

Elisabeth Kübler-Ross sees pain as a gift. "When you look back on the times of anguish, suffering and trauma, you'll see that these are the periods of greatest growth. Looking back you will see that positive things—togetherness in the family, faith, or whatever came out of pain."

"I've always felt that you can't appreciate happiness unless you've known pain and you can't appreciate health until you've suffered illness," said Hubert Humphrey.

"We have a tendency to want to flee death and suffering. They are both realities, but frankly from a psychological or spiritual point of view, we must engage in the suffering of others even as we engage in and face our own suffering, and it is in facing suffering that we as individuals and as groups are ennobled and we really grow as a society," said Monsignor Fahey.

Daphne Krause adds: "It is not adversity or defeat that is the measure of the human being. It is the ability to get up and to go on that is the measure of the human being."

19. They have great personal integrity.

One of the greatest factors unifying the people in this book is personal integrity. The text is replete with examples. Claude Pepper refused to abandon his principles and it cost him reelection to the U.S. Senate. The same is true of Frank E. Moss, whose integrity had been established early in his career. As a young prosecutor, he persisted in prosecuting a polygamist in Utah even though he was advised that it was political suicide to do so. Hugh Downs had the courage to walk away from television at the height of his power, which ultimately resulted in a clamor to get him back on his own terms.

In the same vein, the people in this book believe in living a life of limited regrets. The idea being that at the end of life, they can look back without regretting something they did or did not do. It can also be said that they are consistent in thought, word, and deed; they lived out their beliefs.

20. They have a positive attitude toward aging.

The people in this book share a positive view of aging. They believe that the longer a person lives, the more he or she should be viewed as a victor, not as a victim. Hugh Downs puts it this way:

> When all the myths, injustices, and prejudices are retired, age will be seen in its true light: as a triumph over the forces of decay and dissolution, a time for a well-earned reward and respect, and a time for choice as to one's satisfaction including the right to savor the memories, the friends, the kin, the accomplishments, the honors, skills, techniques, and landmarks that have accumulated in the course of a lifetime. When age is viewed in this light by the whole community, it will be seen that there is no aging problem.

Maggie Kuhn says: "We are not wrinkled babies succumbing to the trivial purposeless waste of our years and time. We are a new breed of people. We are redefining our goals, taking stock of our skills and experience, and looking to the future." Robert Butler says the problem has its roots in the Western view of self, which measures human worth in terms of individual productivity and power. "Old people are led to see themselves as beginning to fail as they age. A phrase that refers as much to self-worth as it does to physical strength." Butler suggests the remedy to the problem is to value people intrinsically for themselves and for what they do for others rather than by their accumulation of material possessions.

Helen Hayes said:

> This is a great time of my life, the best in many ways. I can do what I want, when I want, go where I please, as often and as long as I like. The world is my playground, my workroom, my stage and my responsibility in small measure, too. I have been given much. I owe a great deal. . . . The best part of it is that the miracle of modern medicine prolongs health and life so that "old" does not have to sound like punishment. What we need to have now is for social sciences to catch up with the medicine men.

Monsignor Charles Fahey has written extensively about the need to define the role of senior citizens. He and Robert Butler both suggest that America needs a philosophy of growing old. Fahey says that seniors must contribute to society and that they are particularly suitable to be teachers and judges, custodians of the nation's values. He says that this is the way to build entitlements, adding that, "The strongest entitlements are those of the human heart." "Older people who are hospitable and who open their homes and hearts to others are never alone, but those who are small and selfish and given to immediate gratification are often alone and miserable. They are unconsciously creating isolation for themselves and other people as well."

Through his life and his example, Claude Pepper proved that age is no barrier to achievement. He sincerely believed that with each passing day, he learned something new and thus he became a better person. He wished the same for every senior citizen in America.

21. They do not believe in retirement.

There are two schools of thought on aging; one is the "engagement theory" and the second is the "disengagement theory." The latter view takes the position that seniors have earned a rest and that they should do as little as they can, with emphasis on recreation. All of the people in this book reject this view in favor of the more aggressive theory of aging. Helen Hayes, for example, urges seniors "to retool not retire." She urges them to continue to work, to learn, and to grow. "To rest is to rust," she says.

Claude Pepper agreed, advising seniors, "Keep on doing what you have been doing all along, but maybe at a slower pace."

"A sensible person does not retire. He or she changes activities or actions," says Hugh Downs.

"I don't believe you retire from life, which is what retirement now means," says Maggie Kuhn. "I would like to think of us as helping to heal a sick society whatever way that we can."

"My reflection is that we have to stop putting the elderly in institutions. I think we've got to learn to make greater use of old people instead of making them feel useless," says Virginia Henderson.

"I believe seniors should be activists," says Robert Butler. Arthur Flemming agrees, saying, "I have long felt that non-involvement leads to very rapid mental, physical, and spiritual deterioration, and I think the scientific literature bears me out on this point."

22. They are strong advocates of education.

The people in this book are strong advocates of education, both formal and informal. They believe the school system must be improved in order to give children the best opportunity possible and to keep America competitive in world affairs. They believe in continuing education, but even more, that education should be pursued not just in school, but rather through a lifetime dedicated to learning.

Monsignor Fahey says somewhat tongue in cheek that it is a pity that education is wasted on the young. He says education is desperately needed by old and young alike to help society produce a wise people.

Hugh Downs criticizes the pernicious attitude in American society to the effect that you can't teach an old dog new tricks. "We still cling to the idea that a child has an 'inside learning period' laid in roughly from the age of six to adolescence and then it's over. The formative years should last until the end of life," says Downs, who also believes strongly in self-teaching. "Most things that people think you have to have a teacher for, you can teach yourself."

Pepper, Humphrey, and Moss were three of the strongest advocates for education in the Congress. They supported education as the key element in social mobility. Wilbur Cohen agreed, saying education was the central solution to America's welfare problem. "The vast majority of people on welfare have no education. They can't make change, they can't make a telephone call. We've got to educate these people and train them for jobs."

"Our educational system needs an overhaul and upgrade," says Elsie Griffith. Helen Hayes agrees, quoting Benjamin Disraeli: "The more extensive a man's knowledge of what has been done, the greater will be his power in knowing what to do."

23. They see long-term care as the greatest problem facing America and advocate home care as the best solution.

When asked what were the major issues facing the nation and its senior citizens, the people in this book were unanimous in identifying long-term care. While it is not strictly limited to the elderly, the need for long-term care among seniors is a devastating problem because little exists at present in the form of either private or public help. It was the consensus of the people in this book that this issue should dominate the 1991 White House Conference on Aging. When asked for the best solution to the problem, the group was unanimous in their recommendation of a comprehensive home care program. Claude Pepper, for example, devoted the greater part of the last years of his life trying to win enactment of a national long-term home care program.

All of the people in this book support the concept of home care, although some favor different approaches to the legislation. Most of the people believe that some form of national legislation will be enacted in the reasonably near future. "When the bill is enacted, it will give the whole nation a shot in the arm; it is going to replace despair with hope," said Arthur Flemming.

"Home care is our primary goal," comments Elisabeth Kübler-Ross. "We have moved from institutional care for the dying to a new, healthier way of caring for them in their own environment."

"Science has taught us to lengthen life," says Helen Hayes. "Now we must learn to make a longer life worth living. Older people deserve choices that let us live out our days as we wish. We've seen people making such choices all over America, and we realize what we might have known from the start: For most of us, there really is no place like home."

Hugh Downs expressed similar sentiments:

> There is never anything wrong with getting older or being old but there is always something wrong with being sick, or alone, or broke and discriminated against, or being shunted off in warehouses for the dying when an enlightened culture would tend more toward taking care of its own.
>
> There are societies in the world where home care is so much a part of the culture that they don't think about needing someone to do something about it. Home care is the norm in many parts of the world. Admittedly the techniques and some of the clinical aspects could be enhanced but this is the concept that we need to re-establish in our culture . . . and we are moving in the right direction.

Senator Moss said:

> You have only to ask yourself which you would prefer, to be uprooted and placed in a nursing home or to remain at home with nursing and other medical, therapeutic, and social services delivered to

your door. Home care is much to be preferred from a social policy point of view. It is generally less expensive than institutionalization and it serves the important function of keeping families together.

24. They support some kind of a national health system.

While long-term care was identified as the greatest need and the greatest gap in the American health care system, most of the people profiled in this book believe the entire system needs an overhaul. Long-term home care coverage must be provided immediately, and at the same time or shortly thereafter, some kind of comprehensive system must be put into place.

Virginia Henderson points out that the United States has massive gaps in its health care system and still spends a greater proportion of its gross national product on health care (12 percent) than any other nation. She points out that the Japanese and the Canadians who spend seven percent of their GNP have comprehensive health care systems and better health care statistics than Americans.

"It is tragic that we are only one of two industrialized nations in the world that does not have a national health care system," says William R. Hutton.

"We really have a non-system in America. There exists tremendous gaps in our health care coverage and yet we are paying far more than other nations pay for a comprehensive national system. Something is radically wrong. Health care should be a right for all Americans instead of a privilege for the few," says Frank E. Moss.

"What we have in America is sickness care. We place no emphasis on prevention," says Maggie Kuhn. "Medical students may come in with idealism, but the system drains it out of them. They quickly get caught in pressures to acquire a lucrative practice where they think the dollars are going to flow."

Virginia Henderson has a ready answer for those who do not believe that the public tax dollars should be used to support a publicly funded health care system. She asks the people if they went to public school and when they respond in the affirmative, she notes that she can see no difference between education at the expense of the public or the provision of health care services.

25. They are strong advocates of medical research.

Like Claude Pepper, whose legislation created 12 of the 13 National Institutes of Health, the others in this book are strong advocates of medical research. Robert Butler, the former director of the National Institute on Aging, has a particularly keen interest in this area. He believes that research will soon yield a cure to many diseases, including unlocking the riddle of Alzheimer's disease. When this happens, he believes it will eliminate the necessity of most nursing home placements.

"Research," says Butler, "is the ultimate service because you can prevent people from having a particular disease. It is also the ultimate in cost containment in that you do not have to spend money for treatment."

26. They believe in the importance of role models.

The people in the preceding chapters have been blessed with excellent role models who helped them become the extraordinary people that they are. By the same token, through the exemplary manner in which they have lived their lives, they have become role models for others.

Helen Hayes said that she studied biographies early in life in hopes of finding the key to greatness. She says she was greatly impressed with the people who provided a hiding place for Anne Frank and her family during World War II. "To put your life willingly on the line isn't possible for everyone, but I think everyone must be emulating someone," she says.

Virginia Henderson has her hero in Annie Goodrich. Elsie Griffith admires Lillian Wald. Claude Pepper modeled his life after three educators: C. C. Moseley, George H. Denny, and Roscoe Pound, and later after Franklin D. Roosevelt.

27. They advise seniors to stay active and to take an interest in youth.

Stay active and work with young people is the consensus on what seniors should do. The challenge to older people, says Monsignor

Fahey, is "to participate in the fullness of society, to be truly loving people, to continue to grow, recognizing that a lot of them and a lot of kids and a lot of middle-aged people are going to need help from family, friends, neighbors, and from society. The challenge is to see the whole picture and make an effort diligently to make a difference on behalf of those who share such needs."

Fahey, Downs, Hutton, Kuhn, and others advise seniors to become healing agents in society. "I feel that elderly Americans need to have a role in solving their own and society's problems," says Elsie Griffith. "They need to be involved in coming up with solutions."

"Unlike other societies, the United States has yet to institutionalize a proper role for its older citizens," says Hugh Downs. "So each retiree in America has a challenge of creating his or her own lifestyle. This can be a problem or an opportunity. It should be a period of renewal and of purpose. Most successful are those who have let go of their old roles, opened themselves to broader personal perspectives and who have reached out to grasp new opportunities."

Hutton, Pepper, Moss, and Butler stress the natural affinity between the old and the young and encourage older persons to work with young people as much as possible. "Older people can do wonders with children and children can do wonderful things for old people," says Hutton.

Ratifying this point, Maggie Kuhn says, "I am proudest of what I have done in late life—of the fact that we have forged a successful national coalition of old people and young people working together and that we have moved to bring about a new kind of political awareness building coalitions that transcend special interest politics."

28. They advise young people to choose a career in public service.

There's a broad consensus among the people in this book that young people should be advised to live their lives for the benefit of others. "I have advised young people to fashion their lives and to live in such a way that when they come to the upper ages of life they will be able to look back and see that they did something to make it possible for other people to walk on higher ground, to live a little healthier, happier, and better lives," commented Claude Pepper.

"Learn to be honest with yourself and others. Find some outlet for the goodness within you. Do something that is bigger than yourself, something that benefits everyone. Take an interest in helping people," advises Bill Hutton.

"You must never be so cynical or hurt by loving that you stop caring and build a wall around yourself," says Daphne Krause. "It is better to be hurt, to pick yourself up, and go on loving. Hatred turns in on you and negates you. I believe that more illnesses are caused by hatred and stress than can possibly be imagined. You must have faith in yourself. Never forget every time that you give of yourself, you get back one hundred fold; it is sort of a shot of adrenaline to your mind and spirit," she says.

29. They have a positive view towards government.

There is a broad consensus among the group that government is a positive force, which exists to help people solve their problems. Most people believed with Robert Ball that the argument between liberals and conservatives generally misses the point. It never has been a question of whether the public wants more or less government. What the public wants is *better* government, he says.

"There is an appropriate place for private enterprise in our society, but there are certain things that are so vast that only government is capable of dealing with them," adds Senator Moss. Congressman Pepper made the point this way:

> I've always tried to make government the friend of the people. The government of the United States belongs to the people of this land and whenever their troubles, their disasters, and their needs impel its use, it is available. It is the mightiest institution on the face of the earth, and it can be a hand that will lift up the people if they call upon it.

30. They are unselfish and therefore mature people.

"Human maturity," says Hugh Downs, "is nothing more than

moving along the line from competitive habits to cooperative habits. We must move along this line as a species. We must move along this line as individuals. We must shift from autocentricism to allocentricism—that is from self-centeredness to other-centeredness."

Downs says that salvation may be found in one word. He offers the example of the man who lost his family in an automobile accident. Bereft with grief he asked, "To whom can I turn for comfort?" Downs says the man found salvation in asking, "To whom can I turn *with* comfort?" Downs believes the challenge of a truly mature person is to dissolve the ego shell so that the person become selfless rather than selfish.

Maggie Kuhn agrees:

> We can only survive when we have a goal, a passionate purpose that we're going to devote some time, energy, and thought to. It is important that this objective be beyond ourselves. I'm talking about having a goal that bears upon the common interest and common good. We are the elders of the tribe, and the tribal leaders are concerned about the tribe's survival and not their own.

Elsie Griffith believes that human maturity "involves taking responsibility for the quality of life of other human beings."

"You have to give to people," said Hubert Humphrey. "I don't make a speech. I give a speech. I try to give people a lot of knowledge and perhaps a useful idea or two."

Helen Hayes was asked how she managed to keep each performance of a play fresh night after night. "I focus on the audience for whom this play is opening night. If I thought about myself, the play would have been stale after the tenth performance," she said.

"Whether for the individual or for the nation, self is best served by transcending self," said Senator Moss.

Monsignor Fahey adds: "To the degree that we've become self-centered and selfish, looking for either immediate gratification or to try to wipe away all pain, we become the decadent society."

31. They love life and they love people.

The people in this book have a zest for life. They genuinely love people and there is among them a broad agreement as to the importance of love in society. Claude Pepper and Hubert Humphrey were preeminent examples of people who loved people and no two people were more beloved in return.

"You can change the world with love," says Elisabeth Kübler-Ross. "Most of us are raised with 'I love you ifs.' We try to buy people's love with compliance. That is not love, that is prostitution. Real love has no claims or expectations. It doesn't judge. It listens and respects the individual as he or she is. Real love is unconditional." She also makes the point that most of society's ills are based on the lack of love.

Elsie Griffith, like Senator Moss, believes that the answer to most problems lies in the love, understanding, and caring of one person for another. "It is a matter of one plus one plus one. It has to start somewhere. The most important elements are love and care. It's not so important that we have understanding."

"Somebody once said that there is only one heroism. To know the world as it is and to love it," says Hugh Downs. He quotes Thomas Merton to the effect that, "Power always protects the good of some at the expense of others. Only love can attain and preserve the good of all."

32. They are extraordinarily caring people.

The greatest of all of the common denominators involving the people profiled in this book is the fact that they are extraordinarily caring people. When asked for the single greatest secret in the universe, Claude Pepper said, "Love one another and do unto others as you would have done unto you."

Helen Hayes said, "It all comes down to caring and comforting. Those things we can give each other."

Arthur Flemming adds that, "It involves the common responsibility to love thy neighbor and to help our neighbors achieve their highest possibilities."

Robert Ball says the secret of his success as an administrator of the Social Security program was that he treated his employees with the same respect and consideration that he would have liked had he been in their place.

Wilbur Cohen helped everyone he could along the road of life. Daphne Krause approaches her life as an adventure in caring.

Robert Ball says the secret of his success as an administrator of the Social Security program was that he treated his employees with the same respect and consideration that he would have liked had he been in their place.

Wilbur Cohen helped everyone he could along the road of life. Daphne Krause approaches her life as an adventure in caring.

Hubert Humphrey gave of himself to others. He continued giving irrespective of whether they reciprocated. He gave to those who agreed with him and those who did not. He gave to those who asked and those who didn't. He gave and he kept on giving, even when he was physically exhausted and seemingly had nothing left to give. When asked for the key to success in politics, he said, "You have got to show people that you care about them. The main thing is that you have got to like people."

Summary

Perhaps the examples of Hubert Humphrey, Claude Pepper, Hugh Downs, and all the others whose lives have been profiled in this book will serve to motivate others. With every person who chooses this path, the nation will become a better place. In this way, America will become again what it once was—the most caring nation in the history of the world. If this can be accomplished, then both the country's security and its place in history will have been preserved for the benefit of present generations, and future generations yet unborn.

Afterword

by Frank E. Moss

No anthology of the people who helped raise the lot of the nation's elderly from obscurity and neglect into the bright sunshine of opportunity would be complete unless it included the author of this book. Val J. Halamandaris has done as much as anyone to bring that about. Although he has chosen to stay in the background, he deserves much of the credit for what was accomplished both at the U.S. Senate Special Committee on Aging, where he was closely associated with me, and at the House Select Committee on Aging, where he was Congressman Claude Pepper's senior counsel and closest advisor.

Congressman Pepper chaired the Subcommittee on Health and Long-Term Care of the House Aging Committee for 13 years; I served in a similar capacity in the Senate for 17 years. I am not sure which of us chaired the most hearings. I give the nod to him and he to me. One thing is certain, however: Val did the lion's share of the work for both of us. He did so much work so effectively that people were amazed to find out that I had only one person on my Aging Committee staff. He put together more hearings on the subject of aging, wrote more reports, drafted more bills, and had more influence on the direction of events than anyone before him or since. Although he worked for us, neither Congressman Pepper nor myself had a monopoly on his time. He was constantly in demand to serve other members of the committee because of the quality of his work and the fact that he got results.

Medical World News paid tribute to Val in a 1975 article, saying:

> Working without a private secretary in a supremely unpretentious cubicle on the ground floor of the new Senate office building is a man who if less well known is often more important to the health field than his senatorial employers.
>
> When long-term care legislation is developed, such as bills codifying nursing home patient rights or establishing a loan program to help facilities install fire safety equipment, there's a better than even chance Mr. Halamandaris had a hand in writing it. When one of the committee members delivers a speech, attentive listeners can hear the echoes of Mr. Halamandaris's cogitation.

I placed the article in the *Congressional Record* with a tribute of my own. I said, "No one ever had a more dedicated, more hard working, more talented, or more effective staff member." I said he was among the best in the Senate. Congressman Claude Pepper offered a tribute of his own in 1984, saying that in his more than 50 years of public service, Val was the best and most able person who ever worked for him. The respected columnist, Jack Anderson, had similar words of praise concerning Val's integrity and ability in a tribute to Val which ran in *50-Plus* magazine.

It is hard to convey just how important he was to all of us who served on the Senate or House Aging Committees. Before he arrived on the scene, things could only be described as dull. No one much wanted to attend our hearings. We couldn't get television coverage. Val changed that; he made things happen. He brought a sense of energy and excitement. He gave the senators the information they needed. He knew his subject and when he made a judgment, it was better than money in the bank. He brought to the committee both back-breaking substance and a flair for the dramatic. What had been drudgery became a pleasure. As a result, the media and our colleagues in the Senate began to take us seriously.

One way to show the extent to which Val's work dominated that of the committee is to note that in its entire history, from 1962 through 1977 when he left, the Senate Aging Committee had made one or more of the three network news programs a total of 25 times—22 of which were Val's work. From its beginnings in 1976 through 1982, the House Aging Committee had been featured on the evening news a total of 29 times, 27 of which related to Val's hearings or reports. Hearings, reports, plus news translate into legislation, and one need only to look at the sections in this book that relate to my achievements in the field of aging or to those of Congressman Pepper to get a good feel for Val's prodigious contribution.

As Congressman Pepper noted in his *Congressional Record* tribute, Val is "a great American, a keen lawyer and investigator, and an effective voice for the nation's underprivileged and needy. It is appropriate to acknowledge the many contributions that Val has already made to the constituencies that he has chosen to serve. Over half of Val's life has been spent in service to our nation's elderly both in connection with the Senate Special Committee on Aging, where he spearheaded a number of daring and productive undercover operations, but also with the House Select Committee on Aging where he exposed frauds and abuse in numerous public and private programs serving older Americans."

I concur with Congressman Pepper. Val did extraordinary things during the 20 years he worked for the Congress. He has done even more extraordinary things since then. In addition to being an author, an attorney, and the cofounder of the Center for Health Care Law (a public interest law firm), he is an editor, publisher, a television producer, a trade association executive, a partner in a real estate sales and development company, a museum curator, and a philanthropist. He is a modern-day renaissance man who at a young age has had a very profound effect on our country. The Creative Thinking Association of America recognized this in March of 1990, giving Val their highest award and ranking him with Steven Jobs, the founder of Apple Computer, as one of the people whose work will have the greatest effect on American society for the balance of this century and into the 21st.

Val J. Halamandaris is my friend and protégé. I am proud of all his achievements and confident that impressive as they are, they are but faint harbingers of accomplishments to come.

Early Years

I have known Val for more than 30 years. I met him in 1959, shortly after I began my service in the United States Senate. He had been elected my high school counterpart, U.S. senator and delegate from Utah to Boys Nation, which was held in Washington, D.C. Even then, I could sense something special about him. He had a fire within, a desire to make something of himself, always expressed in terms of helping others.

He soaked up Washington, D.C., like a sponge. He was eager to learn about everything, but it was the Congress that interested him the most. I found him returning to hear debates in the Senate during his free time. I remember he was unusually well informed for a young man his age in both domestic and foreign policy issues.

We became friends. He wrote to me often on his return to Utah and his hometown of Price. Usually, he would ask for information to help him with the high school debate topic. We carried on a lively correspondence, and when I returned to Utah at a later date, I met his parents, John and Merry Halamandaris.

John was a coal miner, big and strong, rough cut and shy, honest as the day is long. He had a heart as big as Texas. Merry was petite and outgoing, one of the most attractive people that I have ever met.

Val's mother told me that when he was born, the superstitious Greek women of the town had read the tea leaves and predicted that Val would become a great man, a powerful champion of the underprivileged. She said Val was named for his paternal grandfather, whose name spelled phonetically was Vlasios. There being no English equivalent, Merry looked around and came up with Val, from Prince Valiant, the crusading knight of the roundtable made famous in the comic strips by Hal Foster. As a boy, Val was always telling Merry about the dragons that he was going to slay and of the wrongs that he was going to make right when he became older.

He was a big kid, six feet tall and 200 pounds at age 15. He had intended to play football because athletic scholarships provided one of the few avenues open for advancement. In Carbon County, if your father was a coal miner, the chances were that you would be a coal miner, too. Val wanted something more and football looked like the way to get it. Unfortunately, he hurt his back when he was 16 and that door of opportunity seemed to close for him.

To her credit, Merry talked her son into using his mind instead of his body. He went into forensics and dramatic arts, and to his own amazement, he excelled in both. Soon thereafter, he was elected student body president of Carbon High School. He made excellent grades and participated in a wide variety of extracurricular activities. What he enjoyed most was writing, sports, and producing advice to the love lorn columns in his student newspaper. The latter was good and funny enough that it was picked up on a regular basis by a widely read columnist for the *Salt Lake City Tribune* named Dan Valentine.

In 1960, Val won an essay contest sponsored by the American Legion on the topic, "What America means to me." He was also selected the Outstanding Youth Leader in the State of Utah.

On several occasions when I returned to my home state for a tour, I took Val along. It was great to watch his growth and development. One of our major fights at that time involved my bill to set aside an area of remote southeast Utah as the Canyonlands National Park. Environmentalists said yes; developers said no. Part of the reason for my tour was to sell my proposal, answer questions, deflate the opposition, and to take the political temperature. Utah's Republican governor came out against my proposal, which made things political. It also meant that my bill faced some tough sledding.

A crucial debate was scheduled in Price between the governor and myself. Because of the press of Senate business, I had to cancel at the last minute. I feared the worst. I was amused to read on the front page of the *Salt Lake City Tribune* that a young boy of 17 had stepped in for me and apparently cut the governor to shreds. Judging by the play the story got, the newspaper editors must have been equally amused. I wrote Val a warm note of thanks.

I was pleased with his choice to attend George Washington University, where I had gone for my law degree. He had gotten some basic courses under his belt by attending the College of Eastern Utah, and as always, he had distinguished himself. He arrived in my office on June 18, 1962, all six feet three inches of him, a 220-pound bundle of energy. He threw himself into every task available. For a while, he ran elevators in the Capitol building. Then he worked in my office as a file and mail clerk. Always, he agitated for more to do. The one area that my legislative assistants were comfortable letting him run with were problems of the elderly. Things were pretty hopeless in those days; the problems of the elderly were multiple and sad, and there was not much we could do to help them. Val took every one of them personally.

I remember he came to see me one day with a troubled look on his face. He had a draft for me to review. He had written a letter to J. Edgar Hoover, Director of the Federal Bureau of Investigation, for my signature, asking Hoover to investigate a particular nursing home because of alleged abuse of the elderly described in a letter that we had received. We did send the letter, but we sent it to the state health department instead. Still, it was a measure of how much he cared. Abuse of the elderly was no casual offense. The perpetrators in his mind were right up there with Al Capone and John Dillinger, and he was ready to make a federal case of the matter.

The timing was propitious. I had been one of those who supported the creation of a U.S. Senate Special Committee on Aging. When we won, I was named Chairman of the Subcommittee on Long-Term Care and of the Subcommittee on Housing for the Elderly. I retained the former for my entire Senate career, which meant that Val would have a great deal more work to do in the area of stemming nursing home abuses.

In 1965, we were successful in winning the enactment of Medicare and Medicaid. It was a banner year for the elderly, but it was a rough one for Val. He wrenched his back, aggravating an old football injury that in turn became complicated by a form of spinal arthritis. He was so racked with pain that he could scarcely go up and down stairs; the slightest touch on his back brought contortions and agony. It hurt me to see him suffering, yet he never let it affect his happy demeanor. The pain continued for years, but it did not stop him from working his way through undergraduate school and from winning his law degree from the Catholic University School of Law.

No one was more pleased with Val's education than John Halamandaris. John never had the chance to go to school beyond the eighth grade. He wanted his sons to have the opportunities he never had. He had a great love for the law and subtly encouraged his boys to move in that direction. John chose to work the graveyard shift in the coal mine, meaning after midnight until about eight a.m. On his return home, he would often forego sleep, choosing instead to take Val and his brother, Bill, into the courtroom to watch the deliberations. Once or twice he also took them into the coal mine. "It did not take a genius to figure out that one was a better way of making a living than the other," said Val.

The Senate Aging Committee

In 1969, I asked Val to accept a position as counsel to the U.S. Senate Committee on Aging. I told him that I wanted my subcommittee to take a good hard look at the problem of nursing homes in America. We were getting entirely too many complaints and it was clear that something needed to be done.

Val took the job with relish, even though it meant being sent off to investigate some of the worst examples of man's inhumanity to man. For example, he investigated a salmonella epidemic in a Baltimore nursing home that claimed 32 lives because of buck passing, insensitivity, and the fact that no one was willing to admit what was going on. There were numerous fires we investigated, including one in Marietta, Ohio, where 30 people died of smoke inhalation because the rubber backing on the carpet produced tremendous amounts of thick, black, noxious fumes. Inevitably, he spent most of his time with what we regarded as the worst nursing homes in America. You have to see the problem close up to understand it, he used to say, and he certainly followed his own advice. To his credit, he did seek out examples of the best and most innovative facilities as examples for others to emulate.

He collected rooms full of information. People did not know what to make of him. Certainly no one would take the time to actually read all that he asked for, but he did. He drove the people at the Library of Congress crazy with his research demands. He engineered original research studies which he undertook himself. He talked colleges and universities into doing helpful studies. He did the same with foundations. He gave the U.S. General Accounting Office more research requests than anyone in their experience. Then he rounded up many of the greatest experts and brought them to testify around a certain set of issues. Finally, when he had gathered all the information that was available on the surface, he told me that we would have to find out pertinent facts that people did not want to disclose to us.

We discussed in some length his views that Congress often tries to legislate in a vacuum. It simply does not have enough information available to make effective judgments. Part of the problem is that vested interests, who are doing well financially, resist any change. They will do whatever they can to keep their machinations from becoming public knowledge. This is even more true when what they are doing is illegal. Neither Val nor I set out to be investigators; we sought the facts and we followed them wherever they led us. We shattered precedent when we elected to use the Aging Committee's subpoena power to compel the production of a document or the testimony of reluctant witnesses. The results were eye-opening.

More than anyone else, Val professionalized the Senate Committee on Aging. He was a crusading young lawyer with a good mind and an appropriate sense of outrage, coupled with a burning determination not only to disclose problems but to do something about them.

Val's hearings inevitably made news. He had the gift of bringing together all the right elements. Always, he remembered the people. He brought them forward first to tell their stories. The second panel usually consisted of a group of experts who could generalize from the particular cases the committee had just heard. Finally, he brought before the committee the bureaucrats or government officials who had the responsibility for enforcing the applicable laws or regulations. Another reason the hearings made news was that he used them as a platform to release reports, not simply to take testimony. He did not believe the valuable time of senators should be used in the tedious task of gathering facts, but rather that they should review what was collected and make policy decisions on the basis of staff recommendations.

What is remarkable, however, is that he did all of this while in pain. He spent most of 1972 in a full body cast. In 1973 and 1974, he wore a Milwaukee brace, a heavy steel contraption that immobilizes the spine from head to hips.

After five years of research, Val took six months in 1974 to produce what many people believe was the best and most impressive series of congressional reports ever written. By himself, he wrote the 12-volume series entitled *Nursing Home Care in the United States: Failure in Public Policy*. The report was a scorching indictment of America's nursing home industry. The research and the mountains of data were so compelling that no one could quarrel with its conclusions, the primary one being that 50 percent of the nursing homes in the United States were substandard with one or more life-threatening conditions.

The first report was signed unanimously by all the members of the Aging Committee and released at a November 1974 press conference before a forest of microphones. The remaining reports in the series were released seriatim throughout 1975. One by one, they made front page news. They called on the nation to formulate a national policy of veneration of the elderly, instead of dumping them out of sight into what President Richard Nixon called "warehouses for the dying."

During this same time, Val was asked to work with numerous other senators. He worked with Senator Edmund S. Muskie, who was Chairman of the Subcommittee on Health, with respect to Medicare issues, including efforts of the Nixon Administration to undermine my legislation, which covered home care under both Medicare and Medicaid. He also worked with Senator Muskie on mental health issues. He worked with Senator Frank Church on issues affecting the elderly as consumers, including health insurance sold in supplementation of Medicare. He worked with Senator Harrison Williams on housing for the elderly and in preparing hearings on income tax overpayments and the elderly. He worked with Senator Edward M. Kennedy on amendments to the older Americans Act and conducted an investigation on New Mexico's dumping of mental patients into boarding homes for Senator Pete V. Domenici. He helped Senator Charles Percy develop hearings and legislation in the area of nursing homes and nutrition.

During the early months of 1975, Val spearheaded one of the most sensitive and highly publicized hearings in which the Senate Aging Committee was involved. We conducted these hearings in New York City, examining the alleged abuses perpetrated by nursing home owners who had become millionaires while spending less per patient per day for food than jails spent to feed prisoners. The allegations included not only poor care, negligence, and abuse, but also massive fraud, political corruption, and the involvement of organized crime in the rip off of Medicare and Medicaid funds.

A central figure in the investigation was a Jewish rabbi named Bernard Bergman. He and his attorney showed open contempt and hostility toward the committee. In one brief appearance, he said he was the victim of the greatest conspiracy since the days of Senator Joseph McCarthy. Needless to say, I did not appreciate the reference. Before we could ask any questions, he left with the promise to reappear. When he failed to appear at a second hearing, the committee issued a subpoena to command his appearance. Finally, both he and his accountant claimed their rights against self-incrimination under the Fifth Amendment of the Constitution. Bernard Bergman later pleaded guilty and served time in Ryker's Island penitentiary.

Val guided the investigation in his usual methodical way. He was fearless. We issued 57 subpoenas, one of which went to the speaker of the New York Assembly, another went to the governor's administrative assistant, and yet another to an organized crime chieftain. Mountains of evidence were collected from nursing homes, banks, and insurance companies. We asked the comptroller general of the U.S. General Accounting Office for help and he assigned a battery of auditors to work with us. In the end, Val went toe to toe with the best New York lawyers that money could buy, and he came out on top. An impressive number of criminals were brought to the bar of justice, and far-reaching federal legislative reforms were put into place that hopefully insured that such wide-scale abuses could never happen again.

As a result of the avalanche of publicity that our hearings generated, including cover stories in such publications as *Newsweek* and *U.S. News and World Report*, most of the 50 states launched their own investigations. They quickly found that what we had documented in New York, Illinois, and California was equally pertinent to Nebraska and Kansas. A sweeping series of nursing home reforms were put into effect among the states, creating new standards and protections for patients.

The hearings and the reports that Val put together did more than anything else to raise the public consciousness concerning problems of the elderly. Reporters discovered the subject of aging. They discovered that the problems were real and that they made good copy. They discovered that the public responded positively to our efforts to institute reforms. The hearings and reports, therefore, fired a ground swell of support for improving not just conditions in substandard nursing homes, but for improving the quality of life for the elderly overall.

In another of his significant firsts, Val helped develop the first hearings on hospice held in America. Together, we developed and supported legislation to provide federal funds to support hospice care. Val later worked with Claude Pepper to get such legislation enacted.

Val worked with Senator Walter Mondale in fighting against mandatory retirement and supporting the establishment of pre-retirement counseling for employees at the workplace.

Val and I worked on hearings that documented that the elderly, who then made up 10 percent of the population, accounted for 30 percent of the victims of crime. We tried to strengthen federal mail fraud and other statutes to create disincentives for those who might be tempted to victimize a senior citizen.

In another of his investigations, Val was called on to evaluate the phaseout of the so-called "202" Federal Housing Administration Program (FHA), which provided direct government loans to church groups and other non-profits at low interest to enable them to build housing for the elderly. Under pressure from the banking industry, FHA had abandoned direct loans in favor of an interest subsidy approach, the so-called 236 program. Under FHA 236, non-profits would borrow money from their commercial banker at the prevailing interest rate and the government would subsidize all but one percent of the interest. Halamandaris proved that political payoffs were being made that resulted in projects being funded. He proved that under the old "202" approach, the government had never had one single failure, while under the 236 program, failures were rampant. What's more, in a typical $3 million project at 9 percent interest, the government would be paying bankers in excess of $9 million in interest over the life of the mortgage. Val termed this give-away program "a welfare program for the rich," noting that the government could make an outright gift of the property to church groups and still save $6 million in the process.

The scandal resulted in the closing of two Florida FHA offices and the prosecution of the director of one office and scores of other officials.

Every effort was made to intimidate Val in order to block the disclosure of facts he had uncovered. One official with the Department of Housing and Urban Affairs (HUD) excoriated Val in order the excuse the FHA director and the HUD under secretary from testimony before the Aging Committee. "Who the hell do you think you are?" said the man. "You find one little crummy case of fraud and you make a federal case out of it. What do you think goes on in this town? This is called politics. You must really be the last of the virgins." Val told him that no man is above the law.

The investigation went forward and some reforms were put into place, although obviously not enough since a dozen years later the same issues surfaced, ably brought to the surface by Congressman Tom Lantos and his Government Operations Committee Subcommittee.

Because of the publicity Val helped generate and because of our growing success in getting our recommendations enacted by the appropriate legislative committees, service on the Senate Aging Committee had become a hot ticket. It soon became the largest committee in the Senate, at one time boasting almost one out of every four members of the body. Our success also led to a steady drumbeat to create a similar committee in the House of Representatives.

Val opened up a line of communication with the offices of Congressmen David Pryor, John Heinz, Claude Pepper, and Ed Koch.

We had invited Ed Koch to sit on the dais with us and participate in our New York nursing home hearings. Koch, who later became mayor of New York City, had become enamored with home care as a better alternative for the care of the disabled and seniors than nursing home care. He developed one of the first and most comprehensive long-term home care bills. He introduced his version in the House and I introduced it in the Senate. It was Congressman Claude Pepper, however, who introduced the bulk of my 48-bill home care and nursing home reform package in the House. We worked very hard behind the scenes with Congressmen David Pryor and John Heinz, who along with Pepper had the goal of creating a House Committee on Aging. The goal was finally reached in 1975.

Val put together the first joint hearing between the Senate and

House Committees on Aging. The subject was home health care. I remember Val laughing at himself. He told me that he had lectured Claude Pepper at length about home care in preparation for the hearing. He said Pepper was too polite to say anything, but an aide told him later that Pepper had introduced the first long-term home care bill in 1942, before Val was born. The Pepper-Moss hearings brought about some modest increases in the Medicare home care benefit, but we won only small victories; the war remained to be won. Pepper continued the fight for a comprehensive long-term home care bill until his last days.

Medicare and Medicaid Fraud

In September of 1975, the Senate Aging Committee received an additional $100,000, which was earmarked to continue an investigation we began in 1974 to examine Medicare and Medicaid fraud. We wanted to see if the widespread frauds we had documented among nursing home owners were equally prevalent among physicians, hospitals, clinical laboratories, purveyors of durable medical goods, and home health agencies. We held 12 hearings between October 1975 and September 1976 and issued six major reports. Eleven of the 12 hearings made front page news across America.

It started with a letter from the executive director of a trade association representing clinical laboratories in Illinois. He charged that Medicaid fraud was rampant and begged us to investigate. Val developed an action plan.

The association executive led us to a doctor who was fed up with being pressured to participate in a scheme of illegal kickbacks in return for having blood and other specimens of his clients tested by Chicago labs. At our behest, he agreed to call up the lab salesman and say he was reconsidering. He asked the salesman to return and reiterate the sales pitch. One of our investigators was there eavesdropping in the closet; another wore a lab coat and pretended to be an employee. The illegal solicitation was overheard, along with a boast that the laboratory was making illegal payments to physicians all over Chicago.

This disclosure led Val and his investigators to the Illinois capitol in Springfield. They visited the comptroller's office and put together a list of all the physicians who used this particular laboratory. This took days and involved hundreds of computer runs. We then had a reasonable expectation that all of these physicians were getting 25 percent of what Medicaid paid the laboratory back under the table in exchange for their referrals. Armed with this information, the lab salesman was confronted, who confessed immediately rather than tell his story before the full Senate in Washington. He said that the lab was forced to make such payment because every other lab was doing so and they simply could not compete if they did not follow suit.

The question then was how to test the premise that other clinical laboratories were involved in similar schemes. Val developed the idea of renting a storefront and pretending to be a medical clinic opening for business. This was done, and a telephone number placed in the window. Within hours, salesmen representing 12 clinical laboratories called at the storefront, which was little more than a desk and a telephone. Eleven of the 12 offered to pay illegal kickbacks from 25 to 55 percent.

Now it was back to Springfield and more computer runs. A profile was developed on the physicians and clinics who dealt with these laboratories. The names of physicians making more than $100,000 from Medicaid were cross-indexed. Some 50 were selected for interview. One bright January morning, Val and his teams, augmented by the Chicago Better Government Association, appeared in the physicians' offices with clipboards, asking innocuous questions about Medicare. Finally, the last two questions asked if the doctors were still using X, Y, Z, or whatever lab. When the shocked doctors answered in the affirmative, the investigators were prepared with a response such as, "I take it then that you are getting their standard rebate of 50 percent off the top on your Medicaid lab billings?" Most doctors admitted they were. Others called lawyers. Still others pointed out that the money they collected was in turn collected by mob figures.

Evidently we were making waves because during the course of our investigation from 1974–76, no less than half a dozen pharmacists, Medicaid "mill" owners, and laboratory salesmen were murdered in Chicago.

When he heard what Val was up to, the governor of the state of Illinois was anything but pleased. He did his best to stop the hearings. He accused me of being out to get him. He said Val was out of control and should be reigned in before he helped elect Republicans in Illinois. The governor even had several of my colleagues call me and pressure me to stop the investigation. He issued press statements saying the Medicaid program in Illinois was as pure as Caesar's wife. He demanded a hearing to which he could send people to tell his side of the story. We agreed to give him a hearing on the condition that he appear in person and testify under oath, and we would notify the press accordingly. Under these terms, he vehemently declined. What he did not know, however, was that Val had called in Mike Wallace and the folks from CBS's "Sixty Minutes." All of those laboratory salesmen who had offered our investigators money under the table were recalled and repeated their offers, which were filmed by CBS through a one-way mirror.

In the end, Val drafted a report, which I released to the public. It contained proof positive that one out of every two dollars that was spent for Medicaid clinical laboratory services in Illinois was being ripped off by the unscrupulous. We turned our report over to Deputy Attorney General Richard Thornburgh in advance of the hearing so that arrests could be made. On February 16, 1976, Mike Wallace went on the air with fascinating footage showing just how vulnerable one government program was at the hands of crooks. The name of the story was "The Clinic on Morris Avenue."

It would be a disservice not to point out that Val and his team conducted a similar investigation in five other states. The report we issued made judgments not only with respect to one state, but nationwide. The other states included New York, California, New Jersey, Michigan, and Pennsylvania. These five states by themselves accounted for the lion's share of Medicaid funds.

The crucial role of Bill Halamandaris should also be mentioned. Val reached out to his brother when we needed help. We were knee-deep in our pursuit of organized crime and its involvement in Medicare and Medicaid. Val needed someone he could trust. Bill agreed to help, but only for six months. Six months became a year. The year that the Halamandaris brothers worked together on the staff of the U.S. Senate Committee on Aging marks the high point in the committee's history. Bill was the perfect complement to Val. They were fire and ice. Bill was so cool that butter would not melt in his mouth. Quietly efficient and with a great eye for detail, he more and more took on the job of chief investigator and field general. While Val hatched the ideas, cleared them through the political process, and wrote the reports, it was Bill who took the greater physical risks. Bill had a way of getting people to give him whatever he asked for whether they knew that they were doing it or not. Val often said that the work they did together in one year equalled or exceeded what he was able to do by himself in the preceding seven years.

Bill's role was highlighted during the investigation of a 2,200 bed extended care facility in Allegheny County. After weeks of investigation and mountains of sworn testimony from employees, it was proven that the hospital was billing both Medicare and Medicaid for the same patients. Allegations about the poor quality of care were documented by committee consultants, including Margaret Cushman, R.N., and Dr. Robert Butler. The result was the federal government stepped in and closed the facility until corrections were made and the money returned. A political backlash was avoided because Val had the foresight to ask for a U.S. General Accounting Office audit. The audit confirmed our findings and neutralized our critics.

Bill also took on the lead role in investigating the trend among the states to dump patients out of their state mental hospitals and into boarding homes. Such facilities offered little in the way of services. Many of them had been nursing homes and could no longer meet federal minimum standards. In writing the report, Val took note of the fact that we had tipped our state mental hospitals on their side, creating instant "psychiatric ghettoes" in our major cities. We pointed out how these patients were often manipulated by operators who wanted to use them to collect federal money under several federal programs, including Supplementary Security Income. We toured boarding homes in several cities so I could see things for myself and I can only say that conditions were appalling.

The greatest of all the investigations that I undertook with the

Halamandarises, however, was an evaluation of "Medicaid mills." Medicaid mills are small clinics located in the ghettoes of our major cities. They differ from normal clinics in that they are owned by entrepreneurs, not doctors. In fact, they hired doctors and gave them only a percentage of the money that they collected from Medicaid. The incentive, therefore, was to cheat and pad the billings. The more the clinic collected, the more the doctor ostensibly would keep. More often than not, the physicians used were foreign medical practitioners. What happened, of course, is that the owner of the mills often refused to pay even the agreed on 25 percent and, if the doctor complained, he or she would be threatened with prosecution for Medicaid fraud. After the physicians signed the bills, employees of the mill often added false charges. Under these circumstances, many physicians working in Medicaid mills were little more than indentured servants. On top of everything else, the quality of care was so wretched that Medicaid clients knew that if they were really sick, the place to go was not to the mills, but to the emergency room of a hospital.

Val and Bill developed a plan to learn to what extent these allegations were true in Medicaid mills nationwide. As always, they tackled the big states. In this case, much of our energy was invested in New York, which by itself accounted for more than 20 percent of all Medicaid funds. The plan was to first collect all the past reports and studies that were available on Medicaid mills. Second, to interview doctors, patients, and clinic owners on a wide sample. Third, to pose as Medicaid clients entering the clinic with Medicaid cards to see what happened. Fourth, it was to pretend to be entrepreneurs interested in buying Medicaid mills in order to learn firsthand of their profitability and of potential financial manipulations.

Hundreds of reports and piles of computer runs were accumulated, thousands of questionnaires were sent out, and dozens of physicians, owners, and state and national officials were interviewed. These interviews were transcribed and the rough outline of a report prepared.

At this point, Val and Bill recruited two Capitol Hill policemen, James Roberts and Scotty McDew, who were detailed to the Senate Aging Committee to assist Val and Bill at my request. All four were given physical examinations by the Capitol physician, Dr. Freeman

Carey. All were pronounced physically healthy. Next, they obtained an old milk truck outfitted with one-way glass positioned to look like yellow reflectors. This was obtained from the Internal Revenue Service in response to our request for a surveillance van. Then, we obtained Medicaid cards from the United States attorney, Southern District of New York. The cards were coded so that all charges would be kicked out of the computer for examination. They presented themselves for treatment in dozens of Medicaid mills in the five states mentioned. This exercise in posing as Medicaid "shoppers" disclosed Medicaid fraud, the dimensions of which few of us had ever imagined.

According to the billings that came into Medicaid, the perfectly healthy Senate investigators were supposedly treated for every disease in the history of man, from arthritis to cancer. Investigators would visit one clinic for a three-minute visit with a general practitioner and leave. The bills would indicate that on that date they had been seen not only by the G.P., but also by the dentist, the podiatrist, the psychiatrist, the allergist, and so on. What is more, they would visit one clinic, and four other clinics in different parts of the city would bill for seeing them, ostensibly on the same day.

Literally thousands of dollars of phony bills were collected. I myself posed as a Medicaid patient for one day. I put on my old clothes and spent a day being "ping-ponged" from specialist to specialist. The whole idea was not patient care, but the generation of income. This experience allowed me to describe Medicaid fraud firsthand to the public.

What we did was extremely risky. We were in the roughest areas of Detroit, Newark, Harlem, Watts, and Chicago. Had we been discovered, there would have been hell to pay. We did have some close calls, such as when Val was discovered outside a clinic waiting to take my picture when I exited. A group of junkies, their pupils big enough to drive a truck through, took exception and they charged at Val, surrounding his car and rocking it from side to side. Val hit the accelerator and escaped just in time to make a perfect diversion for my exit.

What was a great deal more dangerous was Bill's role of pretending to be a buyer of Medicaid mills. He and Val had business cards printed, using a dummy corporation called Total Health Care Industries. Val took the name of Lester Gillis, the real name of mobster "Babyface" Nelson. Bill used Clyde Barrow of Bonny and Clyde fame. They answered ads in the newspaper placed there by people who said they wanted to sell Medicaid mills, taking a physician along for legitimacy. Arriving in a rented limousine and wearing loud suits, they were able to make people comfortable enough to say things like, "Harry, bring the real books." Several of these episodes were taped with a hidden tape recorder provided by the U.S. Attorney's office.

Medicaid mill owners laid out broad gauge extortion schemes. They mentioned the names of politicians who were "on the take." They detailed methods of recovering capital in a hurry, such as "lighting a fire and then collecting the insurance." They told which mafia families had interests and where their territorial lines were.

This entire investigation was brought to a grinding halt because of the innocent error of a clerk on the Aging Committee staff. Val and Bill were operating this investigation on a shoestring. The only people they had were volunteers, college interns, and the two detailed Capitol Hill cops. Through the magic of the phone company, it was arranged that the phone for Total Health Care Industries, a Delaware corporation doing business in Illinois and now a foreign corporation seeking to do business in New York, would be answered on Val's private line in Washington, D.C., at the Senate Aging Committee. Big signs everywhere proclaimed: "Answer: Total Health Care Industries, say Mr. Gillis is out but you will give him the message." A clerk heard the phone ring and dashed madly to pick up the receiver and answered the phone "U.S. Senate Committee on Aging."

Thereafter, there were a series of suspicious events, including a burglary at Val's house where it was obvious to police that the intruders were after something specific. No television, stereos, or other consumer goods were taken. Val imagined what they were after were the tape recordings made of the undercover "buys," which were full of incriminating allegations. The night after the burglary, he and Bill did not return to Val's home on Capitol Hill, but to another family residence. Val had a premonition. He was awake at three in the morning when two men in a red pickup truck stopped in front of the house, one with a crowbar in hand headed for the front door. The other went for the garage. Val awakened Bill, who, thinking fast, flipped on the porch light. The man dropped the crowbar and ran. The man from the garage vaulted into the bed of the truck as it sped away.

The police were called and turned up a two-gallon can of gasoline in the garage. I called Attorney General William Saxbe, who brought in the FBI to watch over our investigators for the next few weeks until their work could be completed.

We released our report to the public in hearings on August 30–31, 1976. The report charged that one out of every five dollars paid out to Medicaid mills was stolen. The report charged that the Medicaid fraud losses in New York State exceeded $1 billion. The report contained conclusive evidence that the state had known of the problem for a dozen years or more, but had done virtually nothing to correct it. It said that those who chose to defraud the system had virtually no risk of being caught and even if they were caught, the odds of successful prosecution were slim. Specific recommendations were made for improvement, including developing a new computer system that could more closely spot fraudulent Medicaid charges.

The story ran on the front pages for the better part of a week. As a result of our work, numerous prosecutions were undertaken and convictions obtained. Legislation long dormant to create the Office of Inspector General to fight fraud in the Department of Health and Human Services passed within a matter of weeks.

One final hearing was held in this series. Val put together the first joint hearing between the Senate Aging Committee and the House Ways and Means Committee. Val directed an investigation to determine whether fraud was widespread in the home health care field. Two egregious examples were found and ultimately the providers were convicted in federal court, but the committees reached the conclusion that this was the one area of Medicare and Medicaid that apparently was free from widespread fraud.

I left the Senate in January of 1977. Val stayed behind, helping Senator Frank Church and Congressman Claude Pepper push through the Medicare and Medicaid Fraud Amendments of 1977, which included many of the reforms that Val and I had suggested. One of these, for example, elevated Medicaid fraud from a misdemeanor to a felony and tightened up definitions to prevent the proliferation of kickbacks. Another amendment created state Medicaid fraud units in an effort to arm the states to prevent these kinds of problems. Senator Church praised Val's work, giving him a generous share of the credit.

The detail of the hearing, reports, and investigations that he undertook along with his brother gives the reader some feel for Val's integrity and scope. He is one of the nicest people in the world, but he can also be among the toughest. It took great courage to do what he did, and the nation is the better for his work. He helped not only to enact new legislation and programs, but to police existing programs and to make sure that federal dollars are being appropriately used for the benefit of the aged.

The House Select Committee on Aging

Throughout 1977, Val had been courted to leave the Senate Aging Committee and join the staff of the House Select Committee on Aging. The Senate Aging Committee was at its pinnacle and it was obvious to all that Val was a major factor in making it that way. Recruiting him would therefore be a real coup. Hiring him would bring some much needed credibility to the House committee and at the same time deprive the Senate of their best man.

To this point, the House Aging Committee had been an object of derision because of its inauspicious beginning. It was staffed initially by people who had been cut loose when the House on Un-American Activities Committee was folded. The first chairman, William Randall, made an effort, but neither he nor his staff knew much about the topic. He served only one term and upon his retirement, Claude Pepper ascended to the chairmanship.

Pepper persuaded Val to join him beginning in April of 1978. Claude Pepper and Val J. Halamandaris were a match made in heaven. They thought alike, they shared the same values, and they genuinely liked each other.

Within a matter of weeks, Val had more things going than was imaginable and what is more, he had a team, made up of Kathleen Gardner Cravedi, Nancy Smythe, and David Holton, to help him. He and Pepper decided that they would take a good hard look at frauds perpetrated against the elderly and see what could be done to help protect seniors.

Research was conducted on land fraud. Hearings were held that disclosed that seniors were fleeced by promoters who sold them land that was non-existent, underwater, or otherwise unbuildable. In a variation on the same theme, Val directed an investigation into frauds associated with the sale of time shares. What was learned was that this new variable of "interval ownership" was not covered by any of the existing statutes designed to bar land fraud. The committee's work in exposing the problem led to legislative reforms at both the state and federal level.

Val launched an investigation into work-at-home schemes, which promised the elderly they could earn big money by sealing envelopes at home in their spare time. Seniors were induced to mail $500 as a down payment; and that, of course, was the last they saw of their money.

From there, Pepper and Val examined so-called business opportunity frauds. For example, seniors would be induced to get in the business of growing plants or earthworms. An up-front investment was always required by the promoters to cover the alleged costs of getting into business. In other words, one had to pay for the small plants or earthworm larvae. When the person had raised these plants or earthworms to maturity, the company allegedly would buy them back at certain pre-agreed rates. The sad part, of course, was that no market for the products existed, and no one ever tried to buy back the mature plants or worms.

An investigation into funeral abuses done jointly with Congressman Edward Roybal pointed up shortcomings in regulations of the Federal Trade Commission. The revised regulations guaranteed full disclosure of the facts in order that the vulnerable family members might make an informed decision instead of being pressured into buying something.

Val and the team conducted research on the number of inpatients in state mental hospitals. They learned that while the number of inpatients, both elderly and young people, had been decreased by two-thirds over the last ten years, the budgets for state mental hospitals on average had increased five-fold. In some states, jobs in state mental hospitals were awarded as political patronage, so there were more jobs than ever, with less patients who needed care and therapy.

They examined nursing home abuses and found that while conditions had improved somewhat in the five years since the Senate reports were issued, major problems remained. When word leaked out that the Department of Health and Human Services (HHS) was considering deregulating the nursing home industry, Pepper and Val scheduled a hearing and then wrote a detailed letter to the secretary of HHS asking that the proposed, watered-down regulations be withdrawn. The strategy worked and the hearing was cancelled.

Hearings were held on organized crime's intrusion into Medicaid and Medicare, which brought fascinating disclosures from top prosecutors from several parts of the country. The Attorney General of the United States, Griffin Bell, testified as to what the Justice Department was planning to do to block the mob's infiltration.

The subject of organized crime also came up in the course of Val's investigation into pension frauds. Val persuaded Jimmy "The Weasel" Fratianno, the self-professed mafia hit man and one-time head of the West Coast mafia, to testify before the committee. Hidden from view behind bullet proof partitions, he gave the Aging Committee a primer on how the mafia muscles in and takes control of pension and employee benefits monies. This hearing was held in conjunction with Senator Sam Nunn's Permanent Investigations Subcommittee of the Senate Government Affairs Committee. The result was pressure on the appropriate agencies, largely the Department of Labor and the Justice Department, of better protection of worker's pensions.

One of the best known of Val's investigations was his in-depth examination into problems in the sale of health insurance to the elderly in supplementation of Medicare.

There are many reputable insurance companies who offer major medical plans that dovetail with Medicare. If they are good, such policies are designed to pay for what Medicare will not. Quite often, however, such policies are limited to only what Medicare covers. In short, they are a rip-off. Even the good policies described above can be a rip-off if a salesman attempts to sell a senior more than one of them.

Most of them contain a clause that says that in the case of duplication, only one will pay. Multiple policies, therefore, are a waste of money.

Val developed an action plan. First, an 11-page questionnaire was drafted and sent over Pepper's signature to all state insurance commissioners. Detailed followup interviews were conducted with five of them. All books, periodicals, and newspapers relating to Medi-gap insurance in the Library of Congress were reviewed. Letters were written to all senior citizens organizations, asking them to ask their members to write to the committee concerning their experience. The files of the U.S. Postal Service were reviewed. Every congressional office was asked to forward their complaints for review. Questionnaires were sent to 250 major insurance companies asking about their experience. Finally, senior citizens were recruited as temporary investigators to test whether agents would use high-pressure tactics in order to induce seniors to buy additional insurance.

Recruiting senior citizen volunteers to act as investigators was a brilliant stroke. The plan was for them to call insurance agents in 10 separate states, asking them to come by for a consultation. The seniors, in fact, had one thing in common: they were all overinsured. When confronted with their multiple policies, a reputable agent should have informed them that they already had more insurance than necessary, rather than try to induce them to make additional purchases. Unfortunately, in 84 percent of the cases nationwide, salesmen tried to sell the senior investigators one or more additional policies. Their motivation, of course, was greed in that they would receive commissions from such sales.

The committee report estimated that $1 billion a year was lost in the sale of worthless or duplicative insurance to seniors purportedly in supplementation of Medicare. To say the hearing and the report received widespread coverage is an understatement.

This hearing marked the ascendency of the House Aging Committee. It proved to any remaining skeptics that it had to be taken seriously. Significantly, the Senate Aging Committee had just conducted hearings on this topic weeks before, which received little in the way of press attention. Reporters were in the position to make comparisons. Several editorials appeared commending the House Aging Committee for the quality of its work. One in the *Miami Herald* criticized the Senate Aging Committee for being timid by comparison.

There was a downside to this aggressiveness, however. One insurance company that sold cancer insurance took exception. They filed not one, but multiple suits against the committee staff, saying that it had violated the rights of insurance agents. Halamandaris saw their real purpose to block the issuance of a second report being prepared on the specific topic of cancer insurance. If they thought a lawsuit would intimate Pepper and Halamandaris, they were mistaken. The report was drafted, circulated, and approved by an overwhelming majority of the committee and issued at joint hearings with the Senate Anti-Trust and Monopoly Subcommittee. More lawsuits followed. A total of eight were filed. It took eight years, but all of these suits were finally dismissed and all the members of the House staff were exonerated and their work commended.

Meanwhile, legislation was enacted creating a federal "good housekeeping seal of approval" for health insurance policies that met certain minimum federal standards.

Another of Val's highly regarded investigations related to medical quackery. As always, Val followed the same pattern. He and the staff gathered mountains of information. They put out the word to the senior citizens network that they were looking for case histories. They reviewed the files in the U.S. Postal Service and the Food and Drug Administration. They corresponded with state and federal law enforcement authorities. They visited interest groups and foundations such as the Arthritis Foundation, the American Cancer Society, and the American Medical Association. Thereafter, Halamandaris and his staff, along with detailees from the U.S. Postal Service, swept through hundreds of magazines. Using fictitious names such as Lester Gillis, they sent away for products based on ads that made questionable claims. Hundreds of products from arthritis to youth "cures" were received in response.

Once received, the products, together with the ad and the representations made for the product, were sent to a specially selected group of blue chip experts for their evaluation. These written evaluations were made a part of the final committee report.

A guaranteed instant face-lift turned out to be a set of facial exercises. A "cure" for impotency was a recipe for Oysters Rockefeller. An arthritis "cure" was a poultice of cow manure. A guaranteed weight loss remedy turned out to be a diuretic pill which when taken causes the body to lose body fluids. Some of the phony products were dangerous, including the kit of untested drugs sent complete with syringes, which was sold as a cancer cure. Another cancer "cure" was a machine that would bathe the subject in red light. Inside the machine was an ordinary light bulb in front of which there had been placed a red gelatin filter. The directions said the product only worked when the moon was full. The patient also had to be naked and facing north in order for it to work.

The report itself is a classic. It runs over four-hundred pages. In addition to being a comprehensive catalogue of phony cures, which the committee concluded cost the nation $10 billion a year, it is a cogent analysis of the failures of the regulatory agencies involved, along with recommendations for reform.

It should be added that Bill Halamandaris helped write this report. In 1980–82, Bill had been working as the Chief Investigator and Director of Oversight for the Senate Aging Committee, which was chaired by Republican Senator John Heinz. Val, during this same time, was Counsel to the Pepper Committee, which was controlled by the Democrats. When Val left Pepper's staff in 1982, Bill moved over from the Senate to take his brother's place.

Val was the lead witness in presenting the committee's report. Bob Hager of NBC News characterized it as one of the most impressive performances he had ever seen. He pointed out that the nation spent $4.60 per person on legitimate research into finding cures for diseases such as arthritis, cancer, and Alzheimer's, while $44 per person was lost on medical quackery. Literally hundreds of these phony products and nostrums had been laid out for review. Halamandaris and Congressman Pepper demonstrated several of these phony products, to the delight of the media.

As a result of this report, legislation was introduced by Congressman Pepper that when enacted strengthened the authority of the U.S. Postal Service in order to keep questionable products from being sold through the mails. Amendments were also made that began to take into consideration the growing trend to make misleading representations for products on television and through the electronic media.

All of the above are but a few of Val's works while at the House Aging Committee. He also drafted a report, entitled *Medicare after 15 Years*. The report evaluates the program's successes and its shortcomings. He helped Kathleen Gardner Cravedi write the first congressional report on the subject of elder abuse. Another report measured the success and failure of state Medicaid fraud units. At the same time, he helped advise Chairman Pepper on strategy with respect to Social Security, mandatory retirement legislation, and a raft of other issues.

Claude Pepper came to rely more and more on Val's seasoned and careful judgment. Val, for example, was one of the few who advised him to take the chairmanship of the Rules Committee. Other staff people who were more interested in hanging onto their jobs than in what was good for Pepper advised him to stay as chairman of the House Aging Committee.

Val had great affection for Claude Pepper. This was shown in the fact that he was single-handedly responsible for getting CBS's "Sixty Minutes" to do a tribute to Pepper. He wrote to his friends at CBS with whom he had worked many times before. In this typical fashion, he did their work for them. Morley Safer received a 30-page memorandum which included pertinent details of Pepper's career and quotes from dozens of his colleagues. The piece that appeared in 1982 pleased Pepper very much, but he did not find out until years later that Val had made it happen. In the same way, Val helped engineer Pepper's second appearance on the cover of *Time* magazine. He wrote to the editors, suggesting that it was time that Pepper was featured in connection with his work on behalf of the elderly. Thus it was that Pepper appeared on the cover of *Time* in 1983 as well as in 1938.

Halamandaris left Pepper in the summer of 1982, for the primary purpose of helping him reach another of his coveted goals—the enactment of a long-term home care bill. After 20 years in the Congress as counsel to both the Senate and House Aging Committees, Val was a very marketable commodity; yet he chose to sign on as the president of a new trade association called the National Association for Home

Care (NAHC), whose total staff would be three, including the president. He did this because he believed in home care right down to his marrow and because he loved Claude Pepper.

Val's accomplishments in the eight years that he has been president of NAHC are testimony to his abilities. Membership in the association increased from 400 to 5,000, the budget from $250,000 to $6 million, and the staff increased from 3 to 50.

In 1987, he cofounded the Center for Health Care Law, a public interest law firm based in Washington, D.C.

He is a skilled writer, having written more than 20 major congressional reports and coauthored a book with me entitled, *Too Old, Too Sick, Too Bad.* He also writes two columns, one called "Caring Thoughts" and the other "Caring People."

He is a publisher of note, having developed two magazines, *CARING*, which is circulated monthly to caregivers and home care providers, and *Caring People*, which pays tribute to people who devote their lives in service to others.

He is a skilled editor who plays a major role in the writing and editorial work in both *CARING* and *Caring People*.

He is a television producer, having developed among other things the documentary film, *Suffer Not the Little Children*, narrated by actress Susan Sullivan.

He is a philanthropist, having worked with me and his brother Bill to create the Foundation for Hospice and Homecare, which raises funds to support educational activity and research in the area of hospice care. He also serves on the Board of the Ankylosing Spondylitis Foundation and helps counsel young people who suffer from the same spinal disease that has afflicted him for so many years.

He is in demand as a public speaker because of his considerable oratorical skills. Over the past eight years, he has averaged more than 30 speeches and traveled more than 100,000 miles a year.

He is a museum curator as a result of an effort to help renovate a former home of abolitionist leader Frederick Douglass in Washington, D.C., and convert it into a museum. The museum will hold the personal effects of Dr. Frederick Douglass and display portraits of other Americans who reflect his caring spirit.

In 1987, Val and his brother Bill came up with the idea to conduct a search for the most caring men and women in America. Their idea was to identify role models for young people who are looking desperately today for someone they can respect. What evolved was the Caring Awards. Every year during the first week of December, the ten most caring Americans are identified and presented with an original work of art, a bronze sculpture by famed designer Frank Eliscu. They are honored in a ceremony in the Senate office building. They are further honored through the preparation of a videotape profile and a written tribute to them which appears in *Caring People* magazine. Each year, over 20,000 governors, mayors, senators, congressmen, Fortune 500 executives, and other notables are asked to nominate the most caring person that they know. As can be expected, competition is fierce and the people are extraordinary. The ten people who are selected are also inducted into the Frederick Douglass Museum and Hall of Fame for Caring Americans.

In order to accommodate these activities, Val, Bill, and I created a non-profit organization called the Caring Institute. Other activities of the Institute include a national photography contest cosponsored by Kodak, called The Art of Caring. Still another program that has been started is called Kids Caring for Kids. It involves children raising money to provide medical care for chronically ill children or to help terminally ill children enjoy a week at Disney World with their families, all expenses paid.

Finally, Val and Bill are working with me and the Association of Former Members of Congress to help create a Hall of Fame for Congress. Virtually every other profession has its hall of honor, but not the Congress. It is an idea that is long overdue and yet until Val came along, no one in the 200 years of this nation's history thought to make it happen. Once again, his emphasis is on creating role models to be emulated by our young people.

Those people who want to know more about what Val and Bill believe need only check the concluding chapter of this book. Their philosophy is accurately reflected in the consensus reached by the extraordinary people profiled in this book. I feel greatly honored to be included among such distinguished company.

I call Val and Bill the "gold dust twins" because they are such a wonderful team and everything they do seems to turn to gold. It is a wonderful thing to see two brothers who are so devoted to each other. By their own definition, they are caring people.

This book features 18 individuals who distinguished themselves in elevating the status of the nation's elderly. I would include the two Halamandaris brothers and make it an even 20. Congressman Pepper would have agreed with me. As usual, he said it best. On Bill's 40th birthday, he said:

> If there is any justice in the world, I am going to come back in my next life as Bill Halamandaris. Imagine being so bright, so personable, so accomplished, and so handsome. I can't imagine another person I should prefer to be.

On the occasion of his 85th birthday, Congressman Pepper told a gallery of notables assembled that Val J. Halamandaris was not only the best employee he ever had, but the best person that he had ever met. This was high praise to be sure, but it was heartfelt. On another occasion, Pepper said of Val that like FDR, he had a soul sweetened by suffering.

I think that everyone who knows him will agree that there is something remarkable about this likeable young man who has already devoted more than 30 years, literally all of his adult life, in an effort to improve the quality of life for the nation's elderly. As the others honored in this book can attest, his contribution has been great. Congressman Pepper summed it up well in a tribute which appeared in the *Congressional Record*:

> Val Halamandaris has demonstrated a deep and lasting commitment to the betterment of our country; he has done much to restore confidence in our government and to earn the respect of the Congress and the people of the United States.

A Selective Bibliography

Following is a list of references that are by or relate to the individuals profiled in this book. The list is illustrative and not exhaustive.

Ball, Robert M. *Social Security, Today and Tomorrow.* New York: Columbia University Press, 1978.

Ball, Robert M., with Wilbur Cohen.*The Report of the Committee on Economic Security of 1935; and other basic documents relating to the development of the Social Security Act.* Washington, D.C.: National Conference on Social Welfare, 1985.

Barrow, Kenneth. *Helen Hayes, First Lady of the American Theater.* Garden City, N.Y.: Doubleday, 1985.

Berman, Edgar. *Hubert.* New York: Putnam, 1979.

Brickfield, Cyril F. *Problems Relating to a Federal Constitutional Convention.* Washington, D.C.: U.S. Government Printing Office, 1957.

———. *State Applications Asking Congress to Call a Federal Constitutional Convention.* Washington, D.C.: U.S. Government Printing Office, 1959.

Butler, Robert N. *Aging & Mental Health.* St. Louis, Mo.: Mosby, 1973.

———. *Why Survive? Growing Old in America.* New York: Harper & Row, 1975.

———. *Sex after Sixty.* New York: Harper & Row, 1976.

———. *The Aging Process.* New York: Raven Press, 1985.

———. *Love and Sex after 40.* New York: Harper & Row, 1986.

———. *Human Aging Research.* New York: Raven Press, 1988.

———. *Love and Sex after 60.* New York: Perennial Library, 1988.

———. *Midlife Love Life.* New York: Perennial Library, 1988.

Butler, Robert N., and Herbert P. Gleason. *Productive Aging: Enhancing Vitality in Later LIfe.* New York: Springer Publishing Co., 1985.

Butler, Robert N., Mia R. Oberlink, and Mal Schechter, eds. *The Promise of Productive Aging: From Biology to Social Policy.* New York: Springer Publishing Co., 1990.

Cohen, Dan. *Undefeated.* Minneapolis: Lerner Publications, 1978.

Cohen, Wilbur J. *Readings in Social Security* . New York: Prentice-Hall, 1948.

———. *Retirement Policies under Social Security: A Legislative History of Retirement Ages, the Retirement Test, and Disability Benefits.* Berkeley: University of California Press, 1957.

———. *Health in America: the Role of the Federal Government in Bringing High Quality Health Care to All the American People.* A special report prepared at the request of the United States Department of Health, Education and Welfare. Washington, D.C.: U.S. Government Printing Office, 1968.

———. *Needed Changes in Education.* College Park: College of Education, University of Maryland, 1970.

———. *Social Security: Universal or Selective?* Washington, D.C.: American Enterprise Institute for Public Policy Research, 1972.

———. *Welfare Reform.* Washington, D.C.: AEI, 1976.

———. *Demographic Dynamics in America.* New York: The Free Press, 1977.

———. *The New Deal, Fifty Years After.* Austin, Tex.: Lyndon Baines Johnson Library, Lyndon B. Johnson School of Public Affairs, 1984.

———. *The Roosevelt New Deal.* Austin, Tex.: Lyndon B. Johnson School of Public Affairs, 1986.

Cohen, Wilbur J., and James N. Morgan. *Income and Welfare in the United States, A Study.* New York: McGraw-Hill, 1962.

Cohen, Wilbur J., and William Haber, eds. *Social Security: Programs, Problems, and Policies; Selected Readings.* Homewood, Ill.: R.D. Irwin, 1960.

Cohen, Wilbur J., with Robert Ball. *The Report of the Committee on Economic Security of 1935; and other basic documents relating to the development of the Social Security Act.* Washington, D.C.: National Conference on Social Welfare, 1985.

Downs, Hugh. *Yours Truly, Hugh Downs.* New York: Holt, Rinehart and Winston, 1960.

———. *A Shoal of Stars.* Garden City, N.Y: Doubleday, 1967.

———. *Rings around Tomorrow.* Garden City, N.Y.: Doubleday, 1970.

Downs, Hugh. *Potential; The Way to Emotional Maturity.* Garden City, N.Y.: Doubleday, 1973.

———. *Thirty Dirty Lies about Old.* Boston: Argus, 1979.

———. *The Best Years Book.* New York: Delacorte Press, 1981.

———. *On Camera: My 10,000 Hours on Television.* New York: Putnam, 1986.

Eisele, Albert. *Almost to the Presidency.* Blue Earth, Minn.: Piper Co., 1972.

Fahey, Charles, and Edward Wakin. *A Catholic Guide to the Mature Years.* Huntington, Ind.: Our Sunday Visitor, Inc., 1984.

Frost, David. *The Presidential Debate, 1968.* New York: Stein and Day, 1968.

Gill, Derek L. T. *Quest.* New York: Harper & Row, 1980.

Hayes, Helen. *Star on Her Forehead.* New York: Dodd, Mead, 1949.

———. *A Gift of Joy.* New York: M. Evans; distributed by Lippincott, Philadelphia, 1965.

———. *On Reflection.* New York: M. Evans; distributed by Lippincott, Philadelphia, 1968.

———. *Twice Over Lightly.* New York: Harcourt Brace Jovanovich, 1972.

———. *A Gathering of Hope.* Philadelphia: Fortress Press, 1983.

———. *Our Best Years.* South Yarmouth, Mass.: J. Curley, 1984.

———. *Loving Life.* Garden City, N.Y.: Doubleday, 1987.

———. *Where the Truth Lies.* New York: Morrow, 1988.

———. *My Life in Three Acts.* San Diego: Harcourt Brace Jovanovich, 1990.

Henderson, Virginia. *ICN Basic Principles of Nursing Care.* Geneva, Switzerland: International Council of Nurses, 1960.

———. *The Nature of Nursing.* New York: Macmillan Publishing Co., Inc., 1966.

———. *Principles and Practice of Nursing.* 6th ed. New York: Macmillan Publishing Co., Inc., 1978.

Henderson, Virginia, with Leo W. Simmons. *Nursing Research, A Survey and Assessment.* New York: Appleton-Century-Crofts, 1964.

Henderson, Virginia, with Yale University School of Nursing Index Staff. *Nursing Studies Index.* Philadelphia: J. B. Lippincott Co., 1963, 1966, 1970, 1972.

Hessel, Dieter T. *Maggie Kuhn on Aging: A Dialogue.* Philadelphia: Westminster Press, 1977.

Humphrey, Hubert H. *The Cause Is Mankind.* New York: Praeger, 1964.

———. *War on Poverty.* Toronto: McGraw-Hill, 1964.

———. *Addresses by Honorable Hubert H. Humphrey, Vice President of the United*

States, on U.S. Relations with Latin America. Washington, D.C.: U.S. Government Printing Office,1967.

Humphrey, Hubert H. *The Challenge of Our Cities.* Washington, D.C.: 1967.

———. *Beyond Civil Rights.* New York: Random House, 1968.

———. *Message to Africa: [Vice President Humphrey's Mission to the African Nations].* A special report prepared at the request of the State Department. Washington, D.C.: U.S. Government Printing Office, 1968.

———. *Revolution and Politics: The Legacy of Independence.* Williamsburg, Va.: Colonial Williamsburg, 1969.

———. *The Political Philosophy of the New Deal.* Baton Rouge: Louisiana State University Press, 1970.

———. *The Urban Crisis.* New York: Da Capo Press, 1971.

———. *Young America in the "Now" World.* New York: New York University Press, 1971.

———. *Observations on East-West Economic Relations: U.S.S.R. and Poland.* Washington, D.C., U.S. Government Printing Office, 1973.

———. *Observations on Soviet and Polish Agriculture, November-December 1972.* Washington, D.C.: U.S. Government Printing Office, 1973.

———. *A Proposal for Achieving Balanced National Growth and Development.* Washington, D.C.: U.S. Government Printing Office, 1973.

———. *The Education of a Public Man.* Garden City, N.Y.: Doubleday, 1976.

———. *Government Regulation.* Washington, D.C.: AEI, 1976.

———. *Hubert Humphrey.* New York: Methuen, 1978.

———. *U.S. Troop Withdrawal from the Republic of Korea.* Washington, D.C.: U.S. Government Printing Office, 1978.

———. *Conscience of the Nation.* Tokyo: Japan-American Cultural Society, 1979.

———. *Hubert H. Humphrey Papers.* St. Paul: Minnesota Historical Society, Division of Archives and Manuscripts, 1983.

Kittredge, Mary. *Helen Hayes.* New York: Chelsea House, 1988.

Kübler-Ross, Elisabeth. *On Death and Dying.* New York: Macmillan, 1969.

———. *Questions and Answers on Death and Dying.* New York: Macmillan, 1974.

———. *Death: The Final Stage of Growth.* Englewood Cliffs, N.J., Prentice-Hall, 1975.

———. *To Live until We Say Good-Bye.* Englewood Cliffs, N.J.: Prentice-Hall, 1978.

———. *Living with Death and Dying.* New York: Macmillan, 1981.

———. *Remember the Secret.* Millbrae, Calif.: Celestial Arts, 1982.

———. *Working It Through.* New York: Macmillan, 1982.

Kübler-Ross, Elizabeth. *On Children and Death*. New York: Macmillan, 1983.

———. *AIDS*. New York: Macmillan, 1987.

Levitan, Sar A. *Towards Freedom from Want*. Madison, Wisc.: Industrial Relations Research Association, 1968.

Manfred, Frederick Feikema. *Prime Fathers*. Salt Lake City: Howe Brothers, 1988.

Martin, Ralph G. *A Man for All People: Hubert H. Humphrey*. New York: Grosset & Dunlap, 1968.

Moss, Frank E. *The Water Crisis*. New York: F.A. Praeger, 1967.

———. *Initiatives in Corporate Responsibility*. Washington, D.C., U.S. Government Printing Office, 1972.

———. *Staff Report to the Federal Trade Commission on the Ad Substantiation Program, Together with Supplementary Analysis of the Submissions and Advertisers Comments*. Washington, D.C.: U.S. Government Printing Office, 1972.

Moss, Frank E., and Val J. Halamandaris. *Too Old, Too Sick, Too Bad*. Germantown, Md.: Aspen Systems Corp., 1977.

Pepper, Claude. *Analyses of the Impact of the Proposed Fiscal Year 1982 Budget Cuts on the Elderly*. Washington, D.C.: U.S. Government Printing Office, 1981.

———. *Ask Claude Pepper*. Garden City, N.Y., Doubleday, 1984.

———. *Pepper, Eyewitness to a Century*. San Diego: Harcourt Brace Jovanovich, 1987.

Polsby, Nelson W. *The Citizen's Choice: Humphrey or Nixon*.Washington, D.C.: Public Affairs Press, 1968.

Robbins, Jhan. *Front Page Marriage*. New York: Putnam, 1982.

Ryskind, Allan H. *Hubert; an Unauthorized Biography of the Vice President*. New Rochelle, N.Y.: Arlington House, 1968.

Shearon, Marjorie O'Connell. *Wilbur J. Cohen*. Chevy Chase, Md.: Shearon Legislative Service, 1967.

———. *Wilbur J. Cohen: The Pursuit of Power*. Chevy Chase, Md.: Shearon Legislative Service, 1967.

Sherrill, Robert. *The Drugstore Liberal*. New York: Grossman Publishers, 1968.

Skeist, Robert J. *To Your Good Health!: A Practical Guide for Older Americans, Their Families, and Friends*. Chicago: Chicago Review Press, 1980.

Solberg, Carl. *Hubert Humphrey*. New York: Norton, 1984.

Westman, Paul. *Hubert H. Humphrey, The Politics of Joy*. Minneapolis: Dillon Press, 1978.

Zehnpfennig, Gladys. *Hubert H. Humphrey, Champion of Human Rights*. Minneapolis: T. S. Denison, 1966.